A Colour Atlas of
Minor Surgery

Edited by

William F. Walker

DSc, ChM, FRCS(Ed), FRCS(Eng), FRSE

Consultant Surgeon
Ninewells Hospital, Dundee and
Honorary Reader in Surgery at
University of Dundee,
Scotland

Wolfe Medical Publications Ltd

Published by Wolfe Medical Publications Ltd, 1986
Printed by Royal Smeets Offset b.v.,
Weert, Netherlands
ISBN 0 7234 0810 6

This book is one of the titles in the series of Wolfe Medical Atlases, a series which brings together probably the world's largest systematic published collection of diagnostic colour photographs
For a full list of Atlases in the series, plus forthcoming titles and details of our surgical, dental and veterinary Atlases, please write to Wolfe Medical Publications Ltd, 3 Conway Street, London W1P 6HE

Contents

Acknowledgements 5
Contributors 5
Introduction 7
Local anaesthetic drugs 8
Sebaceous cyst (back) 9
Sebaceous cyst (scalp) 11
Ganglion 13
Lipoma of back 15
Biopsy of temporal artery 17
Excision of gland of neck 20
Excision of thyroglossal cyst 22
Parotid duct stricture 25
Tracheostomy 27
Circumcision 30
Frenuloplasty 34
Vasectomy 36
Undescended testis 38
Excision of cyst of epididymis 41
Lord's operation for hydrocele 43
Repair of a baby's inguinal hernia 47
Epigastric hernia 52
Repair of direct inguinal hernia 55
Inguinal hernia repair under local anaesthesia 58
Appendicectomy 62
Fistual-in-ano 66
Haemorrhoidectomy 67
Closure of a colostomy 71
Pilonidal sinus 73
Varicose veins 77
Aspiration of breast cyst 81
Fine needle aspiration of breast for cytology 82
Disposable needle biopsy of discrete solid tumour 83
Open biopsy of breast under general anaesthesia 85
Drainage of breast abcess 87
Subareolar mammary duct excision for duct ectasia 88
Microdochectomy 92
Localising technique for impalpable breast lesions 97
Lower axillary clearance *without* mastectomy 100
Palmar fasciectomy 103
De Quervain's stenosing tenovaginitis 106
Removal of head of radius 107
Bunionectomy 109
Keller's arthroplasty 112
Ingrowing toe nail 115
Trigger fingers 118
Corneal foreign bodies 120
Procedures on the eyelids 121
Entropion 123
  Ffook's modification of Wies procedure 123
  Modified Wheeler's procedure 125
Ectropion 128
  Cautery 128
  Wedge resection 129
Procedures on tear ducts 130
  Syringing (lacrimal sac washout) 130
  Probing 131
  Three-snip procedure for spastic occlusion 133
Plastic surgery 134
  Basic principles
    Placing the scar
    Sutures
    Shape of excision
    Grafts and flaps
    Scar revision
Placing the scar 136
Suture removal and wound healing 137

(CONTINUED)

Excision biopsy of suspicious lesion in the leg 138
Excision biopsy of a mole on the face 139
Excision of a larger lesion on face leaving curved scar 141
Shaping excision, removal of 'dog ears' 144
Wound repair 146
Biopsy of pyogenic granuloma 148
Tattoo excision 149
Cutting and preparing split thickness skin graft 150
Application of split skin graft – tie over (bolus) dressing 153
Application of a split thickness graft by staples/sutures 155
Full thickness skin graft to repair a defect from excision of basal cell carcinoma of eyelid 157
Local flap repair 160
Cross fingers flap 161
Wedge excision of a small lesion of lip 163
Vermillionectomy 164
W wedge exision of malignant lesion of lower eyelid 165
Triamcinolone injection of hypertrophic scar 167
Scar revision – W plasty 168
Scar revision – Z plasty 169
Scar revision – excision 171
Perineal warts 173
Labial warts 175
Excision of labial cysts 176
Bartholin's cyst 178
Acute Bartholin's abcess 179
Excision of the vaginal cysts 181
Cervical cysts 183
Pendunculated labial and vulval benign tumours 184
Cervical polyp and cervical erosion 185
Removal of large cervical polyps 186
Dilatation and curettage 188
Pilonidal sinus 190
Lichen sclerosis 190
Leukoplakia 191
Leukoplakia of cervix 191
Cervicitis 192
Laparoscopy 194

Index 197

Acknowledgements

Grateful thanks are due to the Department of Medical Illustration of Ninewells Hospital and Royal Infirmary, Dundee who undertook the photography and to the Department of Medical Illustrations of University of Aberdeen who did the photography in the Orthopaedic section. I should also like to thank the individual photographers and theatre staff of the various hospitals for their skill and patience.

Figures **2**, **3** and **4** in the section on Laparoscopy (pages 194-195) are reproduced with the kind permission of Searle & Co., San Juan, Puerto Rico and Professor Melvin R. Cohen.

Contributors

J A Coleiro, MD, FRCS
Consultant Ophthalmic Surgeon, Ninewells Hospital, Dundee

A Lawson, MD, FRCS (Ed), Ninewells Hospital, Dundee
Senior Registrar in General Surgery, Royal Infirmary, Dundee and Ninewells Hospital, Dundee

M H Lyall, ChM, FRCS (Ed)
Consultant General Surgeon, Ninewells Hospital, Dundee

P McCollum, MB, FRCSI
Registrar General Surgery, Ninewells Hospital, Dundee

K Mills, MA, BSc, FRCS
Consultant Orthopaedic Surgeon, Grampian Health Board

A M Morris, FRCS (Ed), FRCS (Eng)
Consultant Plastic Surgeon, Royal Infirmary, Dundee

N B Patel, MD, FRCOG
Consultant obstetrician and Gynaecologist, Ninewells Hospital, Dundee

P E Preece, MD, FRCS (Ed), FRCS (Eng)
Consultant Surgeon, Senior Lecturer, Ninewells Hospital, Dundee, (Breast Surgery)

William F Walker, DSc, ChM, FRCS (Ed), FRCS (Eng), FRSE
Consultant Surgeon, Ninewells Hospital, Dundee and Honorary Reader in Surgery at University of Dundee, Scotland

Introduction

Minor surgery, as defined in this book, refers to cases which are dealt with mostly by surgeons in training and, of course, as training reaches towards the higher levels the operations will grow in complexity. Minor surgery is therefore within the compass of senior house officers or registrars.

It should be emphasised that all operations are carried out on patients who do not regard them as 'minor', are quite concerned about the outcome and sometimes frightened and need reassurance.

All operations have a capacity to 'go wrong' and should therefore be carried out with meticulous attention to every detail. Operations are assumed to be carried out in a hospital or some such suitable environment.

Anatomy

The operator must be fully aware of the anatomy of the part being operated on, so that damage to surrounding structures are avoided. This is one of the most important fundamental precepts of surgery and must be observed at all times.

Anaesthesia

Local anaesthesia should be within the amount recommended and the use of adrenaline with it, which lessens the dose required, should be considered carefully. Regional or extensive nerve blocks or general anaesthesia should be given only by an experienced anaesthetist. All drugs may affect the very young and the old differently from the other age groups. The after-effects of any drug used must be considered when the patient is being discharged, especially so the possible effects on drinking, driving, and use of heavy machinery within the next 24 hours.

Local anaesthetic drugs

Dosage

The dose for each patient must be individualised. The young and strong can tolerate larger doses than the elderly and emaciated. Usually the weakest effective solution should be used. Remember to ask the patient if any allergic reactions have occurred from a previous administration.

		Maximum dose
Lignocaine (xylocaine)	40 ml 0.5 per cent	= 200 mg plain solutions
	20 ml 1.0 per cent	
	70 ml 0.5 per cent	= 350 mg with adrenaline
	35 ml 1.0 per cent	

Drugs

Those drugs in common use vary from country to country.

Local Anaesthetic plus Vasoconstrictor

Vasoconstrictor drugs e.g. Adrenaline, are added to prevent a rapid rise in blood levels of anaesthetic, to prolong anaesthesia, and to produce a relatively bloodless field. Therefore, they are especially useful in lengthy vascular areas.

CAUTION

1. **Be careful in patients with previous reaction to anaesthetic drug;**
2. **Therefore, exercise extreme care in choice of drug;**
3. **Do not give more than recommended dose;**
4. **Monitor the patient for 30 minutes after injection;**
5. **If reactions occur, apply a tourniquet to limit absorption and slowly release tourniquet;**
6. **Do not inject into inflamed or infected tissue because of rapid absorption.**
7. **Adrenaline should NOT be added to injections in digits or appendages.**

Sebaceous cyst (back)

These arise from the sebaceous glands of the skin. They are most common on head, neck and back. They are attached to the skin and may exhibit a punctum. **The patient should be warned that recurrence is possible after excision, especially if any part is left behind.**

1

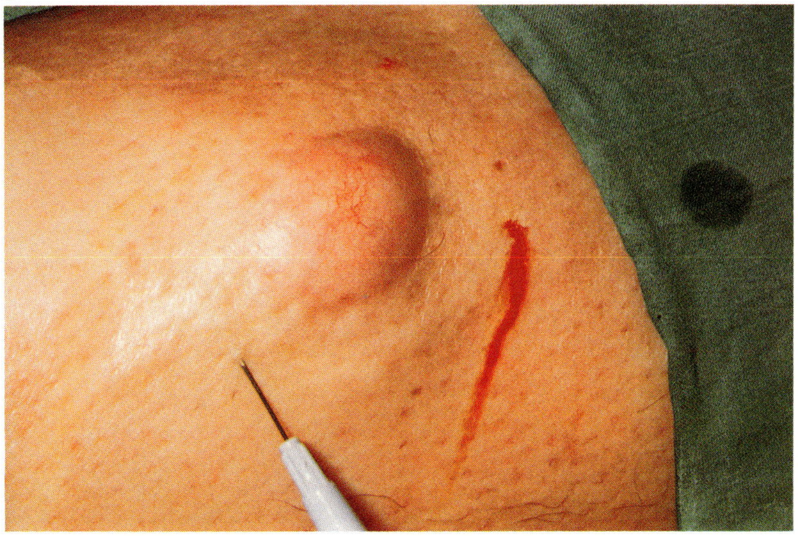

1 **Local anaesthetic 1 per cent with adrenaline is most commonly used** and is infiltrated round the cyst and given sufficient time to have an effect.

2 **In this reasonably small cyst about 2.5 cm in diameter, a simple incision is made over the cyst** and the edges peeled off the underlying cyst.

3 **Tissue forceps or skin hooks may help the retraction** and a further forceps pulling on the cyst may delineate the adjoining tissue to be dissected off.

4 **It is preferable not to rupture the cyst** and gauze dissection may aid the sharp dissection.

2

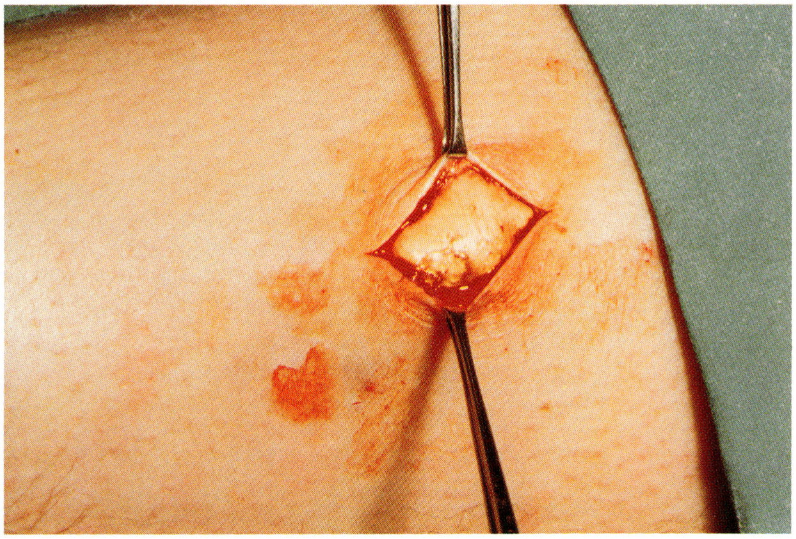

3

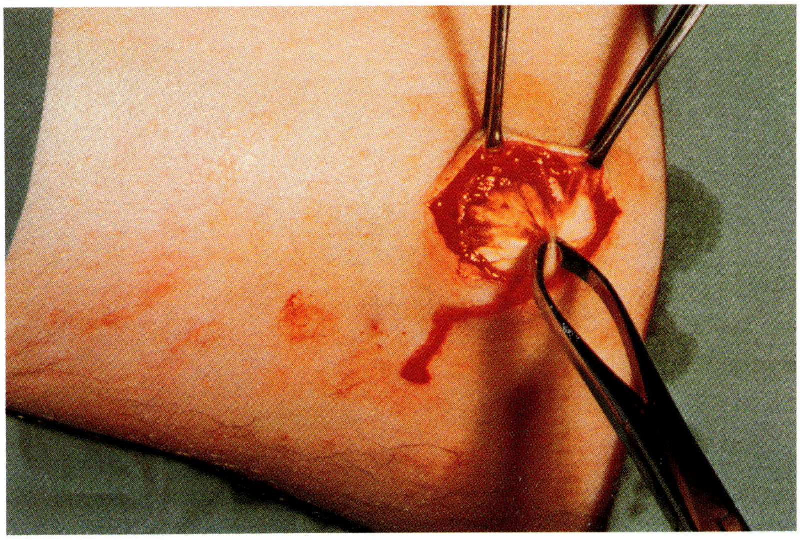

4

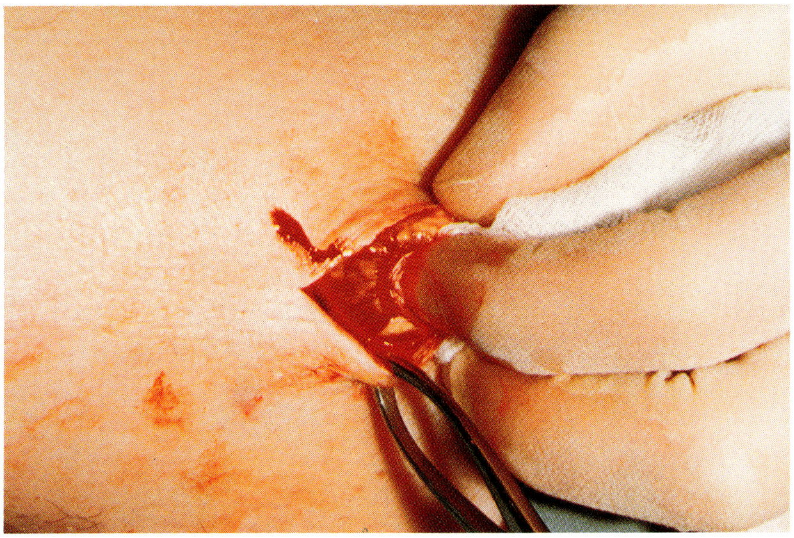

5

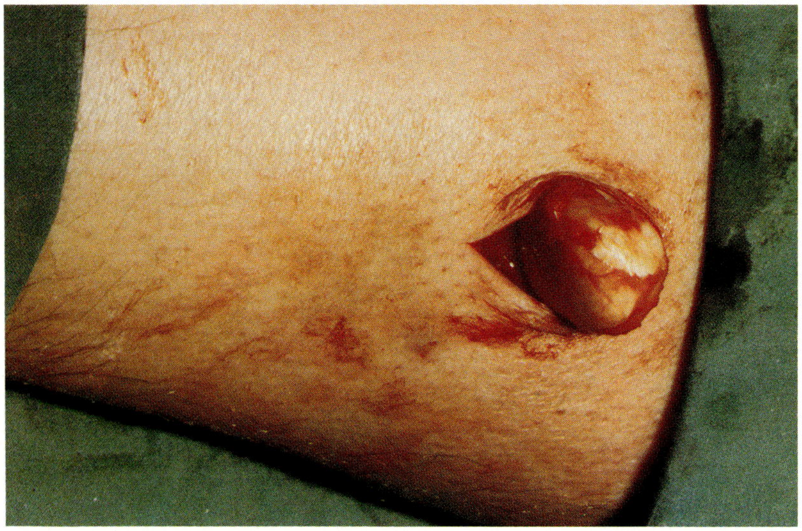

6

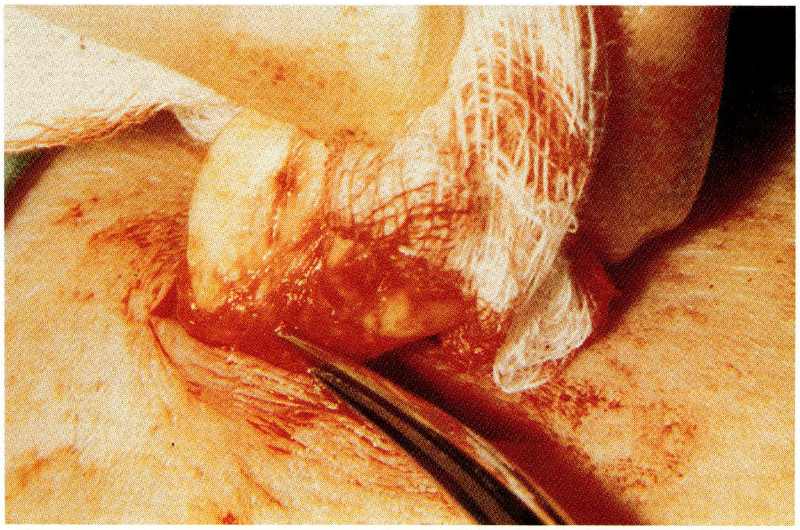

7

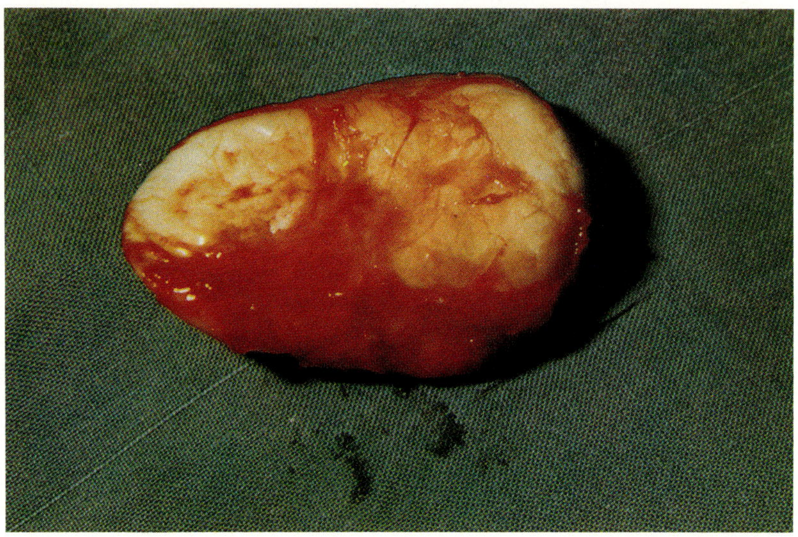

5 With this the cyst can be well mobilised with its yellowish-white contents.

6 Again using gauze to grip the cyst, it is pulled upwards and the final holding tissues underneath are divided.

7 Complete excision of the cyst without rupture is the accomplished object. If it is ruptured, the cyst wall should be entirely removed in pieces to prevent recurrence.

8 Skin is sutured using mattress approximating sutures. Dressing should obliterate dead space.

Caution: Note that unless done cleanly and with minimal trauma, infection may occur.

8

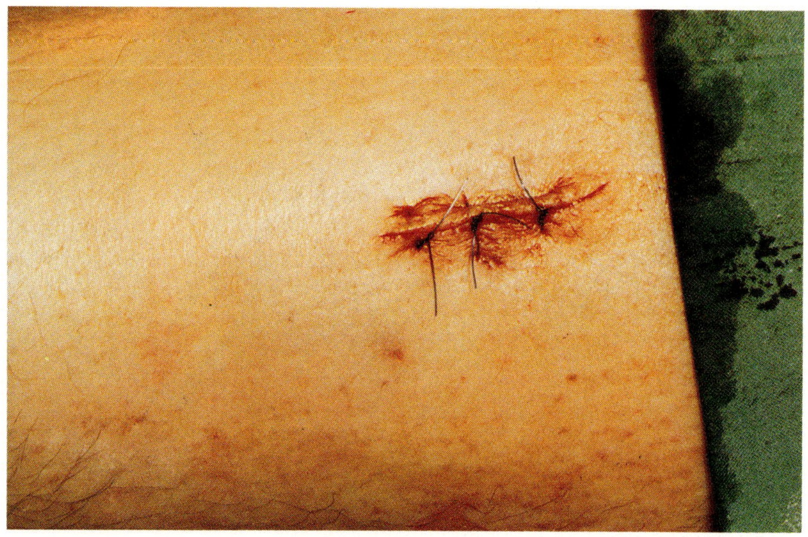

Sebaceous cyst (scalp)

1 In the scalp the cyst tends to be more prominent as it cannot bulge backwards into the softer tissues which are minimal in the scalp.

2 There is thus an excess of skin and an elliptical incision is used removing the redundant skin with the cyst.

3 Traction on the skin ellipse helps to move the cyst from side to side and allows all round sharp dissection.

1

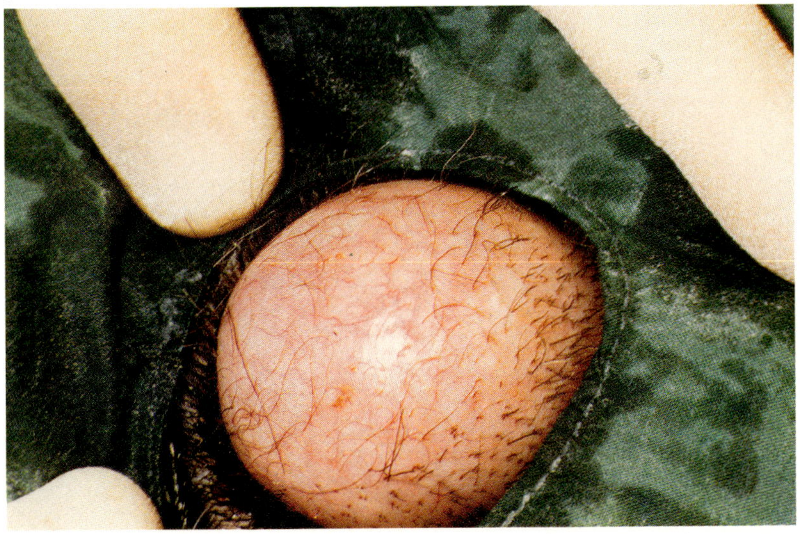

3

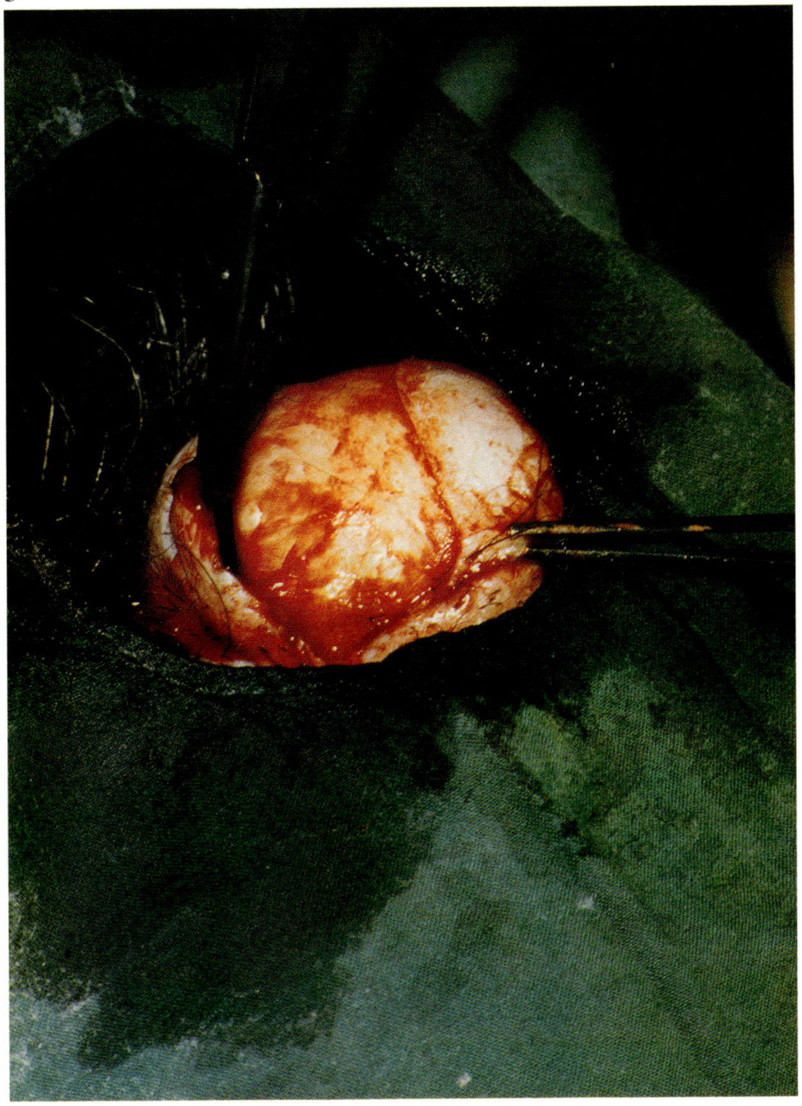

2

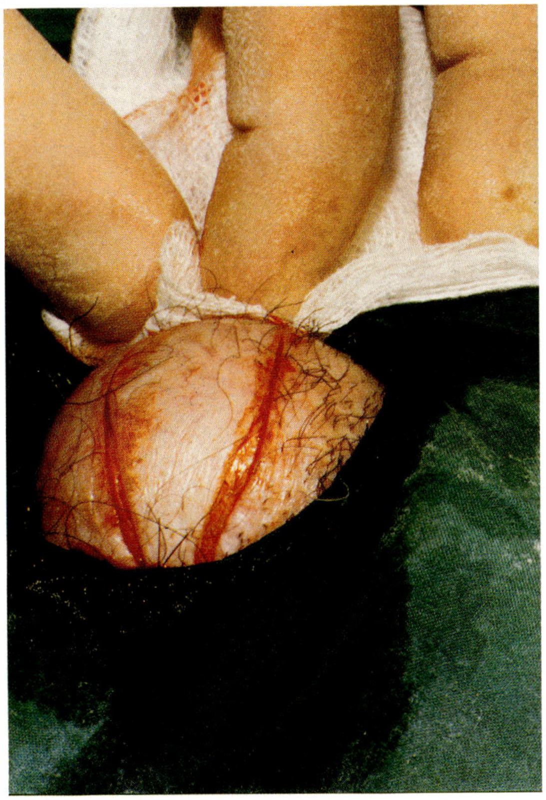

4

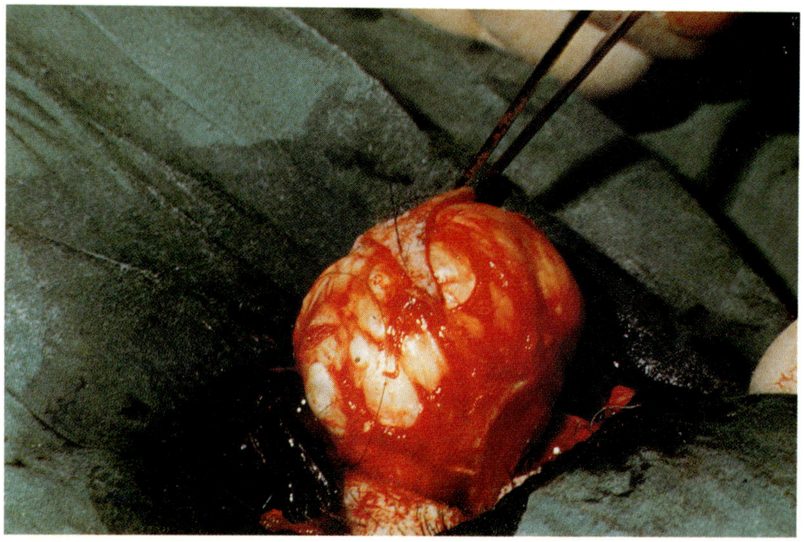

4 It remains to dissect out the deeper tissues again with help of traction.

5

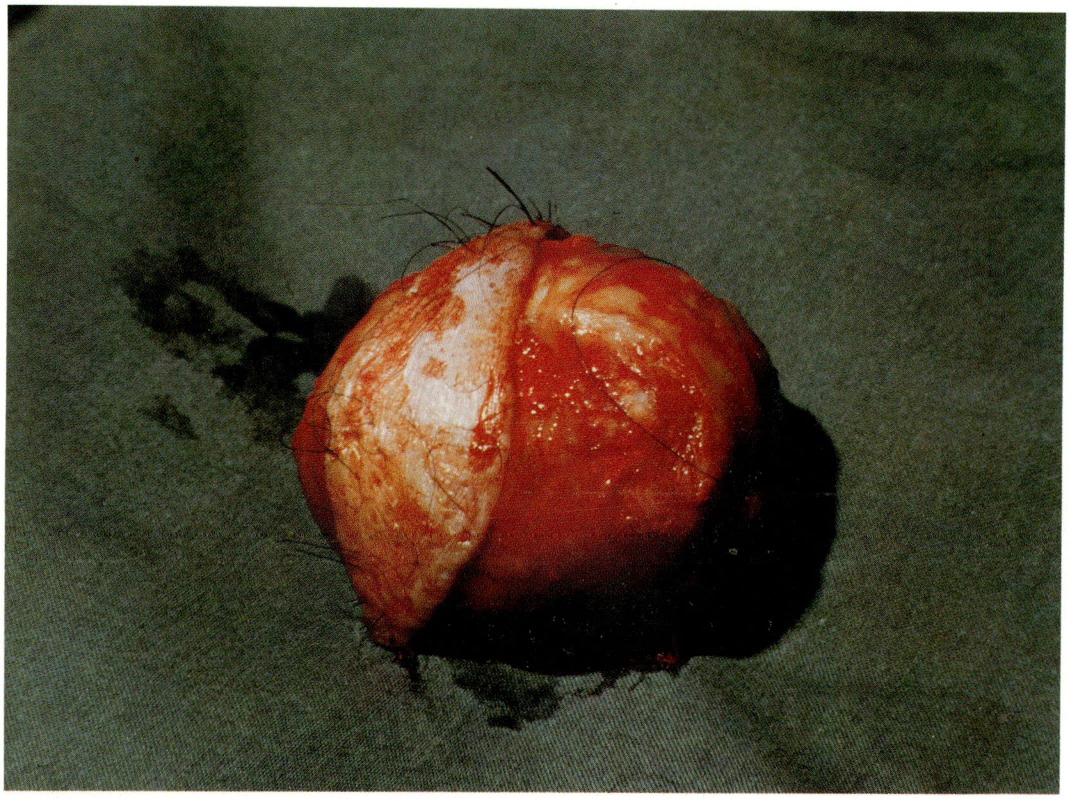

5 Complete excision has been attained.

6

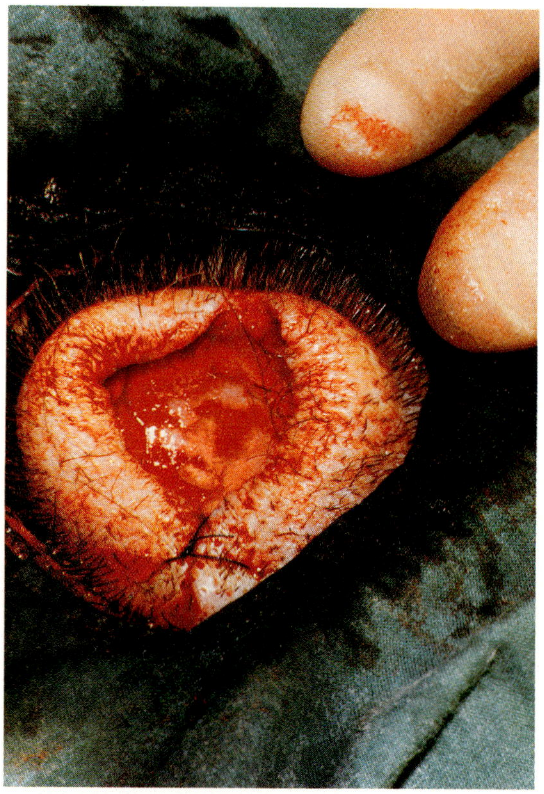

6 This leaves the gap, often with bleeding points which must be tied or cauterised; the first suture has been inserted.

Ganglion

A ganglion is a cystic swelling containing a thick gelatinous like fluid and is found near joints and tendons. The exact cause is not really known. They may in some areas become tender with pressure; in other areas they are painless but sometimes unsightly. **In operating it is important to look out for nerves which could be damaged and because they are related to joints, it is often necessary to remember this when making the incision i.e. in skin-crease lines.**

1

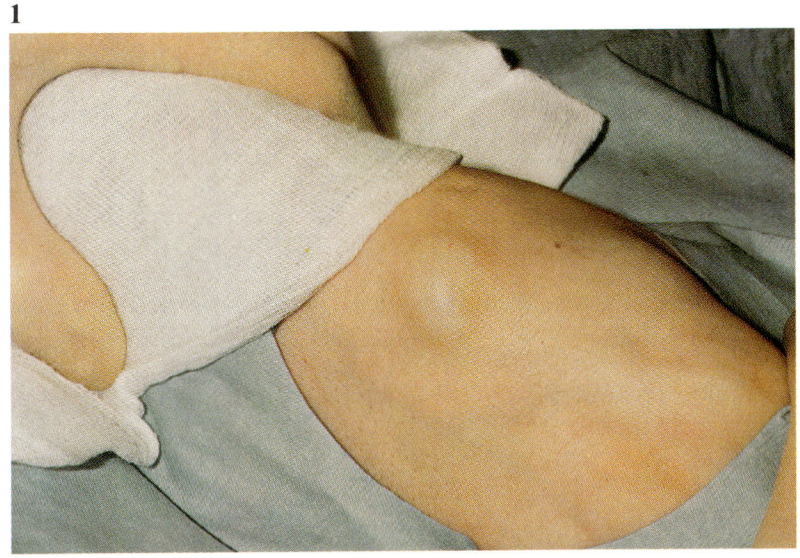

1 A common site of ganglion is in the back of the hand or wrist as seen here. A tourniquet can give a bloodless field for operation under general anaesthesia. Alternatively local anaesthesia may be used.

2

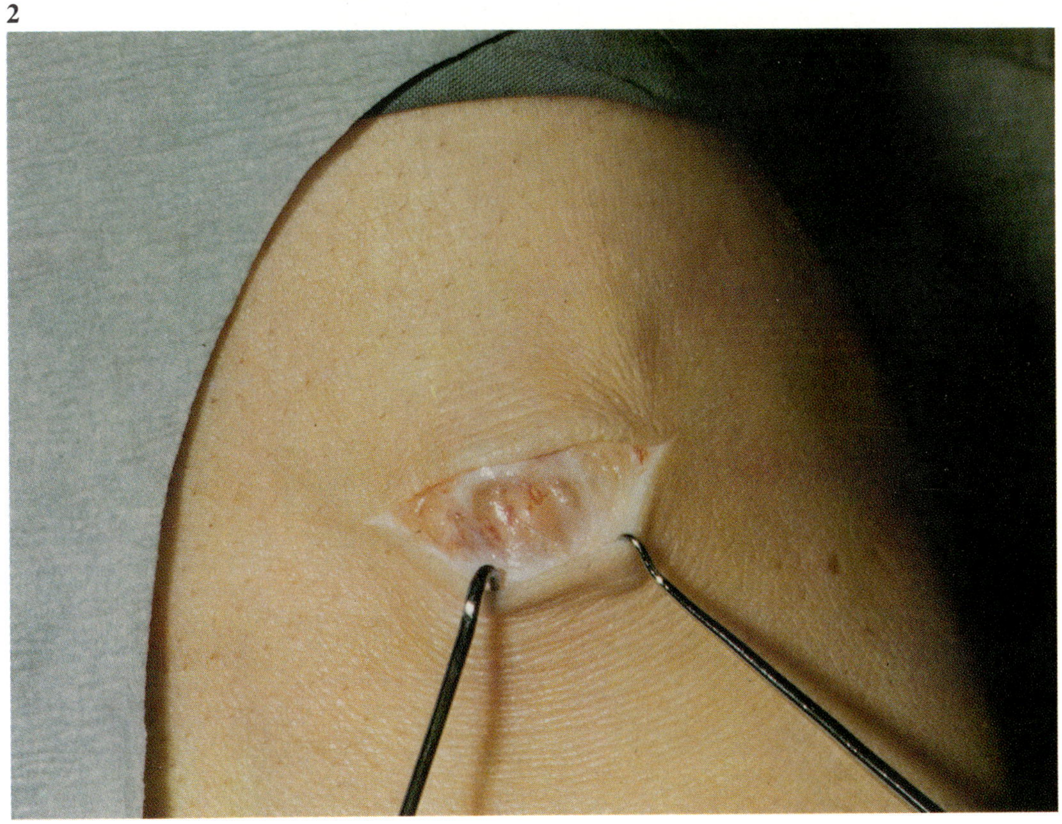

2 Under general anaesthetic and a tourniquet the ganglion was exposed. Note use of skin hooks to minimise skin damage.

3

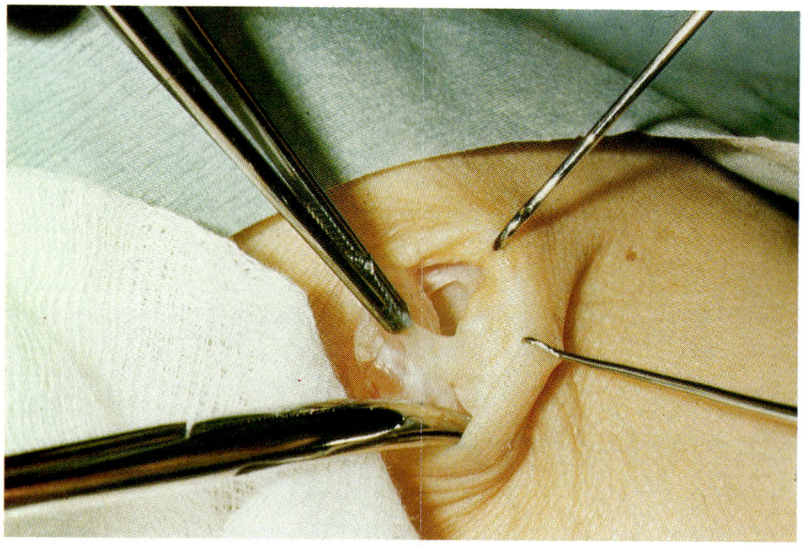

3 The cystic mass is being dissected out from tendons and, if necessary, joint capsule. During dissection be on the look out for nerves and vessels. The latter, if not tied, will lead to bleeding or haematoma.

4

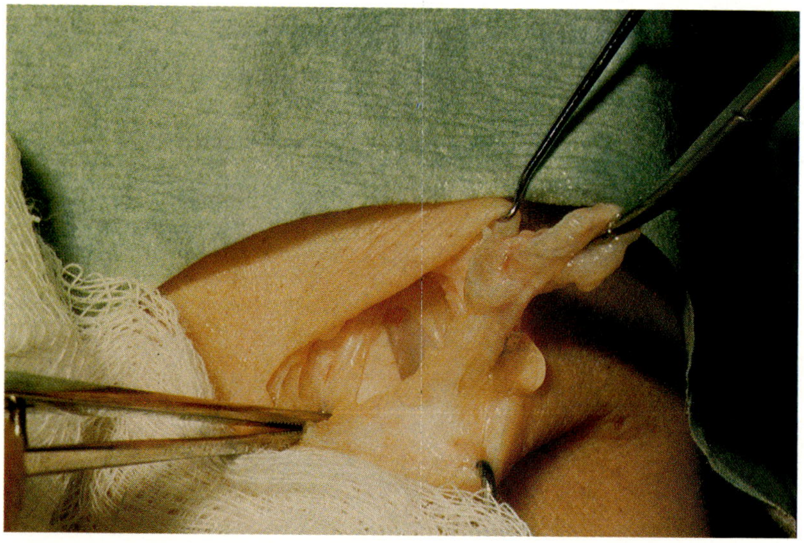

4 In this area the ganglion extended down to a tendon sheath from which it was excised.

Note: It may communicate or be attached to joint capsules and require ligature of communications and suture of capsule.

5

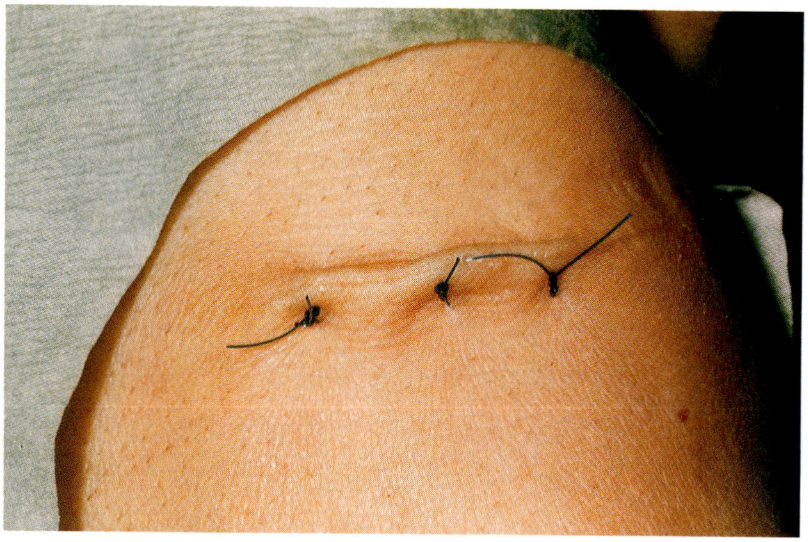

5 Wound was closed with Prolene.

Lipoma of back

Lipomas are fatty tumours arising in subcutaneous fat areas usually in the arm and the back. They can occur in any fat area in the body and occasionally can be malignant as a Liposarcoma. It is wise to send the tissue to the pathology department for analysis.

1

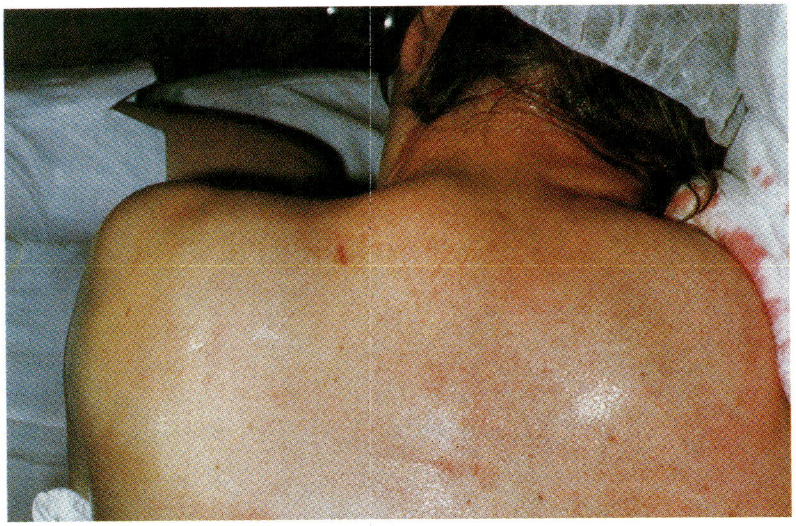

1 Lipoma was present at junction of the base of the neck and the back.

2

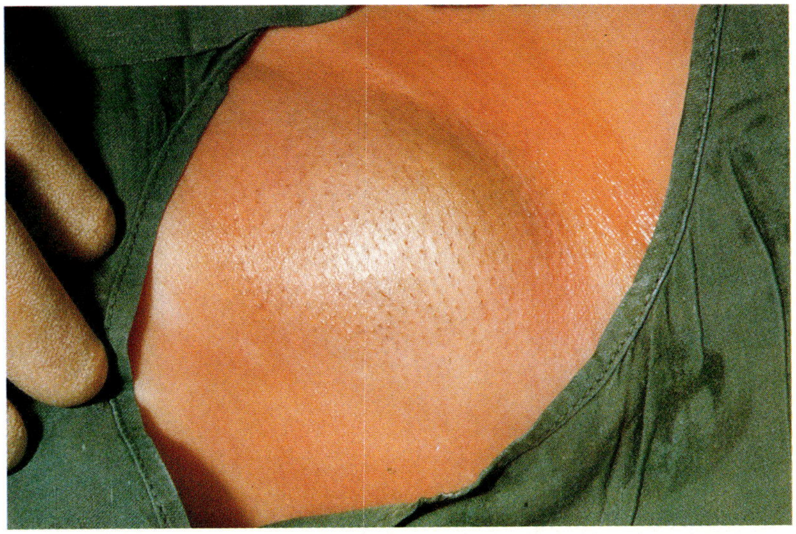

2 In very large ones general anaesthesia may be kinder to the patient. One per cent lignocaine was infiltrated round this lipoma.

3 Before cutting it is essential to test for the success of the local anaesthesia.

4 The skin is incised over the lipoma in the line of skin-crease held between finger and thumb of other hand. This accentuates the bulk of the lipoma.

3

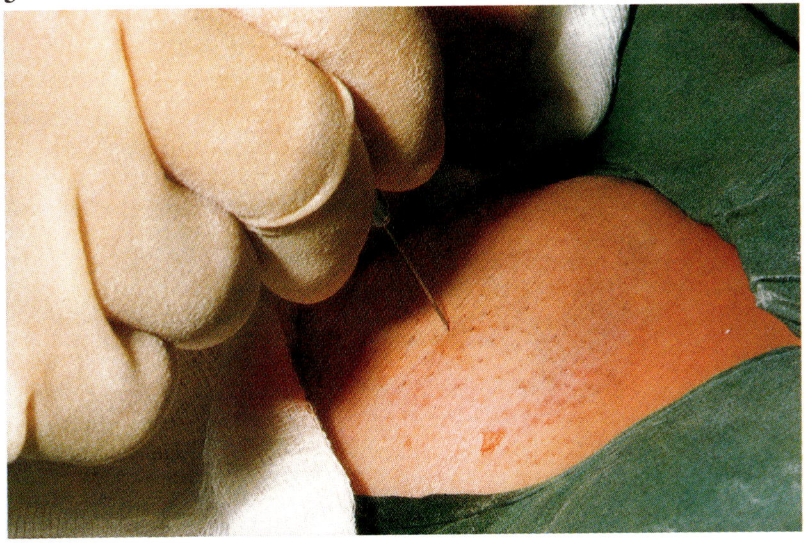

4

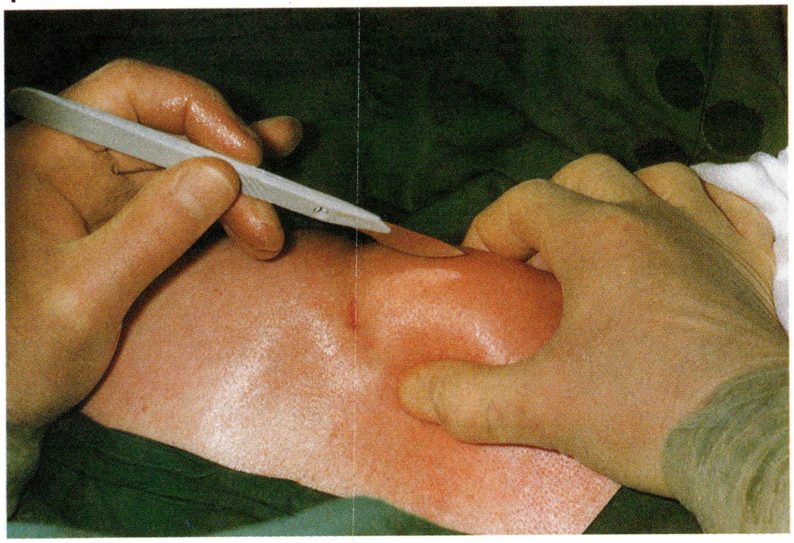

5

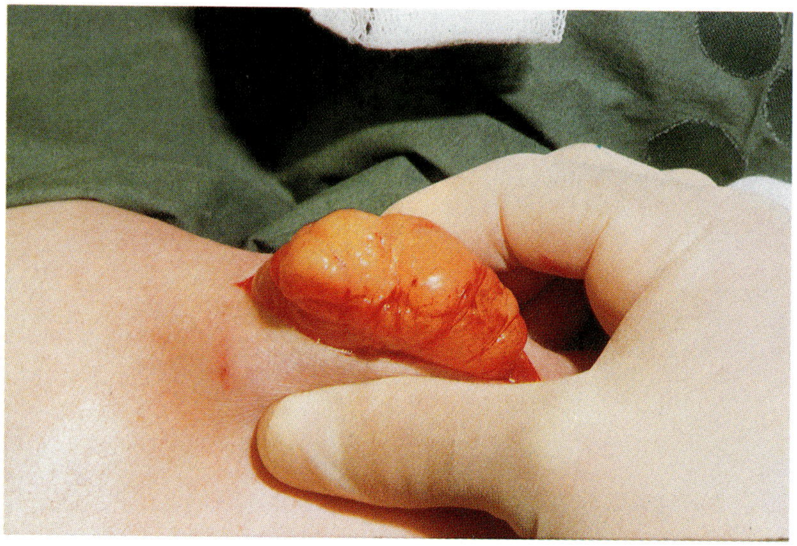

5 Gentle to moderate pressure can almost extrude the fat which can be further dissected out using scissors round the margins.

9

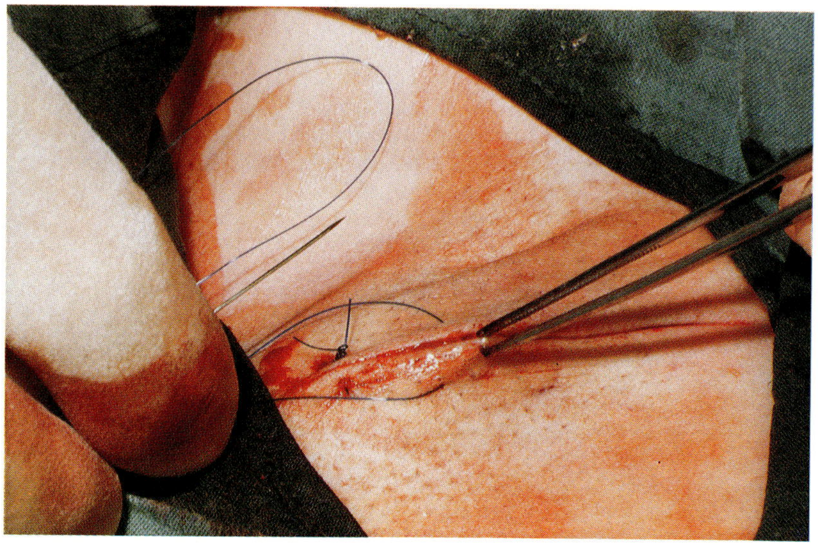

9 Skin is closed with interrupted Prolene mattress sutures.

6

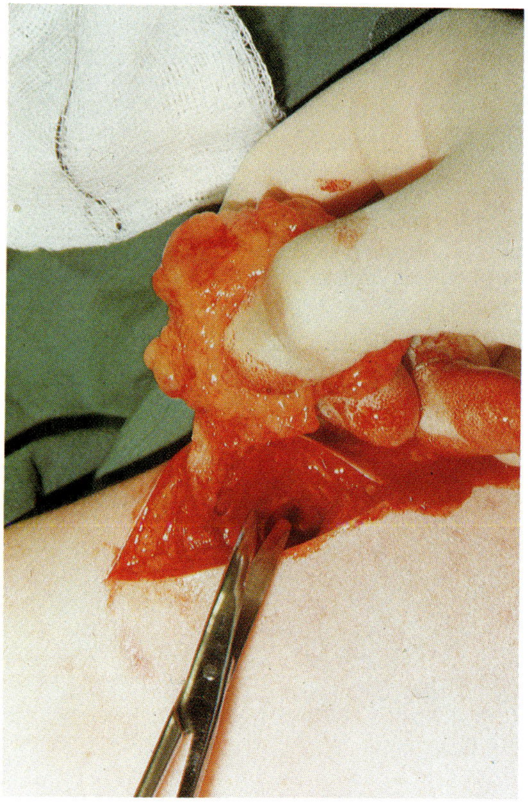

6 Final touches with the scissors completed the removal.

7

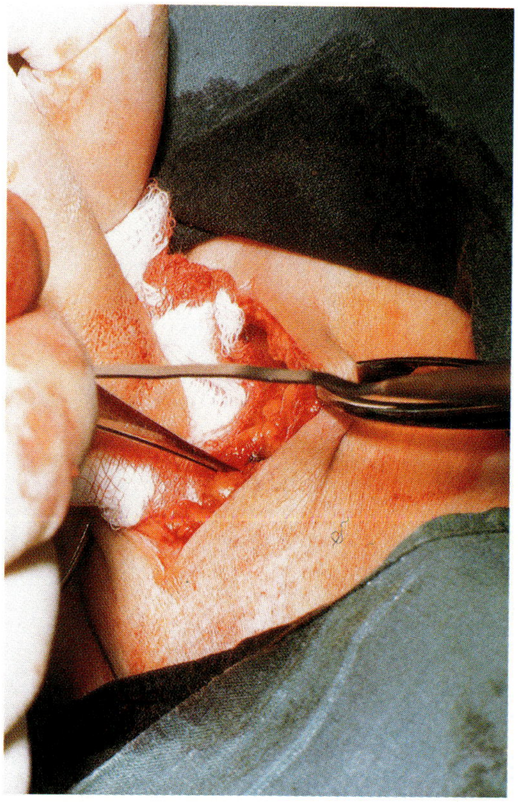

7 Diathermy may be used to stop the bleeding.

8

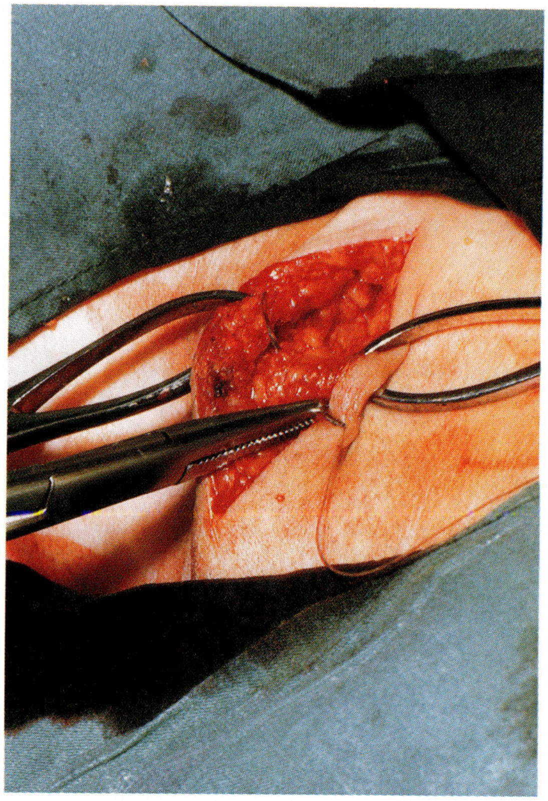

8 Deep catgut sutures may help to approximate the skin margins and obliterate the dead space. A suction drain and/or a pressure dressing may be required with large lipomas.

Biopsy of temporal artery

This procedure is required for the diagnosis of temporal arteritis.

1

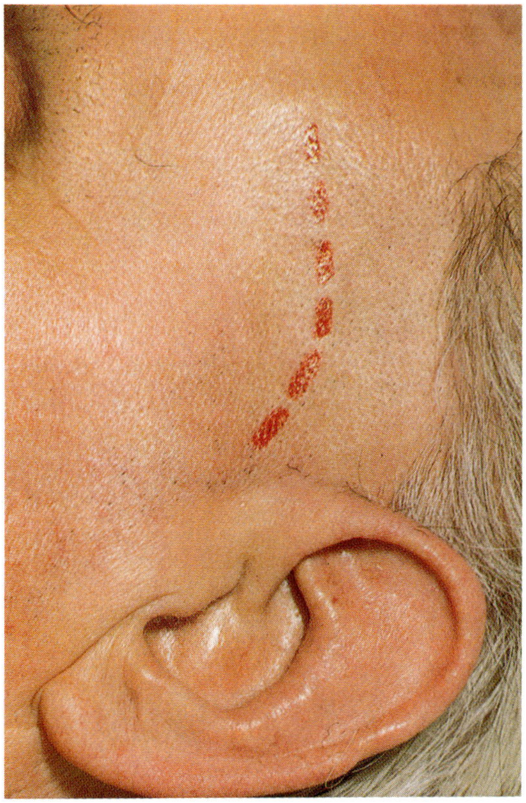

2

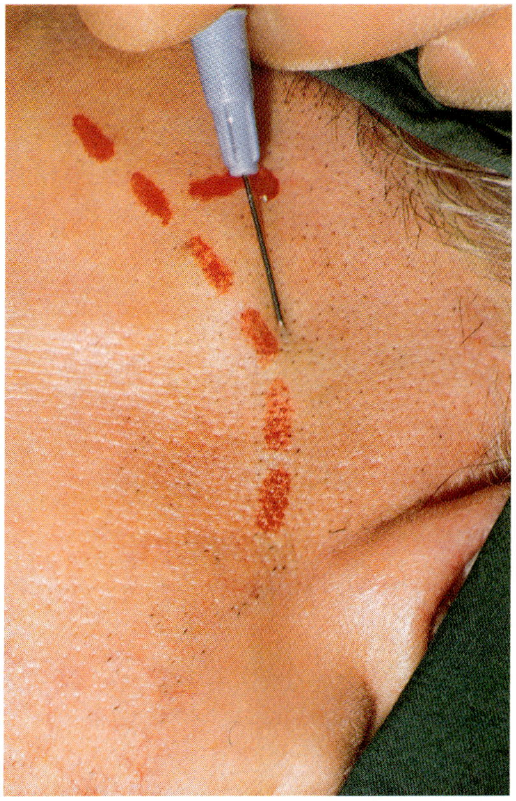

3

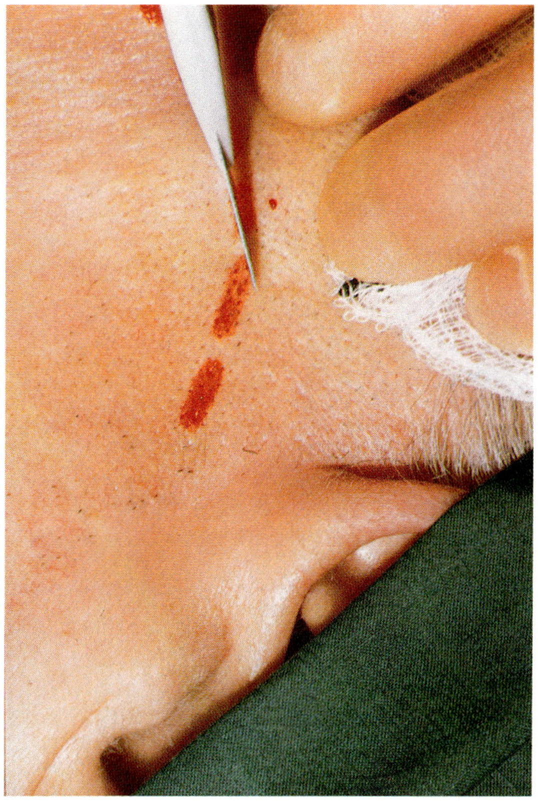

1 The artery can be palpated as it passes upwards in front of the ear, gradually sweeping forward into the forehead. The line of the artery is outlined prior to injection of local anaesthetic.

2 A few millilitres of one per cent lignocaine are sufficient and are injected in the line of the artery, care being taken to avoid injection into the vessel. This is done by aspiration before injection.

3 A short incision about 1.5-2 cm is all that is required. The edges of the wound are separated by skin hooks.

4

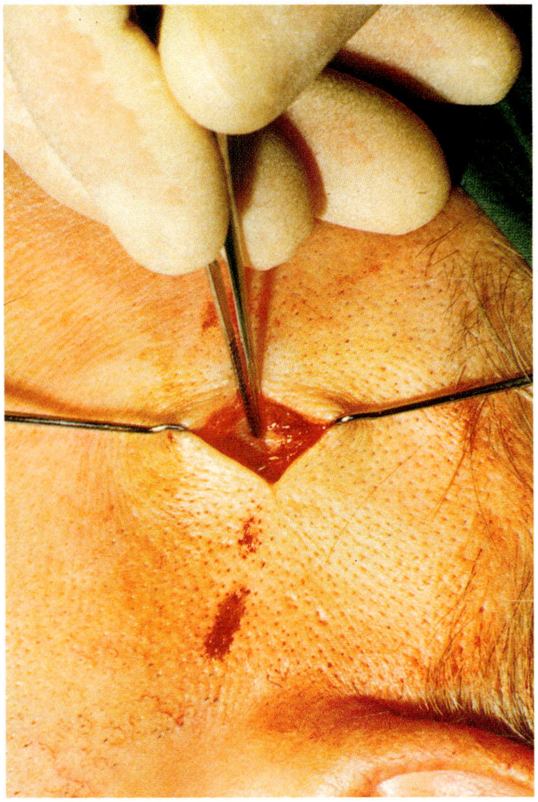

5

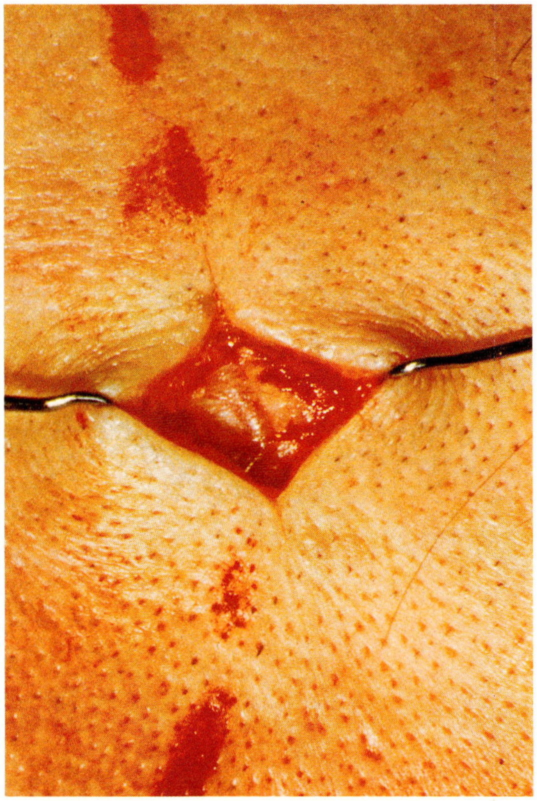

4 The artery is just visible in the wound.

5 The artery is easier seen when the superficial fascia is dissected out.

6

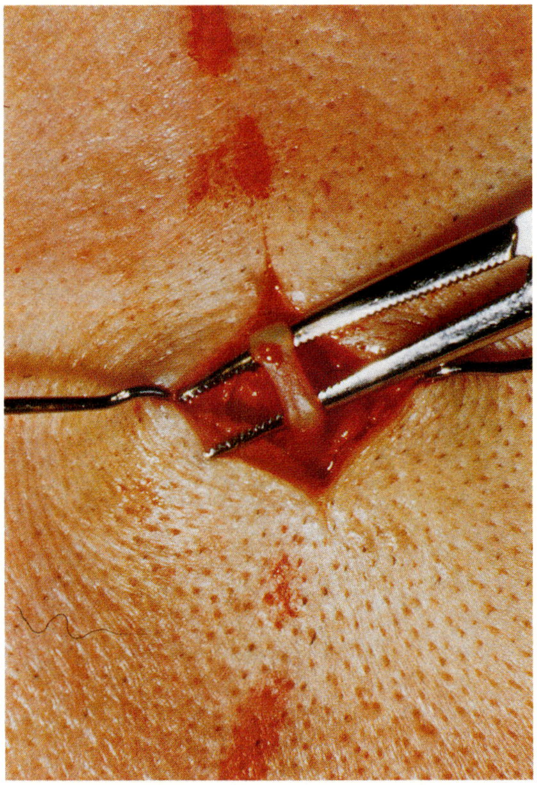

7

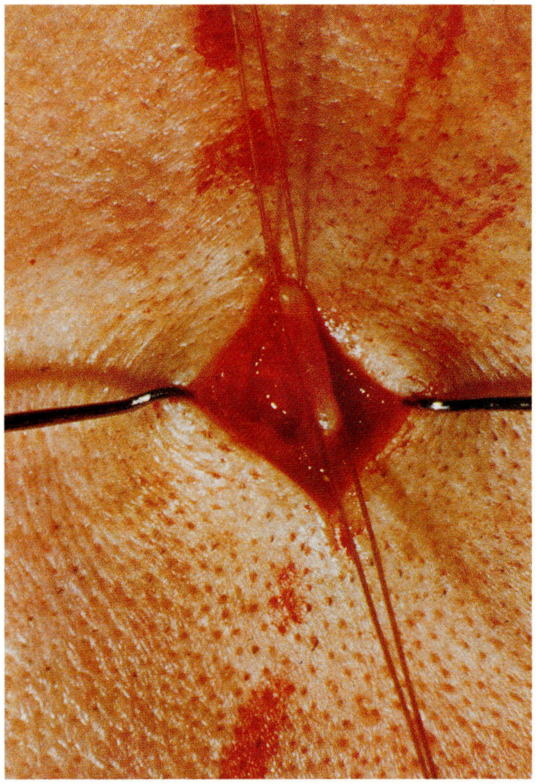

6 A length of the vessel is isolated.

7 Catgut sutures are placed round the vessel and tied.

8

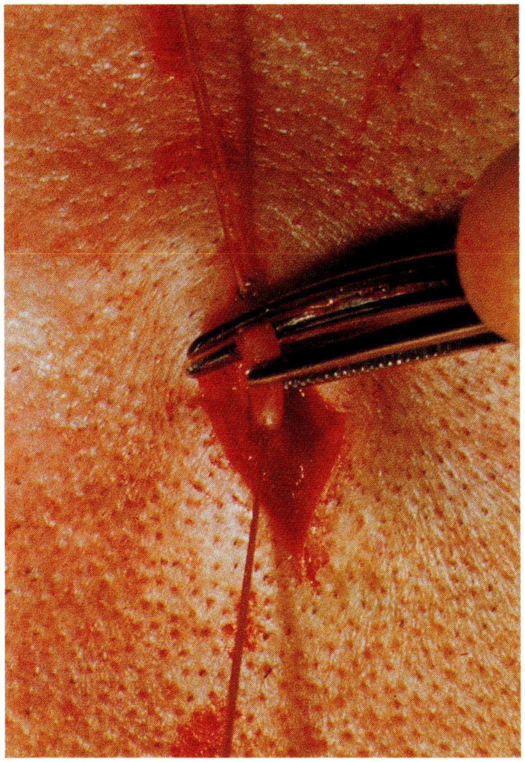

8 About 1.5 cm of the artery is excised for histology.

9

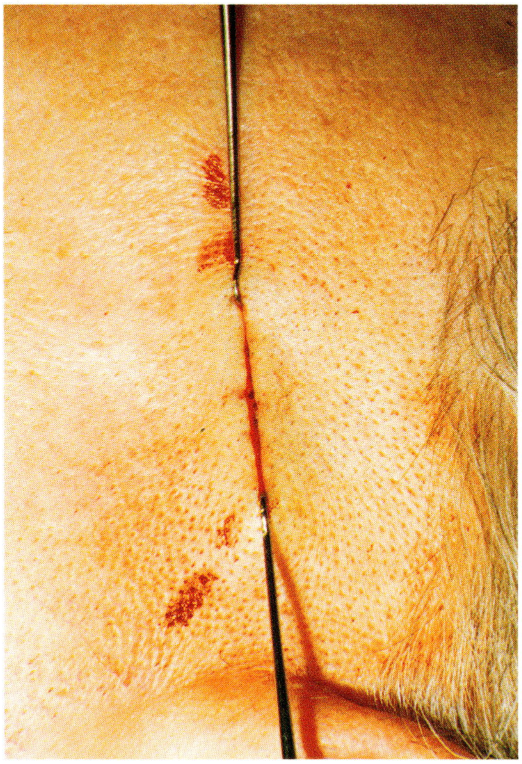

9 Traction on skin hooks at either end of the wound will facilitate fine closure.

10

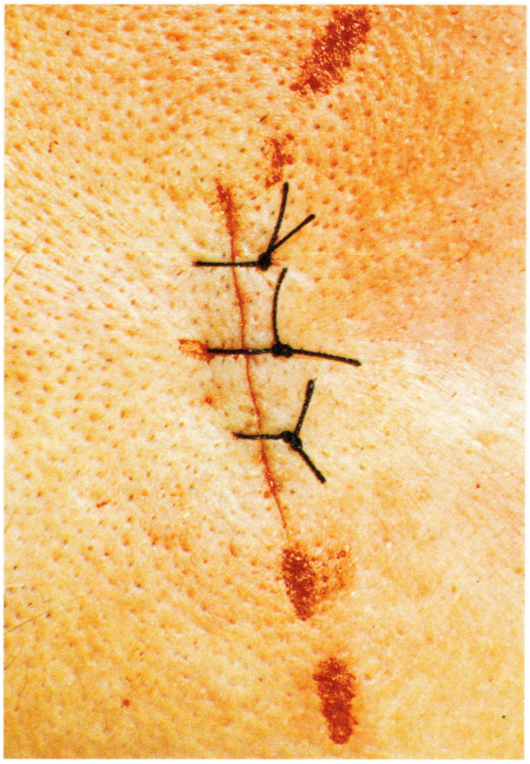

10 This is done by simple skin sutures.

Excision of gland of neck

This is usually required to establish diagnosis: to exclude tuberculosis or reticulosis in the child or adult, and secondary carcinoma in the adult and elderly.

1

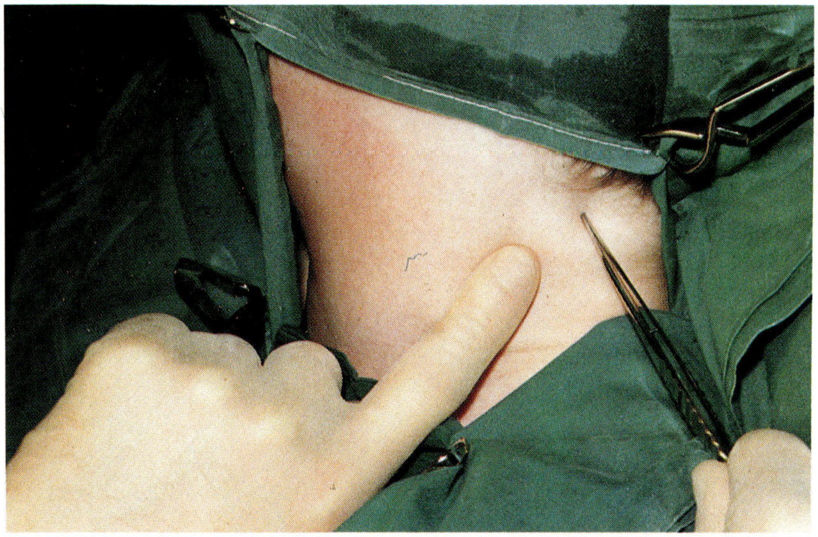

2

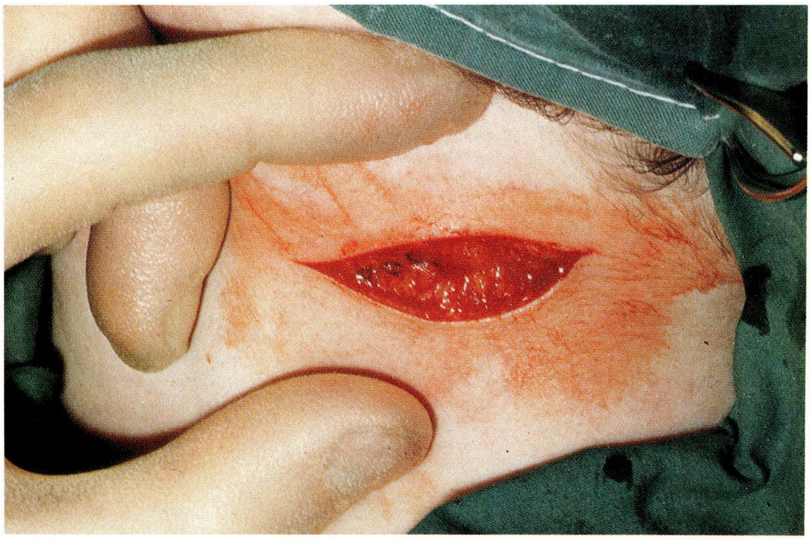

1 The gland in the upper part of the anterior triangle of the neck is outlined by two blue spots and finger and forceps.

2 Under general anaesthesia an incision is made over the swelling in the line of a skin crease.

3 Gradual deepening of the incision and careful haemostasis will reveal the swelling. Nodes present in the internal jugular chains will require retraction of the sternomastoid laterally.

4 Further dissection brought the enlarged gland into view and allowed removal.

Caution: Take great care with the deep surface: look out for blood vessels and nerves.

3

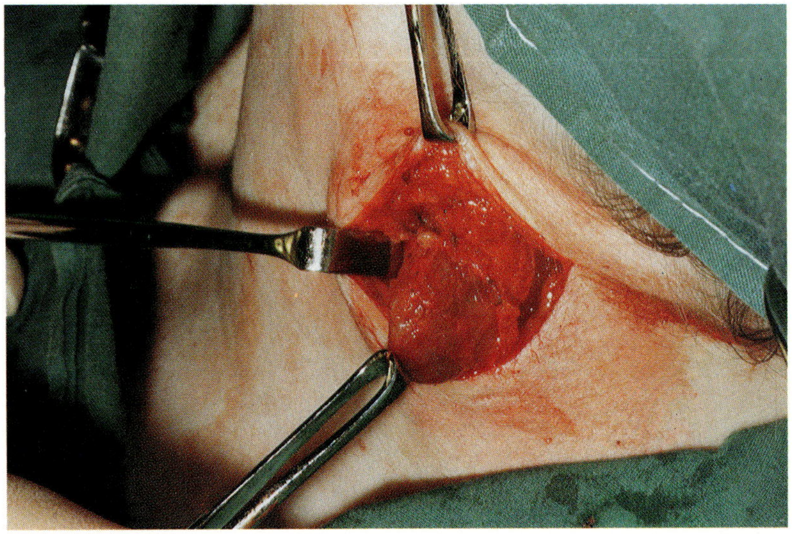

4

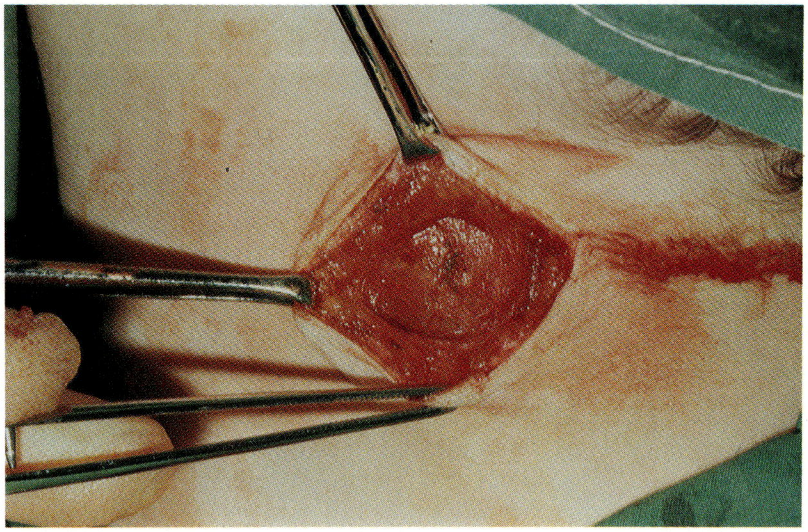

5

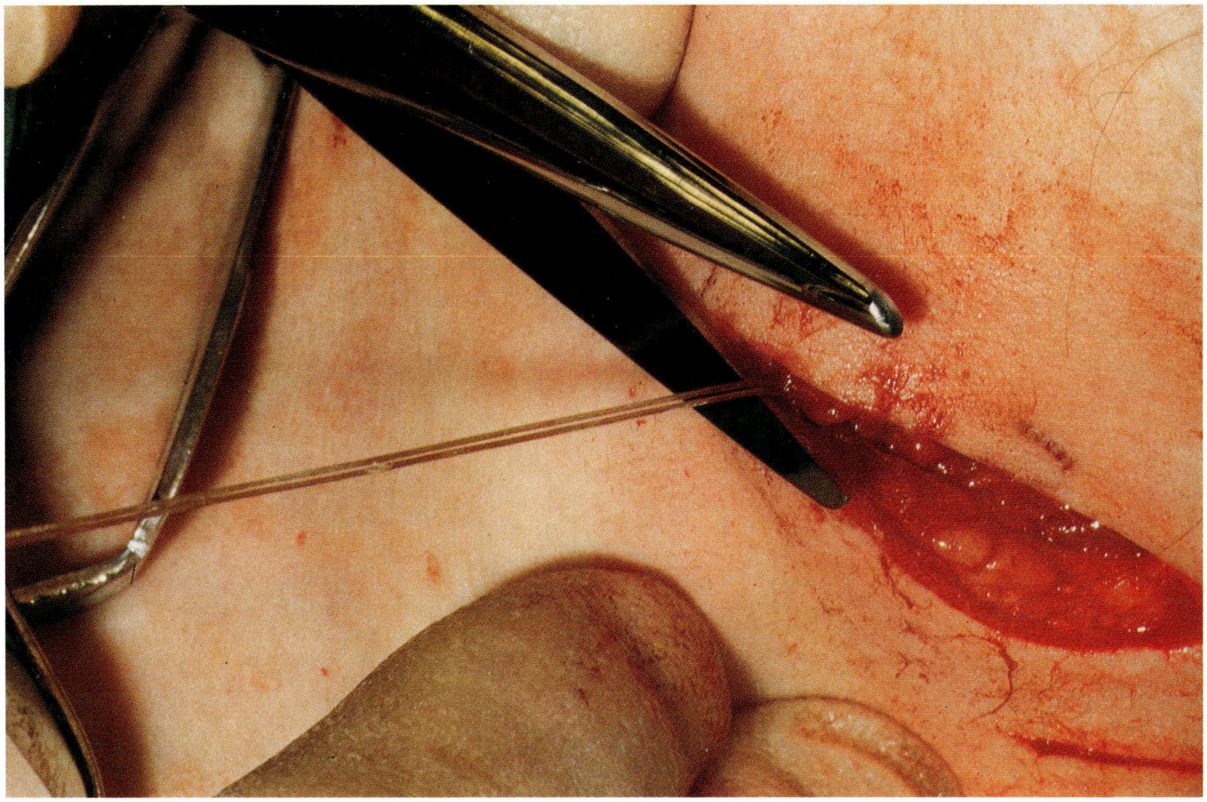

5 The deeper layers are sutured by interrupted catgut stitches which will help to bring the edges of the skin more neatly together.

6

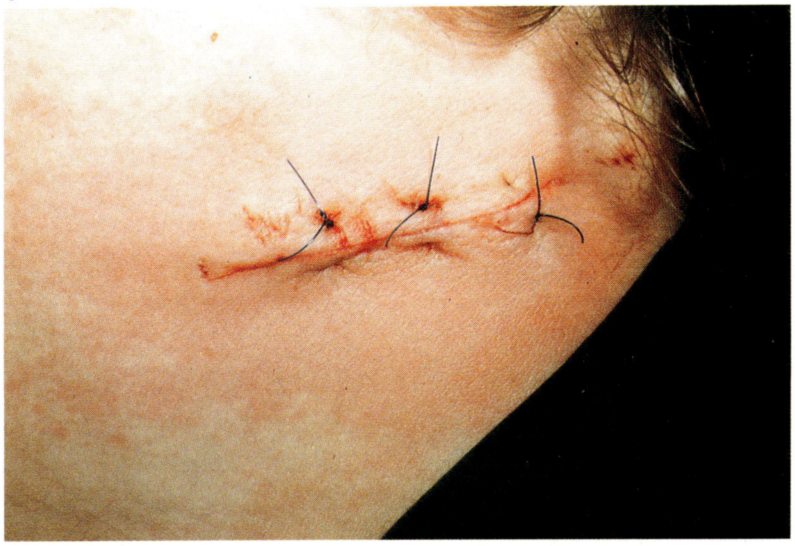

6 The skin is closed with interrupted Prolene stitches.

Excision of thyroglossal cyst

A thyroglossal cyst is a cystic space developing along the line of descent of the thyroid which develops as a bud, pushing down from the floor of the pharynx and presents as a midline swelling in the neck. It characteristically moves up when the tongue is protruded, showing the relationship between the tongue and the thyroglossal cyst and tract.

1

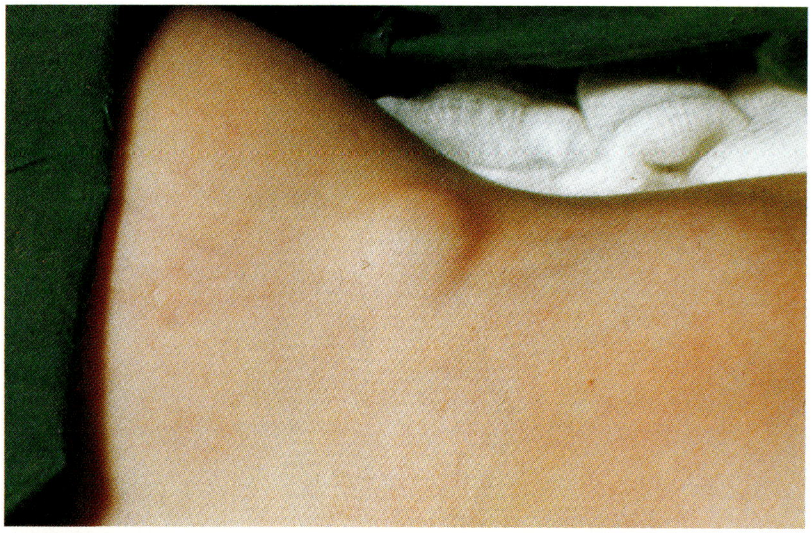

2

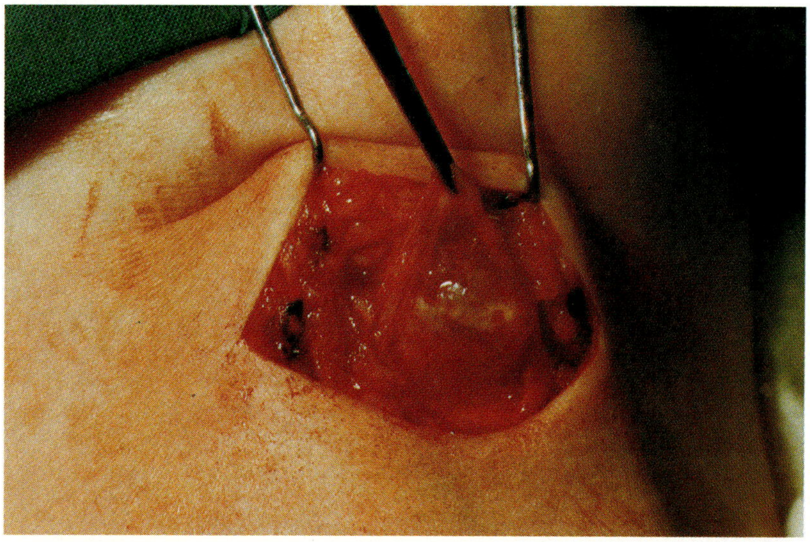

3

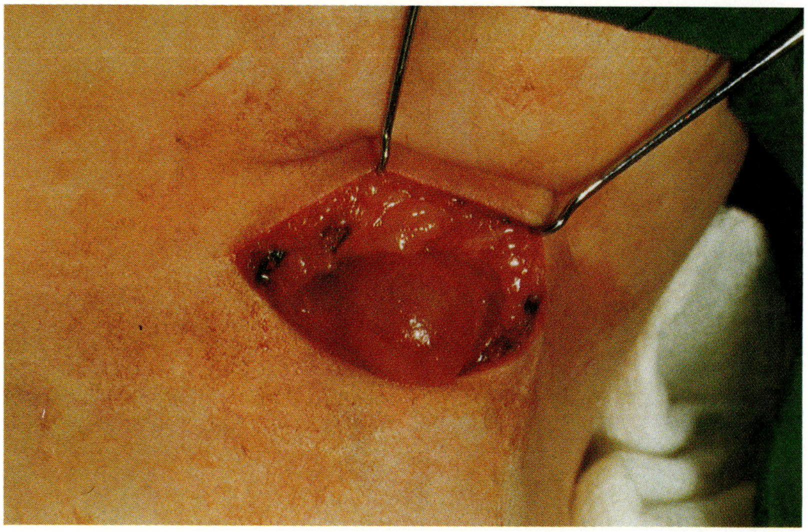

1 A lateral view showing the smooth swelling just below the region of the hyoid bone.

2 Under general anaesthetic a transverse incision is made across the cyst and the skin reflected. On division of the platysma the cyst comes into view.

3 Dissection all round isolates the cyst and the tract which lies behind and at the upper pole. Vessels are ligated or coagulated. Note the use of skin hooks rather than tissue forceps. The hooks are less damaging to the skin.

4

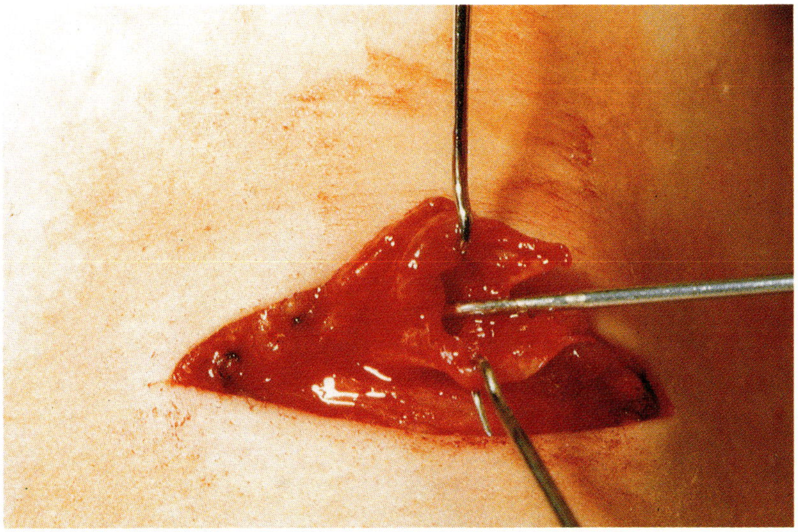

4 The cyst was opened and a probe inserted along the thyroglossal ducts to determine its length and direction.

5 The duct is being dissected out to the hyoid bone, behind which it passes just to the left of the midline.

6 On lifting the duct up there appears to be a broad stem. This however is narrowed down by dissection.

7 The narrowing in the duct is visible. The probe would go no further than the lower border of the thyroid bone and it was obvious that there was no upward prolongation.

5

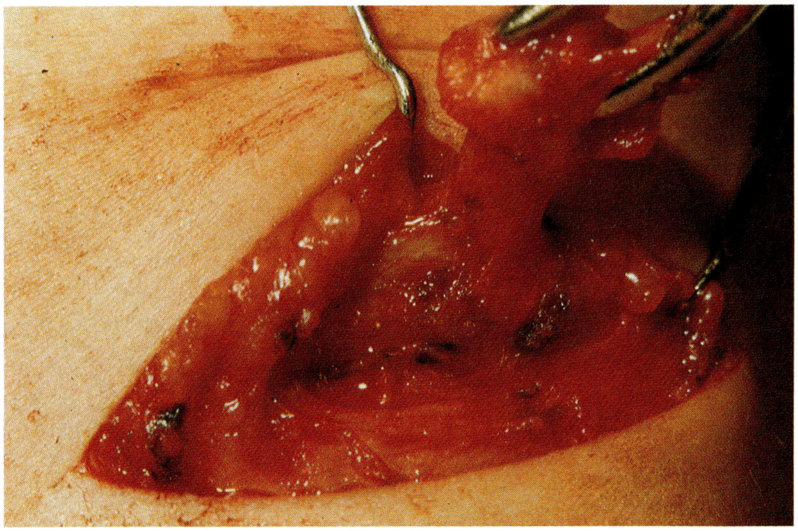

6

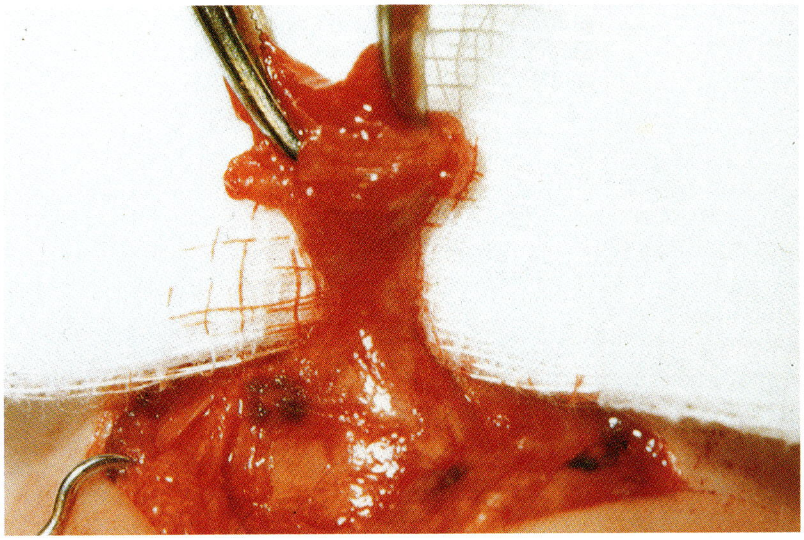

7

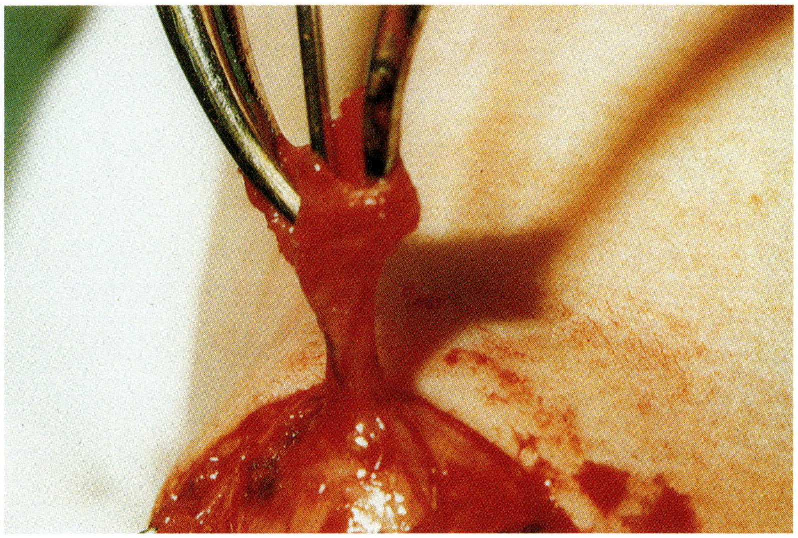

8

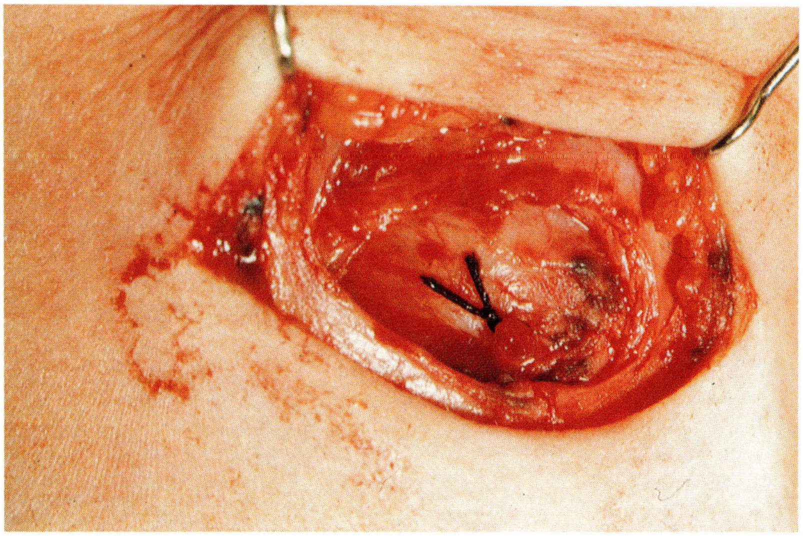

8 The duct was then cut off flush and tied. If there was a further prolongation of the duct the middle part of the hyoid should be resected and the duct followed upwards towards the base of the tongue. If any duct is left a further recurrence is possible.

9

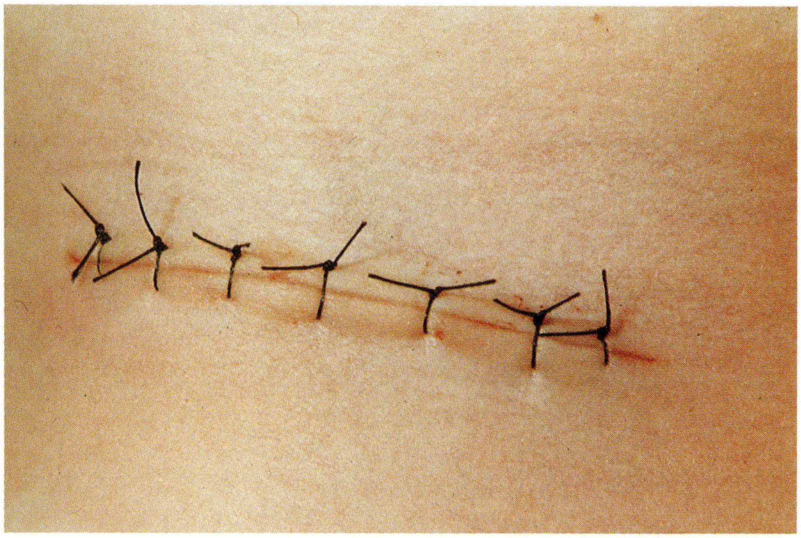

9 The platysma is sutured with catgut and the skin closed.

10

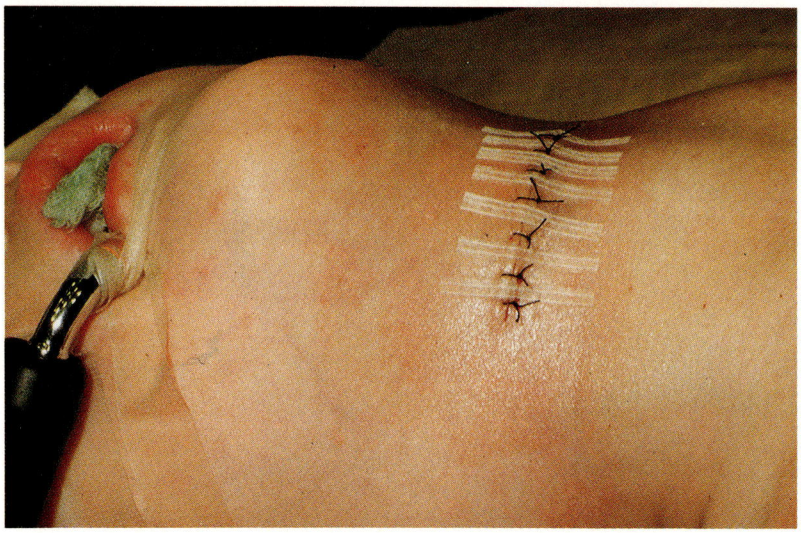

10 Steristrips can be added to ensure smooth coaptation of the wound edges. Stitches can be removed in two to three days and steristrips left for a further four days.

Parotid duct stricture

Operations on the parotid duct are usually for dilatation of the duct to allow passage of a stone or a plastic operation to keep the duct open following a stricture.

1

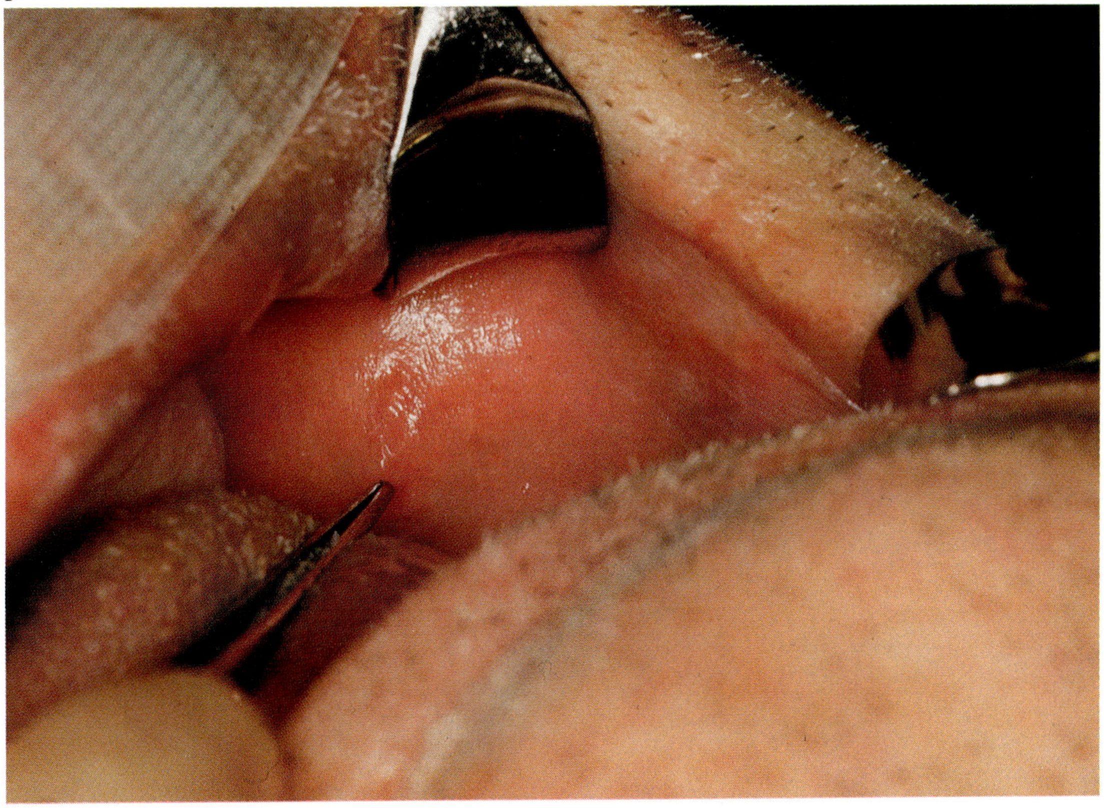

1 The duct orifice is located on the cheek opposite the second premolar tooth of the upper jaw. If the patient is edentulous, as here, its presence may be detected by pressure on the gland and the duct to express pus or secretion. The opening is demonstrated by the forceps.

2

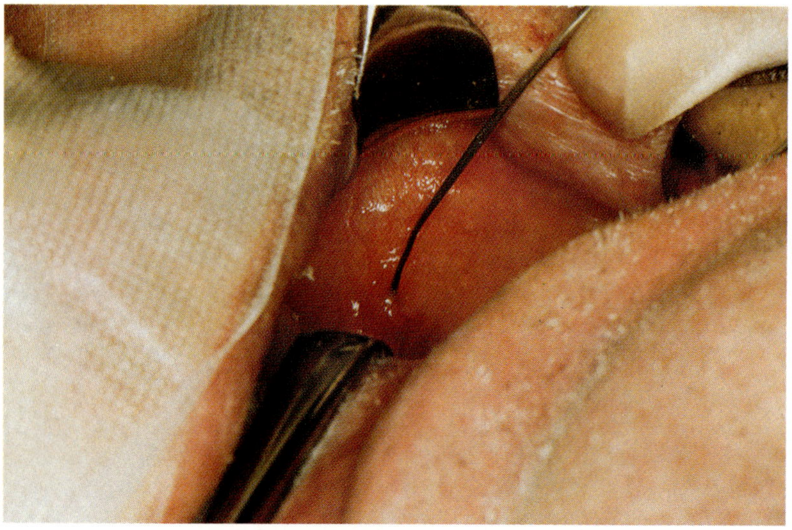

2 **A probe is inserted into the duct to confirm its presence** and a little viscus secretion can be seen at the orifice, which can be further gradually dilated by Nelaton dilators.

3

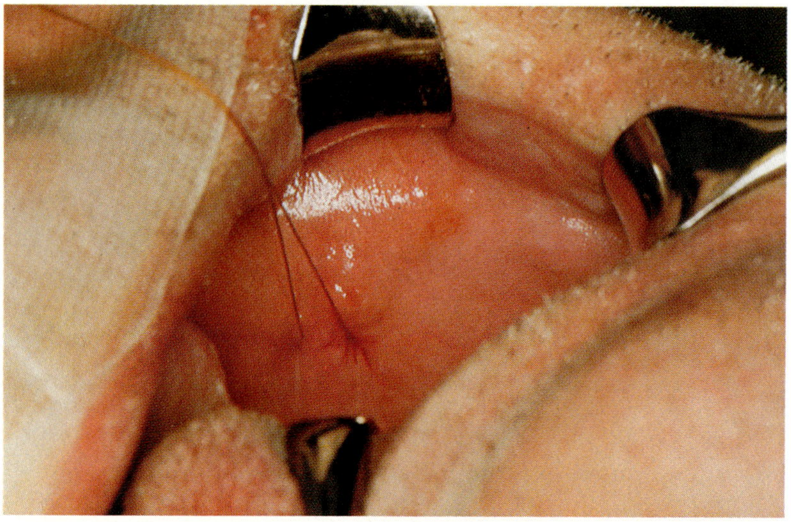

3 **A sling was placed round this duct proximal to the stone** to prevent it going back towards the gland on manipulation. The orifice of the duct is visible on the right of the sling.

4 **Because a stricture was present the duct was cut with scissors** back to the stone and stricture which was laid open.

5 **The lining of the duct was stitched to the mucosa to keep the duct open** and prevent post-traumatic fibrosis, and stricture.

4

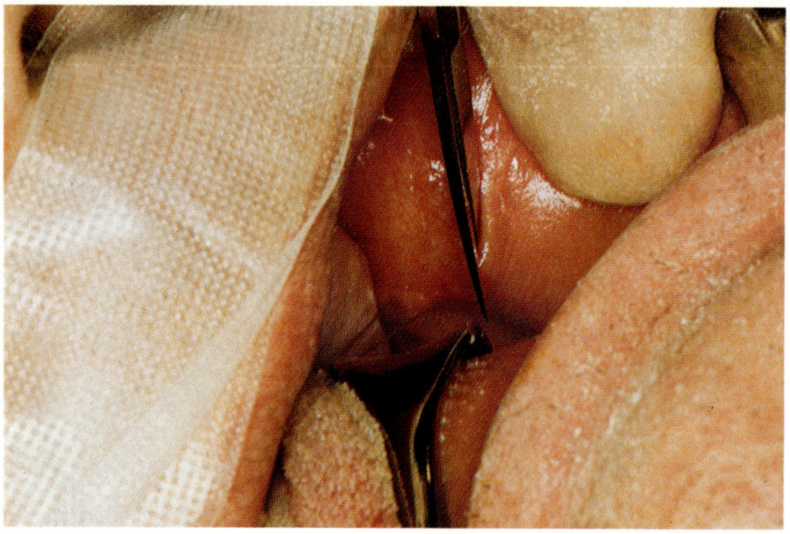

5

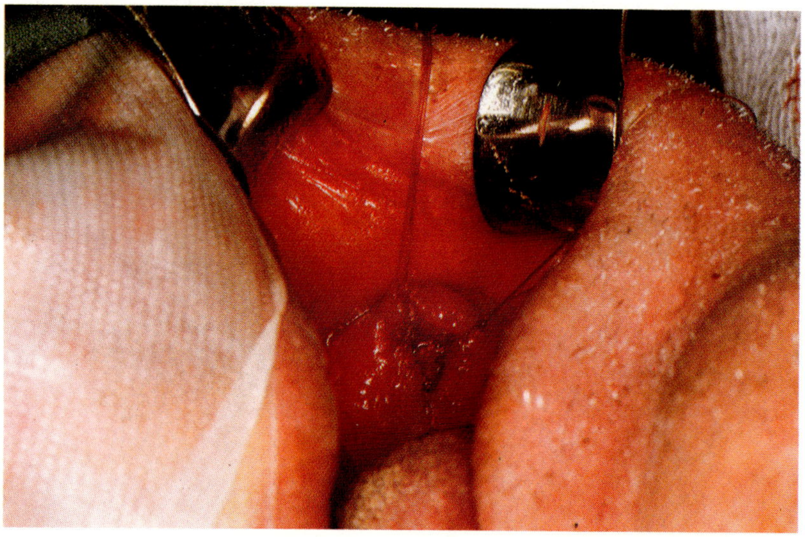

Tracheostomy

The incision is made in the line of the neck creases, transversely 2.5 cm above the sternal notch and at least 5 cm long, with a small firm sand bag beneath the shoulders to hyperextend the neck and the patient towelled as for thyroidectomy. **In the case of acute obstruction of the airway the neck veins may be very distended and a vertical midline incision would produce less bleeding.**

In an emergency situation a cricothyroidostomy would be faster and safer.

1 Before starting at all, assemble, dis-assemble and test tube and ensure fit with anaesthetic tubing will be possible. Is suction available? Use low-pressure seal tube.

1

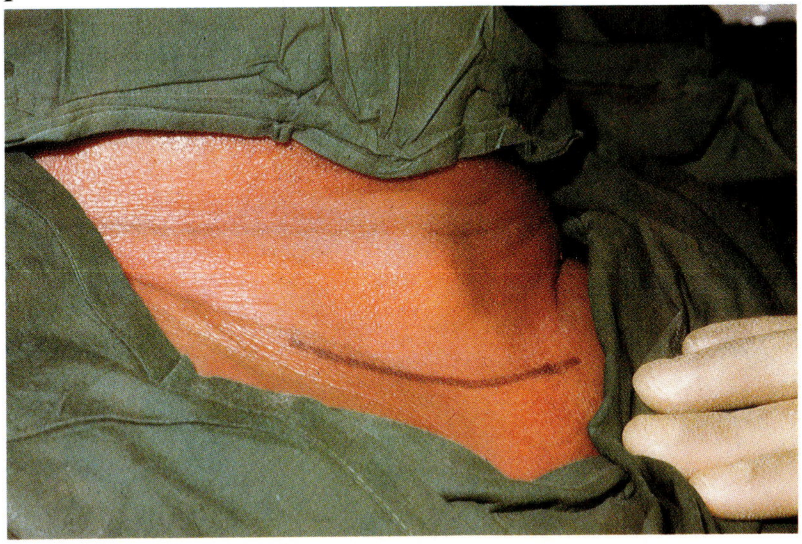

2 The platysma is incised in the line of the incision, which can be conveniently held open with a Joll's retractor. Superficial veins, particularly those joining the anterior jugular veins, are ligated with fine braided non-absorbable suture material such as 3/0 Nurolon and divided between the ligatures.

2

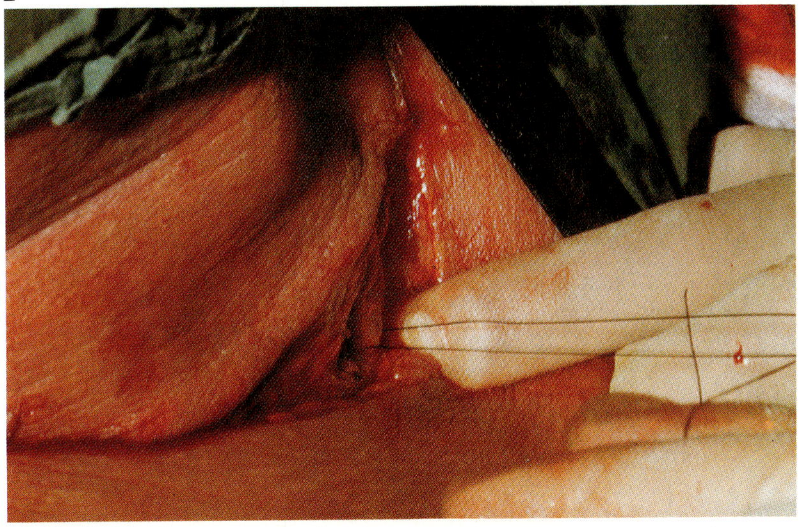

3 The deep cervical fascia is incised vertically in the midline, this incision being deepened with scissors to separate the strap muscles.

3

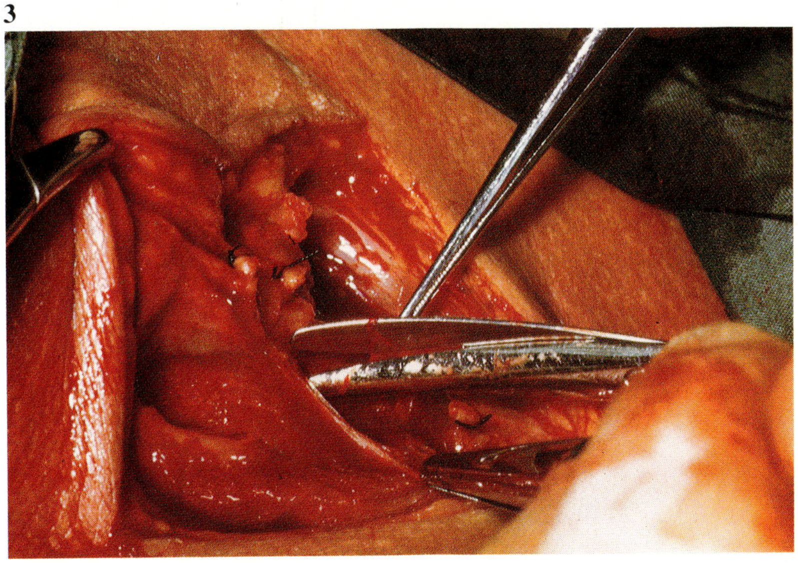

4

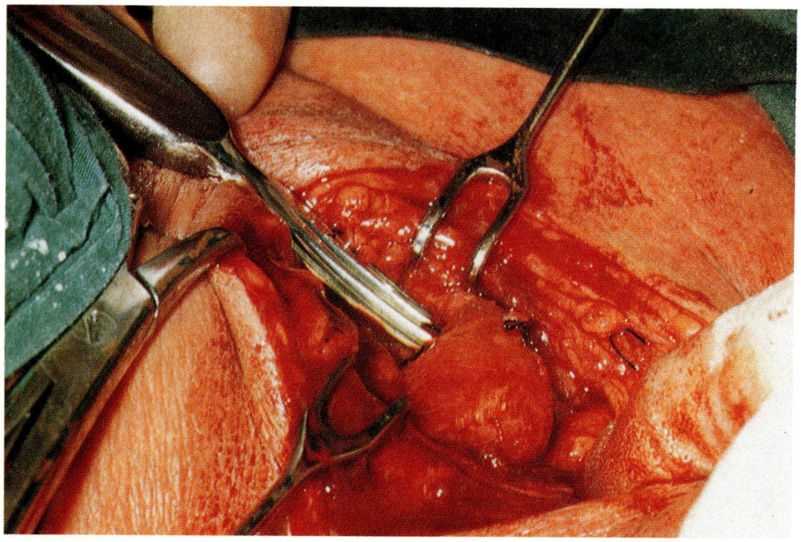

5

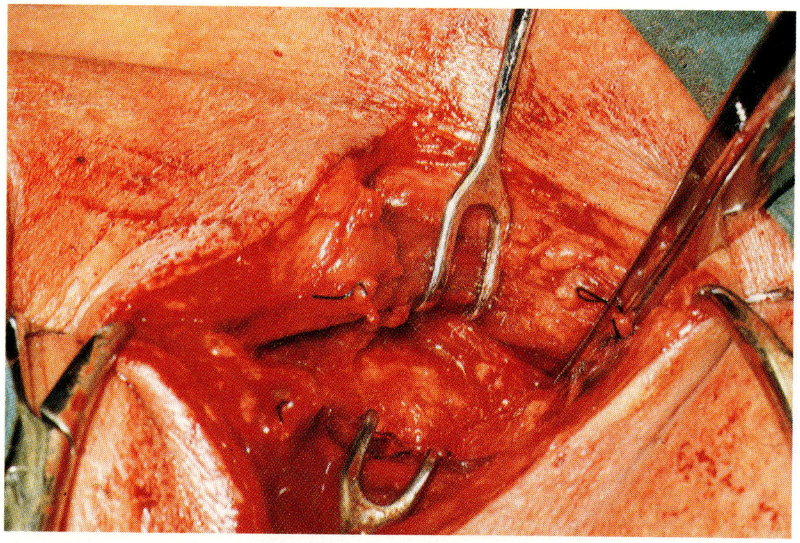

4 The pretracheal fascia is divided revealing the isthmus of the thyroid. Applied to the front of the trachea, the flat Kocher's dissector is convenient for elevating the isthmus, which is then divided between clamps and ligated.

Note: The thyroid isthmus may be usually displaced.

5 Small double hook retractors are used to hold open the space between the strap muscles, exposing the upper three cartilagenous rings of the trachea, now cleared of thyroid isthmus.

6 The size and cuff of the tracheostomy tube selected earlier are checked. A single hook steadies the cricoid in preparation for incising the trachea.

7 A scalpel is used to incise longitudinally the second and third or third and fourth cartilagenous rings of the trachea, anteriorly. By this means, a disc of anterior wall of the upper trachea of appropriate size to accommodate the selected tube is excised.

An alternative technique is to make an n-shaped incision in the trachea with base downwards. The elevated flap is then stitched to the lower end of the wound, thus allowing for easier reposition of the tracheostomy tube (after Bjork).

6

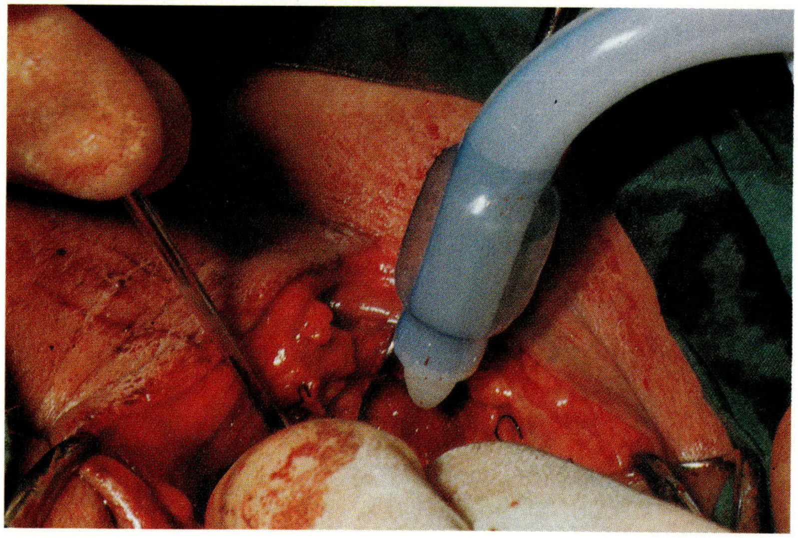

7

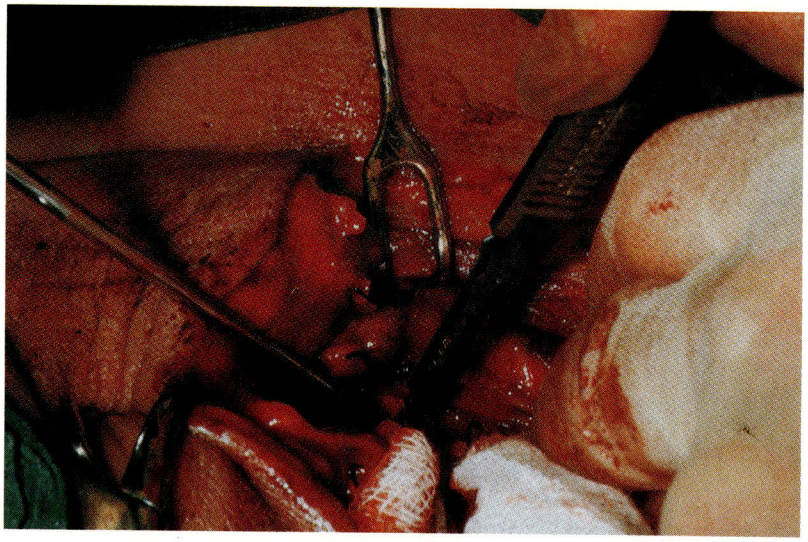

8 The selected, tested, tracheostomy tube is inserted by the surgeon as the anaesthetist pulls the endotracheal tube (ETT) upwards.

Note: The ETT should be removed no further than the upper end of the opening in the trachea, so that if a problem occurs with placement of the tracheostomy tube, the tube can be rapidly and easily re-advanced. Only when the tracteostomy tube is in, tested and known to be correct should the ETT be finally removed.

8

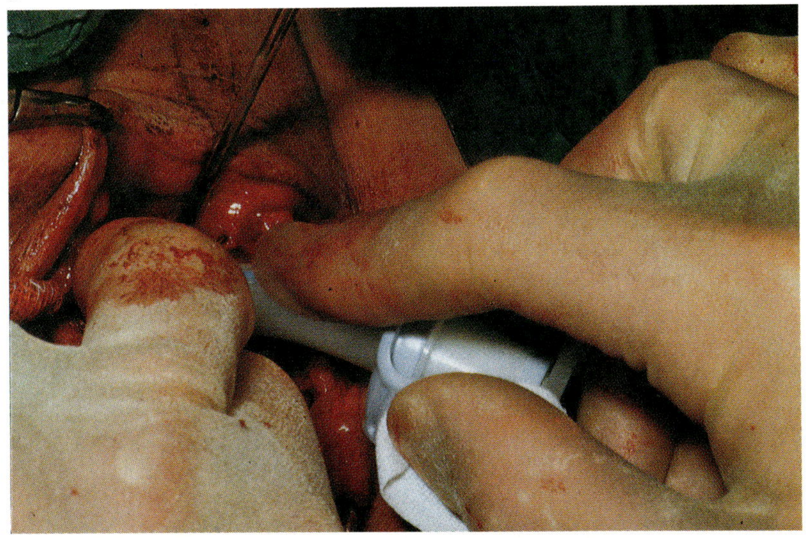

9

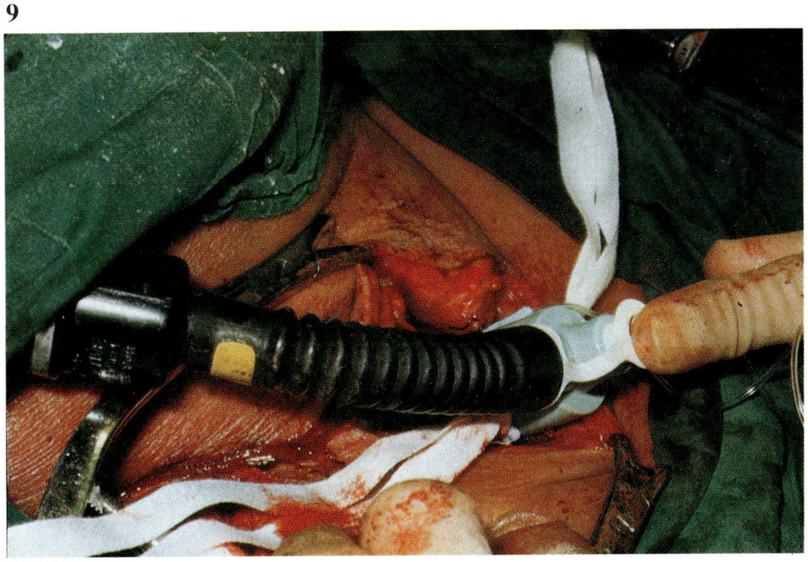

9 A sterile catheter mount is connected to the tube, and the patient reconnected to ventilation.

10

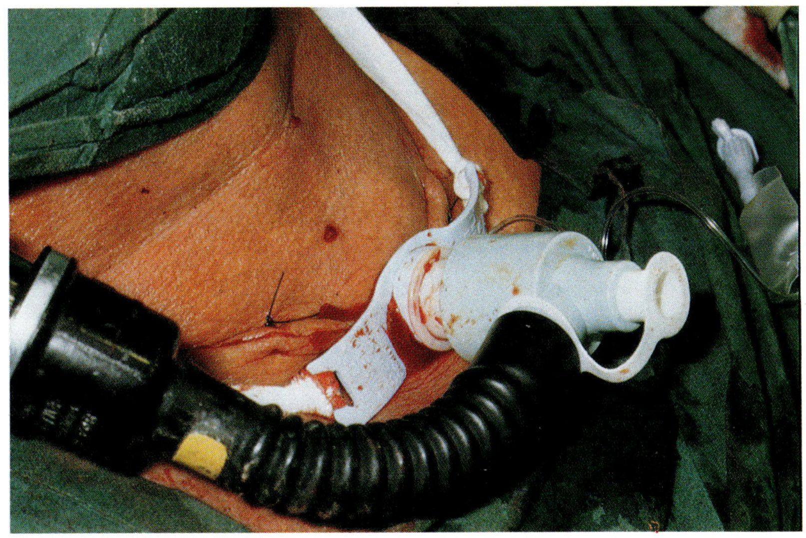

10 The wound is closed on either side of the newly sited tracheostomy tube with a few interrupted monofilament mattress sutures, and the tube tied securely in place by tapes passed around the neck. These sutures are not obligatory.

Circumcision

1 The probe is seen entering a very tight phimosis.

Note: Diathermy must not be used in any part of this operation.

1

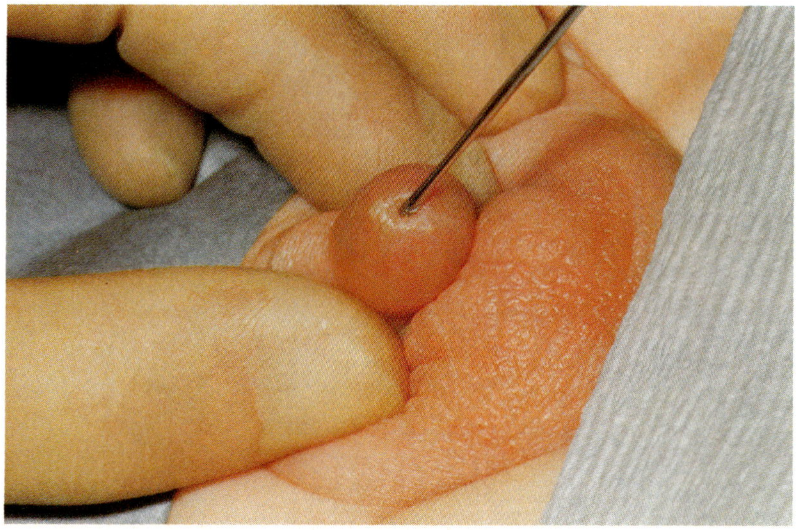

2 After probing it is easier to insert the tip of a haemostat and dilate the opening.

2

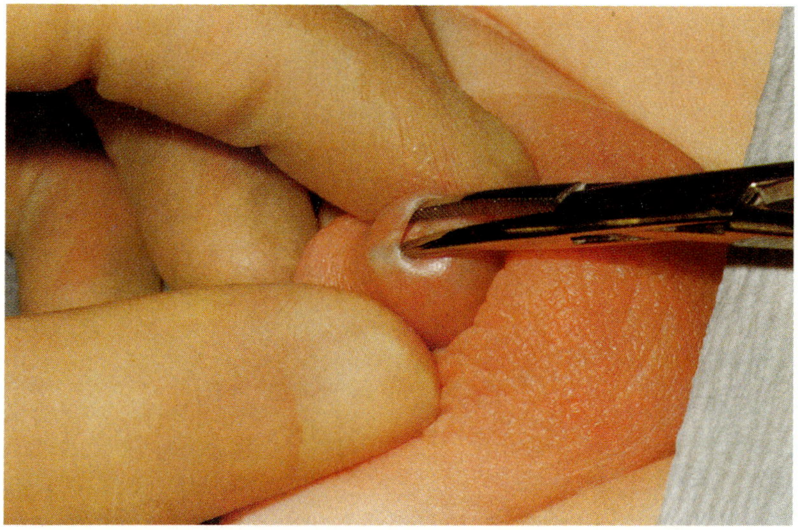

3 This allows retraction of the prepuce and a display of the prepucial adhesions which must be broken down by dilatation or by gentle pressure with a gauze swab.

4 The glans is shown totally devoid of the adhesions and with a well-marked sulcus.

3

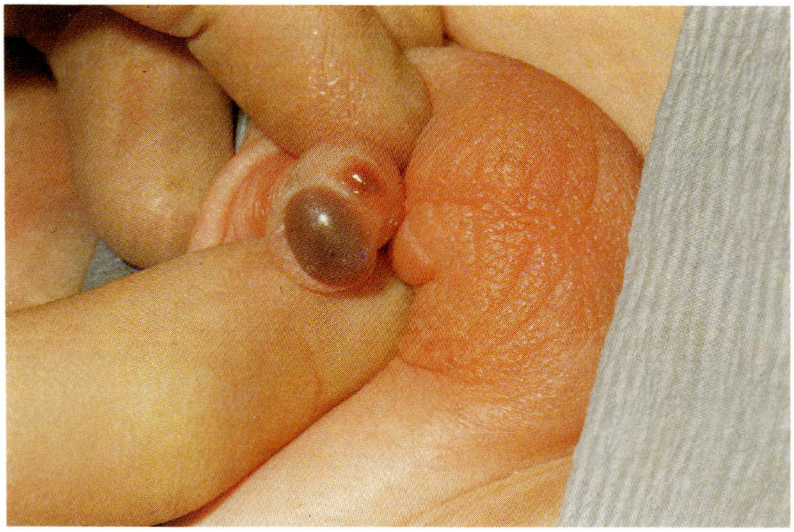

4

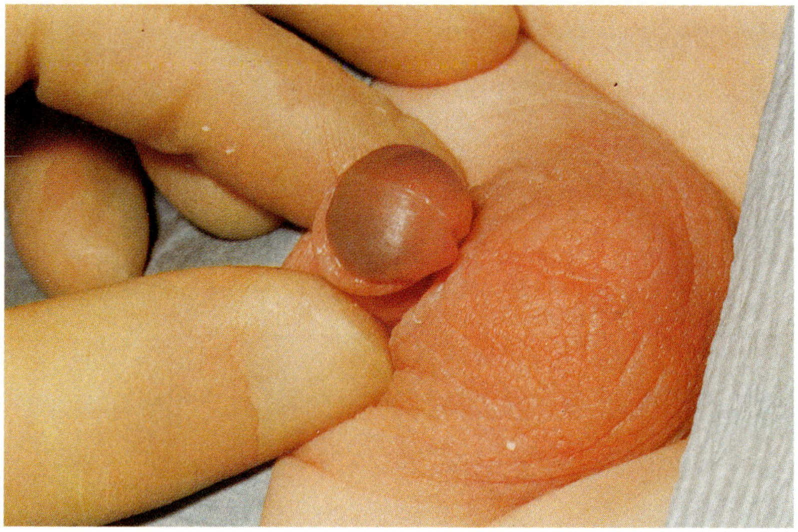

5

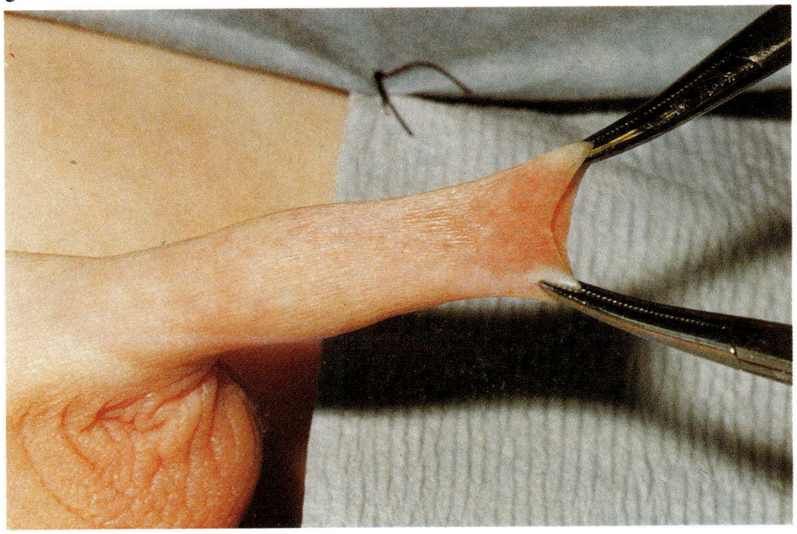

6

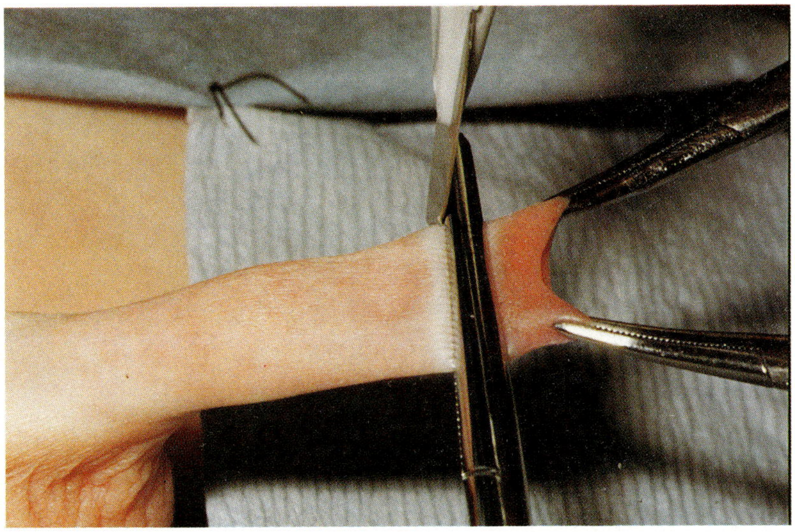

7

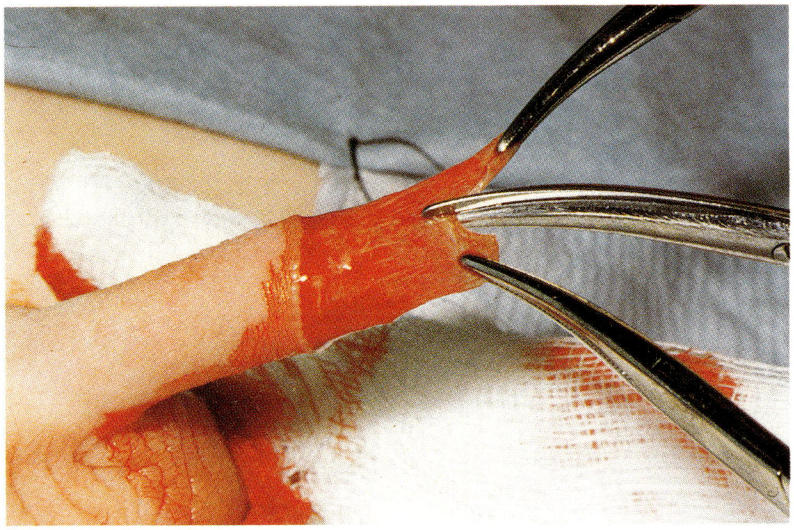

8

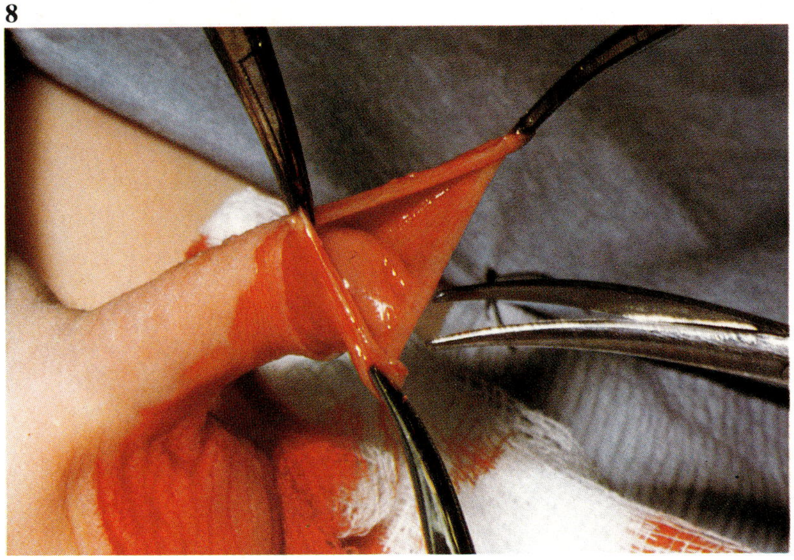

5 The prepuce is now drawn forward to its full extent by haemostats. At this point a number of choices are available: one is to continue as shown in the next few illustrations; the other is to do a dorsal slit down the mid-glans position and then cut sideways. The vital points are not to cut the tip of the glans penis and not to cut off too much skin.

6 An artery forceps is then placed across the prepuce distal to the glans and the prepuce is divided proximally to the forceps. Care must be taken to avoid injury to the tip of the glans. This can be avoided by feeling the glans with the finger and thumb and keeping it clear of the scalpel. Alternatively a bone distal forceps can be used, instead of the forceps, and the prepuce divided distally to it.

7 The skin now retracts exposing the serous or inner layer which is divided down towards the sulcus but stopping short by about 10 mm.

8 Haemostats are placed at the inner layer at the midpoint, another at the frenum and two others midway between.

9

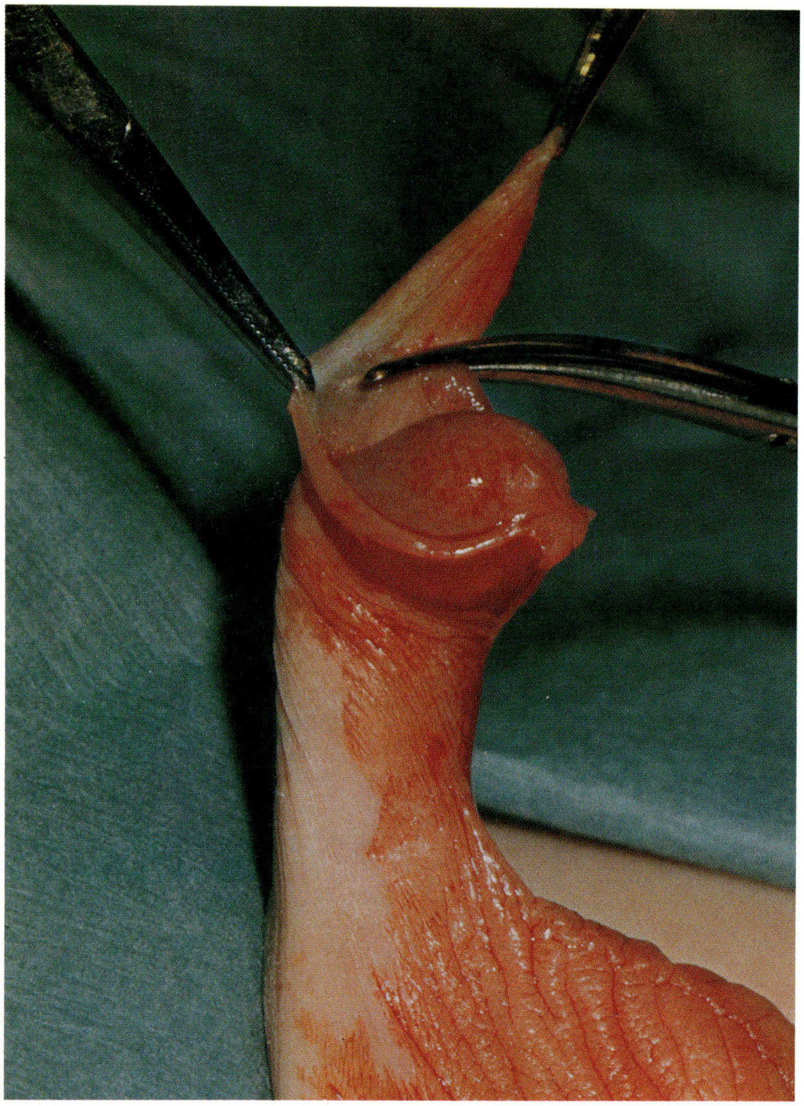

9 **The serous layer is then trimmed** leaving about 10 mm margin all round.

10

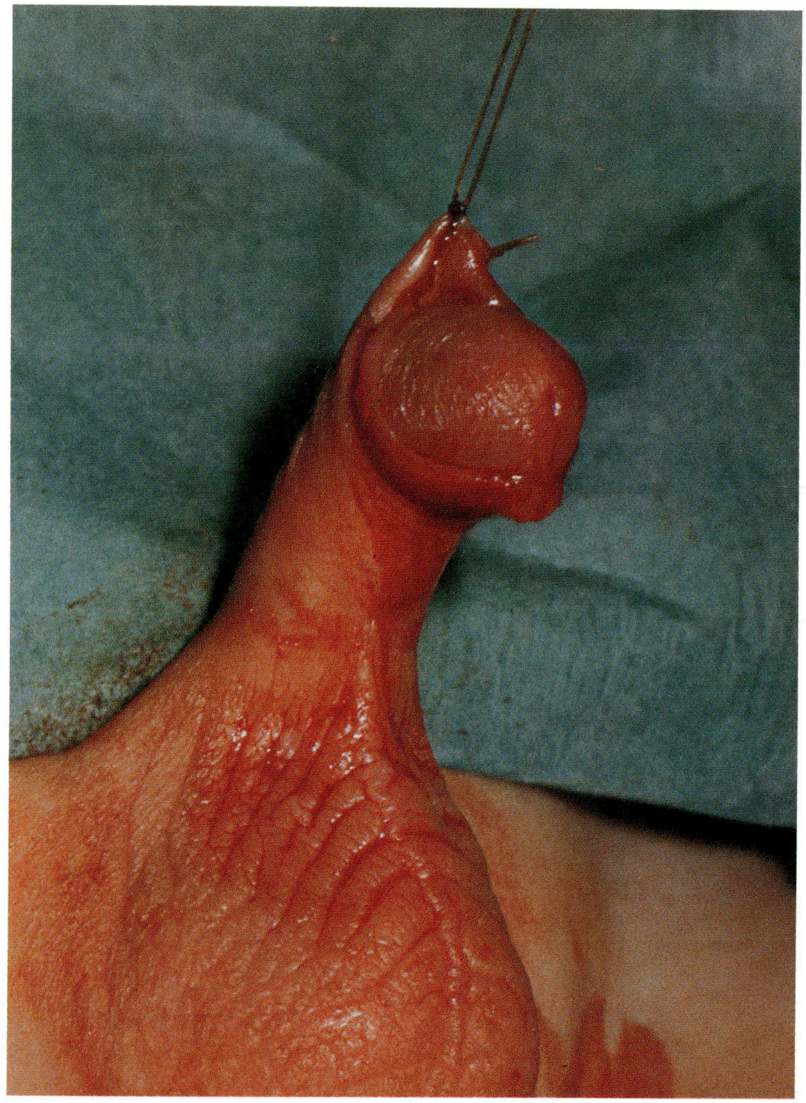

10 In trimming, vessels are cut and need to be carefully sought and tied off with catgut. Do not use diathermy in this area.

11

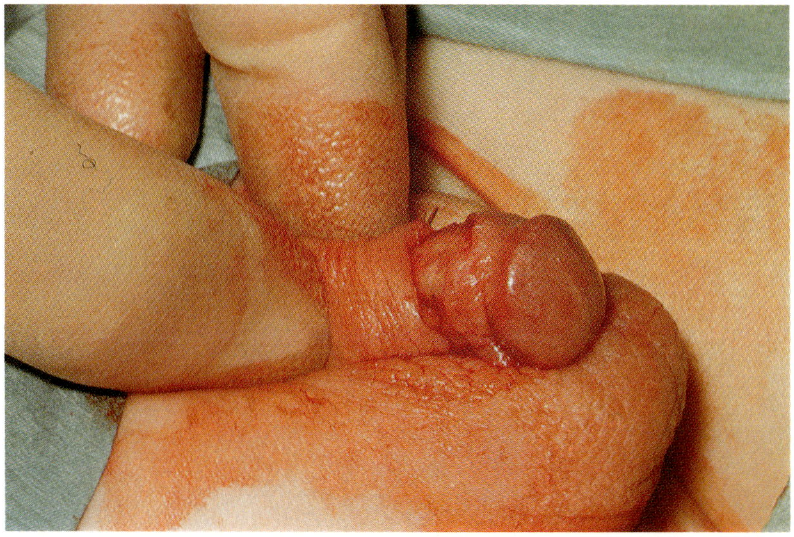

11 Sutures of absorbable material, 3/0 catgut as here or Dexon or Vicral, are inserted starting at the mid-dorsal area and extending round at frequent intervals approximating skin to serosa.

12

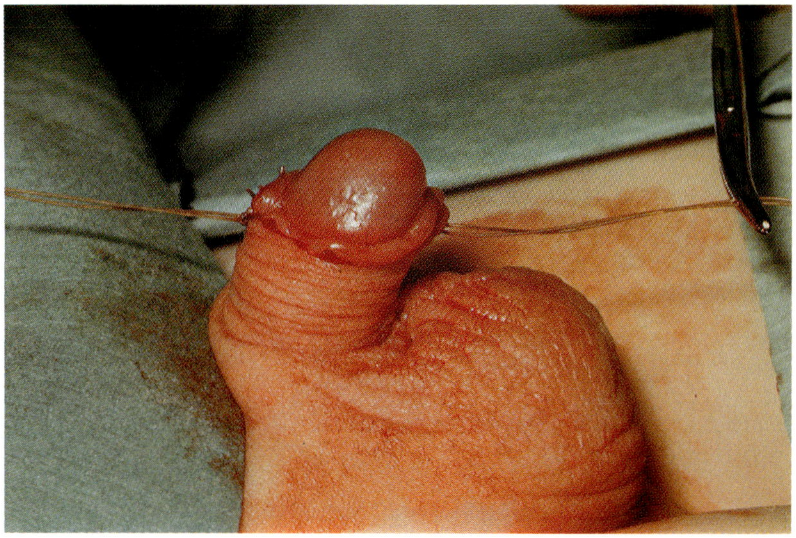

12 A three-in-one suture is indicated at the frenular area – skin, frenum and skin again, to make sure that there is no bleeding from the frenular artery.

13

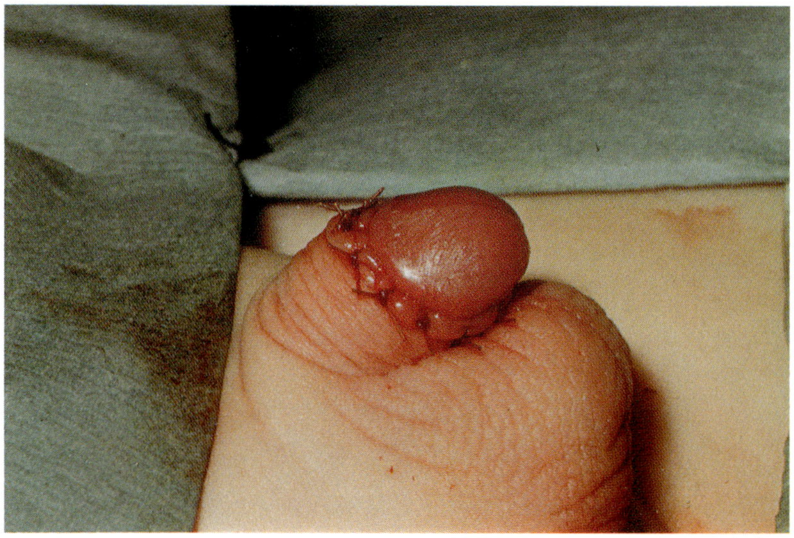

13 Operation is finished. All bleeding has ceased. A Vaseline dressing covered with gauze is applied.

Frenuloplasty

This operation may be required when thickening of the frenum has occurred, possibly because of repeated trauma. The procedure is usually carried out under general anaesthesia, but it is possible to use a local anaesthetic.

1 The side view shows the tightness of the frenulum, limiting the movement of soft tissues.

2 The frenulum is thickened and shortened and was traumatised easily at intercourse.

3 The fibrosed frenulum is divided at its mid point.

1

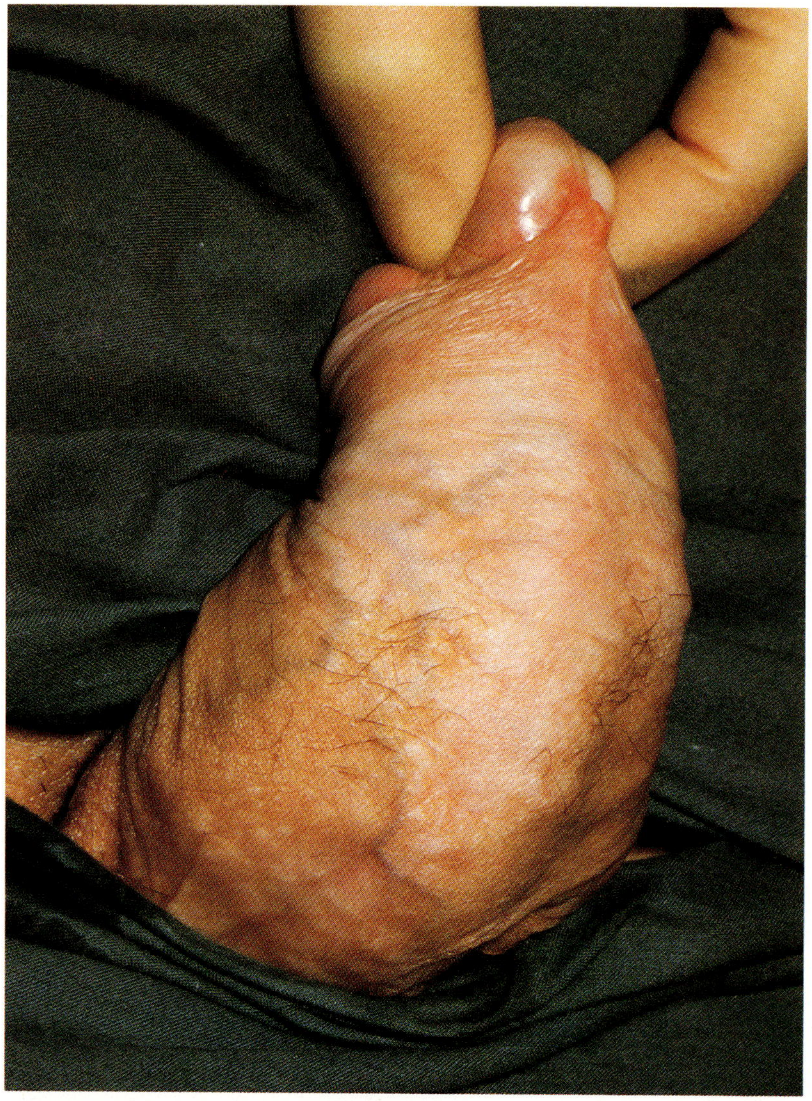

2

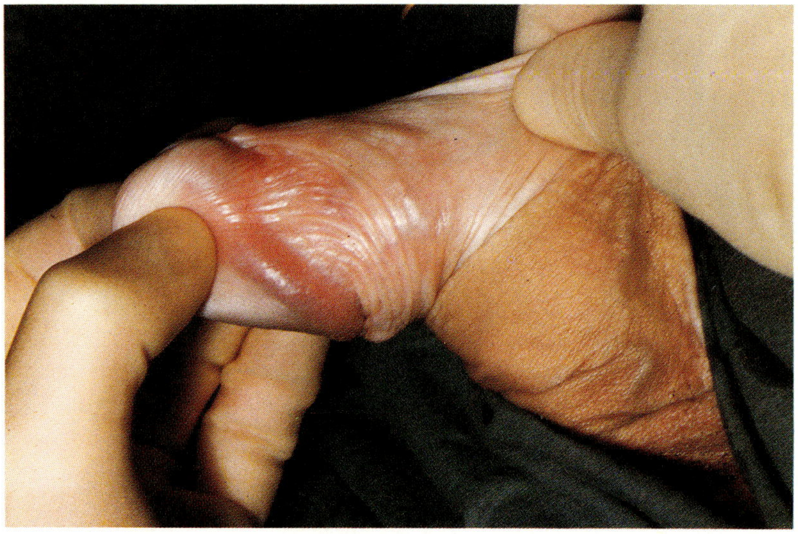

3

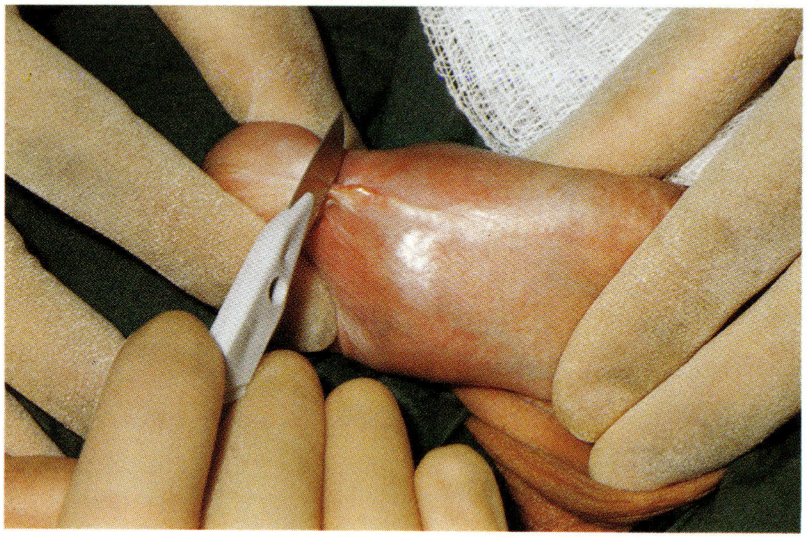

4

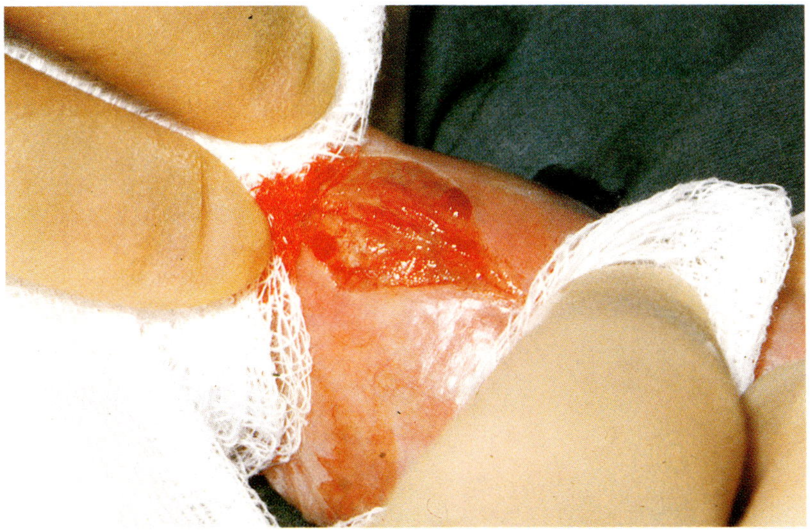

5

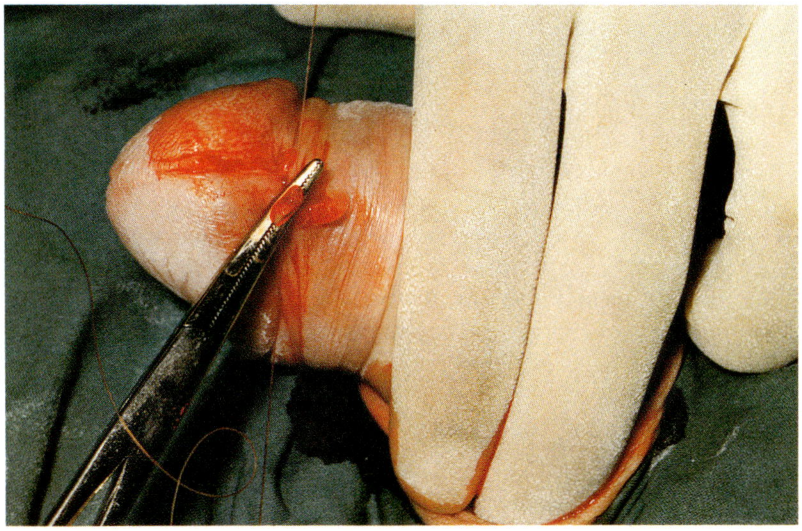

4 Once the skin is divided the frenular vessels can be seen in the midline and the straight incision elongates to a diamond shape.

5 The vessels are divided and tied with catgut.

6 A view of the area after ligation of the vessels.

7 The diamond area is converted into a linear one by suturing with catgut.

8 The end result allows the glans penis to straighten out and make erection easier.

6

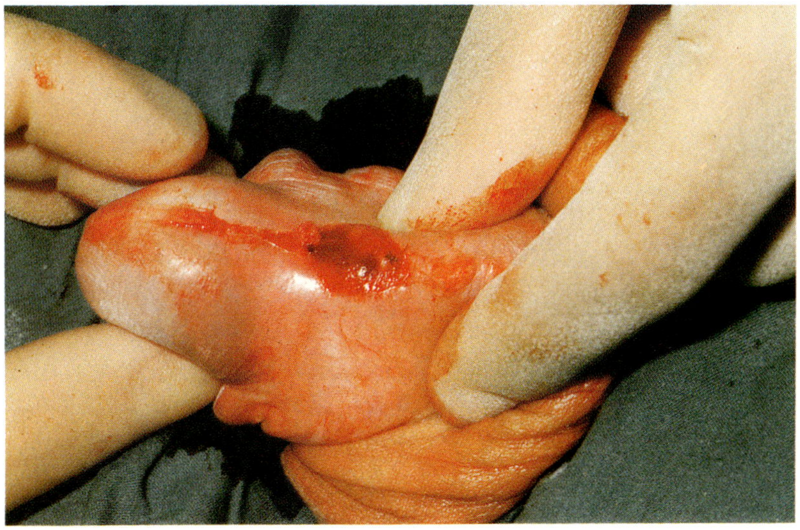

7

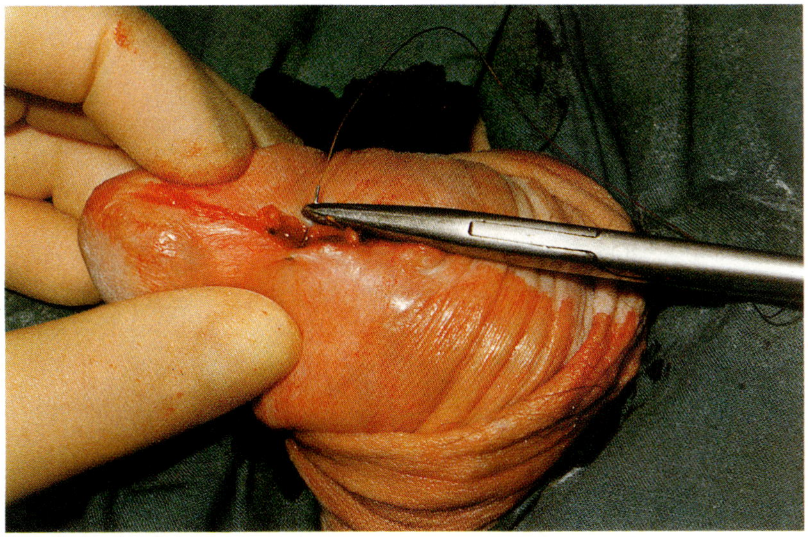

8

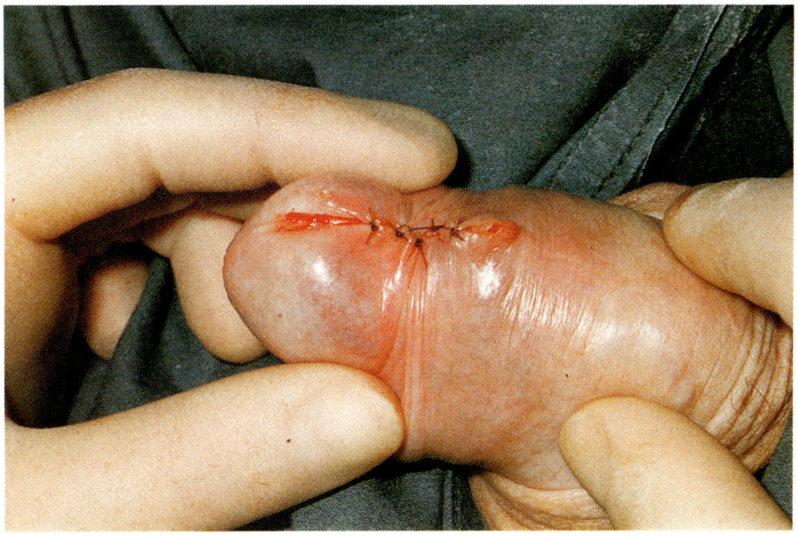

Vasectomy

This procedure can be carried out under general or local anaesthetic. The latter is perfectly satisfactory and is used throughout the world. **There are, however, occasions when patients under local anaesthetic may feel sick or develop cardiac arrhythmias, especially when undue traction on the cord and vas deferens is used.** In an anxious patient general anaesthetic would be kinder, especially in those with a rather small but bulky scrotum.

1

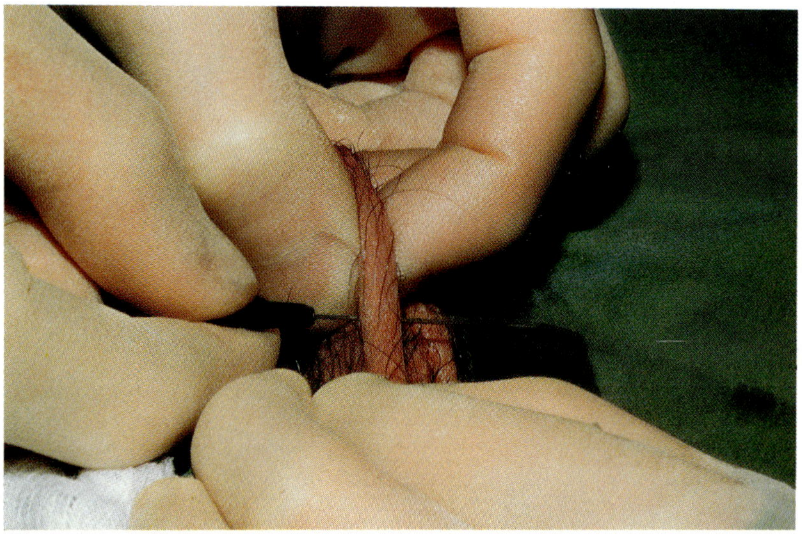

1 The vas deferens can usually be felt easily in the scrotum and isolated between finger and thumb.

2

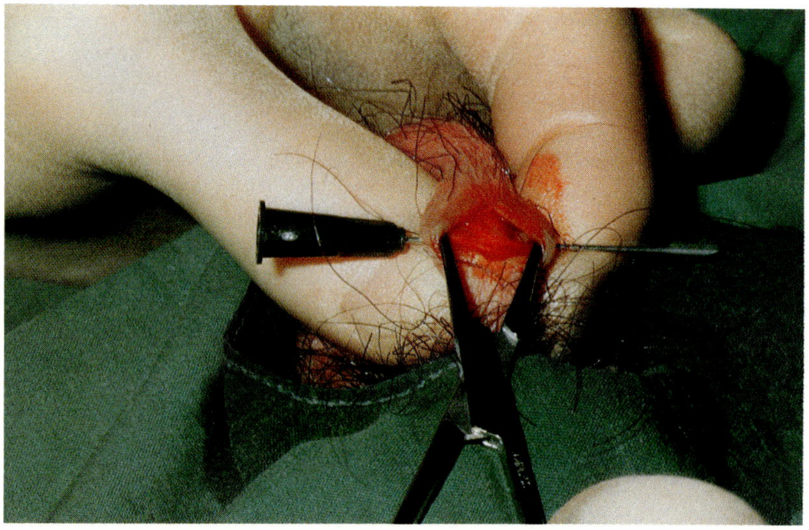

2 If local anaesthetic – one per cent Lignocaine – is used it can be infiltrated round the vas and into the skin and the needle finally pushed through the skin behind the vas and out through the skin on the other side.

An alternative technique is to anaesthetize in the midline and via a central transverse incision secure the vas on either side of the septum.

3 The vas is easily isolated from the other tissues using a sharp pointed pair of scissors which is replaced by artery forceps.

4 The vas is gradually isolated in greater length.

5 About half an inch of the vas is removed for histology to confirm the tissue.

6 The cord is now doubled back and fixed by a non-absorbable suture to prevent it joining up again. The skin is closed with catgut and the same operation performed on the other side. It is better **not to** diathermy the vas as it makes reconstruction, if desired in the future, difficult. The patient should be warned that several months must lapse before sterility occurs and that check-samples of semen will be needed.

3

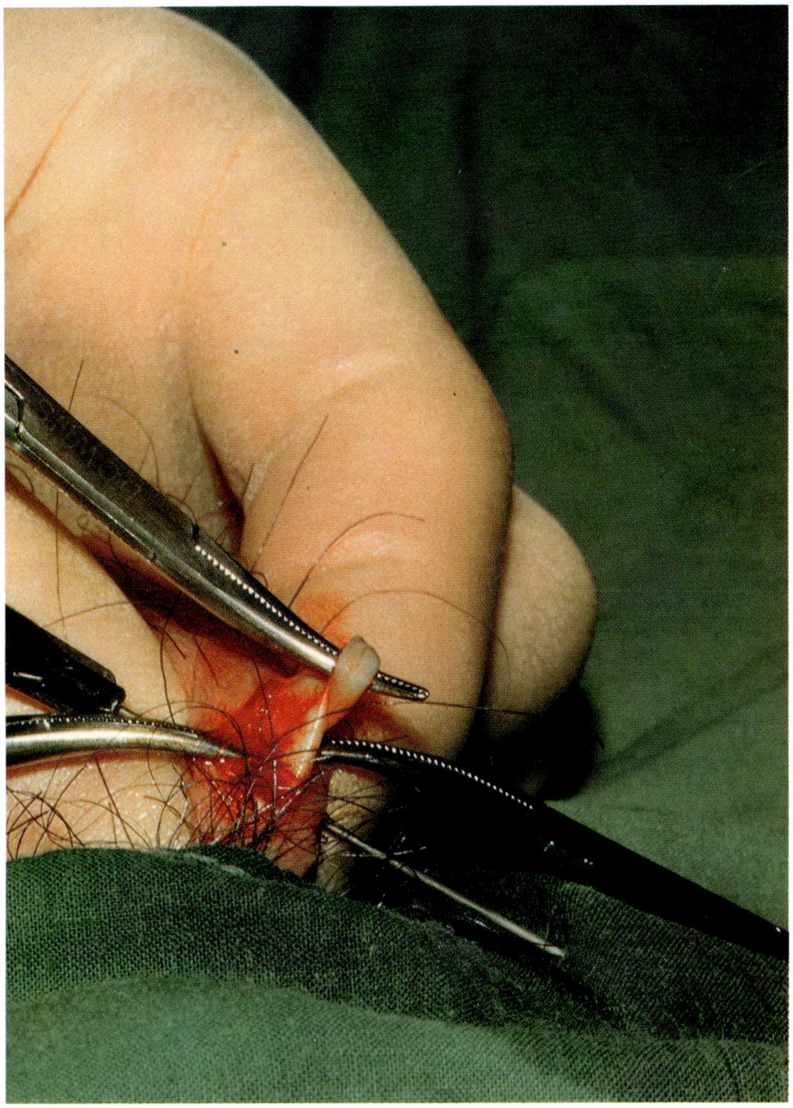

4

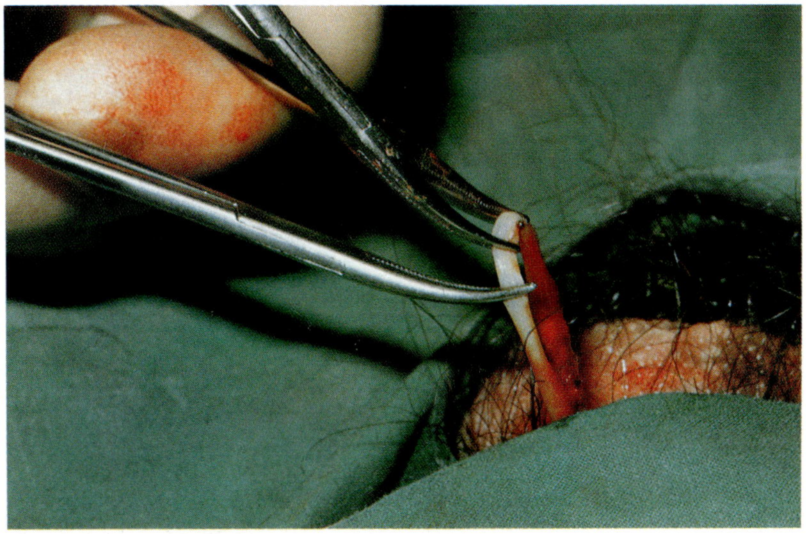

5

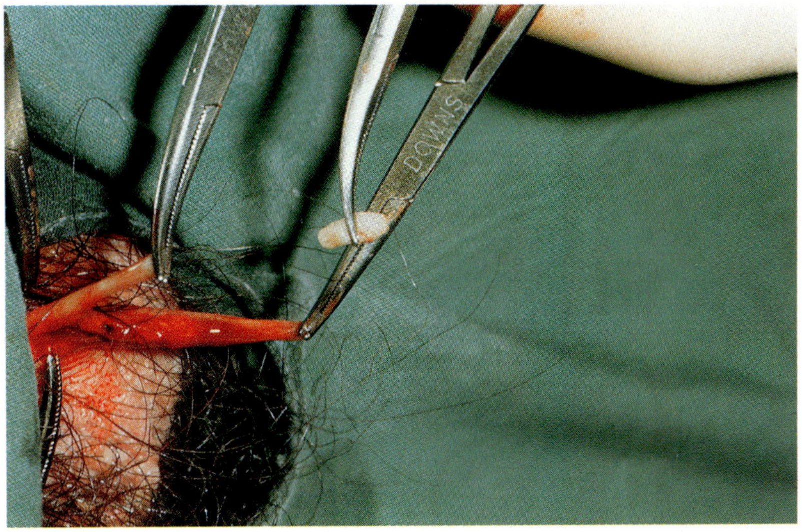

6

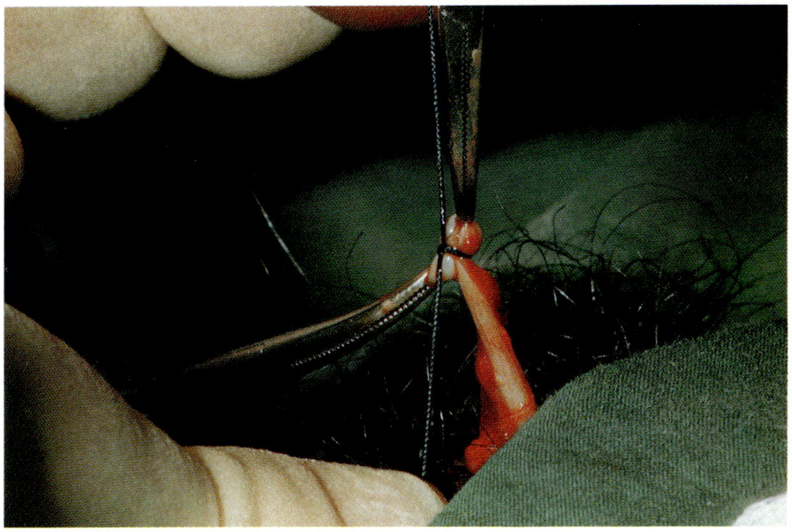

Undescended testis

1

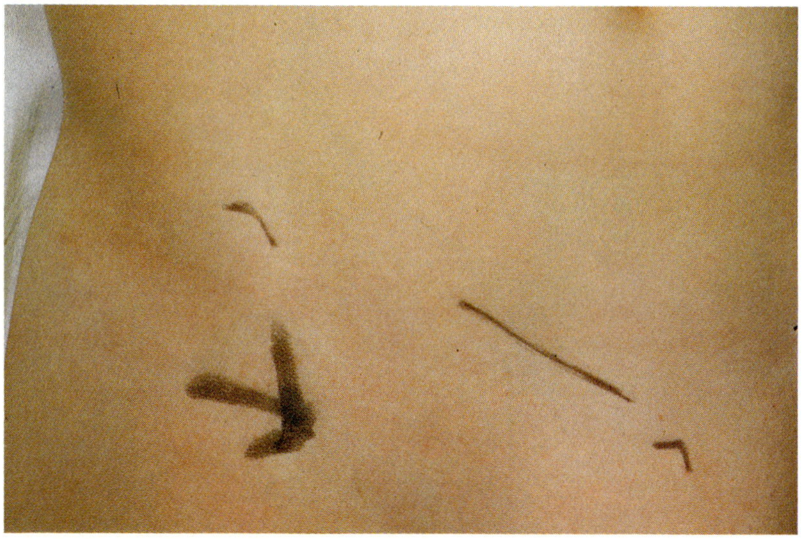

1 **The marks indicate by arrow the side to be operated on:** the anterior superior iliac spine, the pubic tubercle and finally the line of incision over the inguinal canal. **This procedure should be undertaken only if the testes are palpable; otherwise, the junior surgeon may be embarking on a major procedure.**

2

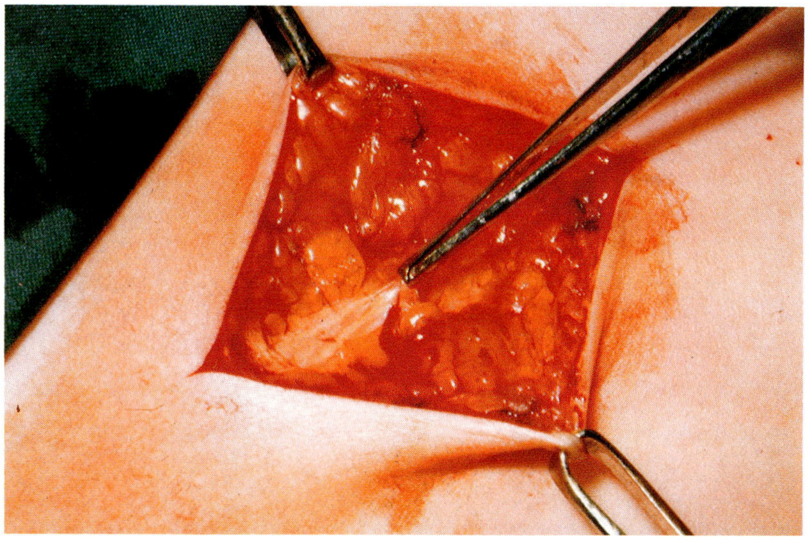

2 On incising the fatty layer, the deep [Scarpa's] fascia forms a well-defined layer which has to be incised carefully as the testes may be injured.

3

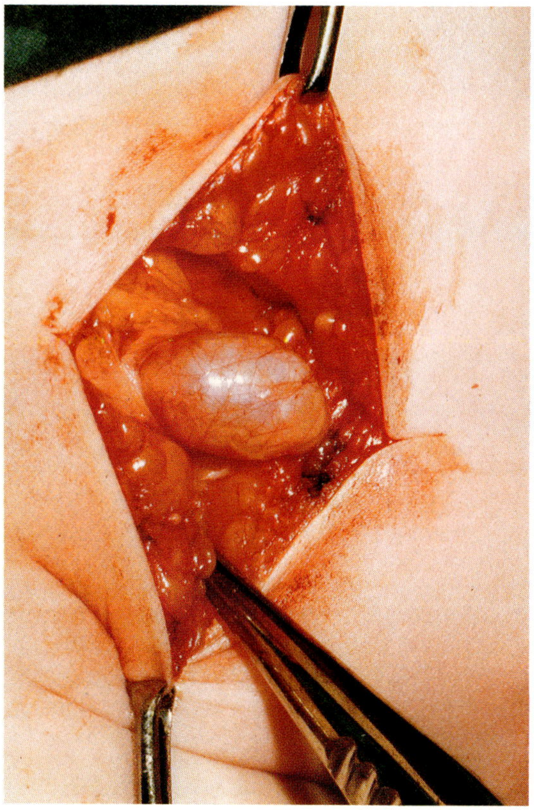

4

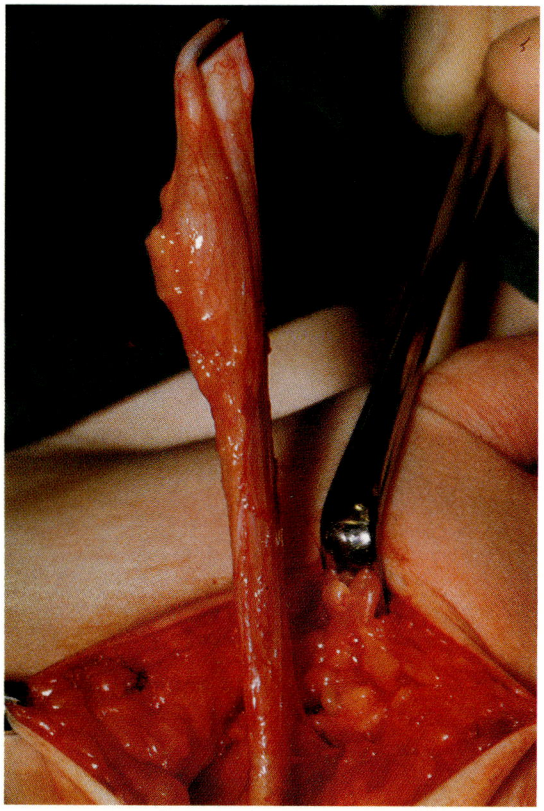

3 The testis can be seen lying in the superficial inguinal pouch.

4 The tunica vaginalis testis is held up by forceps and the spermatic cord is dissected out by dividing fine tissue backwards through both rings. A patent processus vaginalis was present.

Note: Avoid diathermy because of possible damage to vas.

5

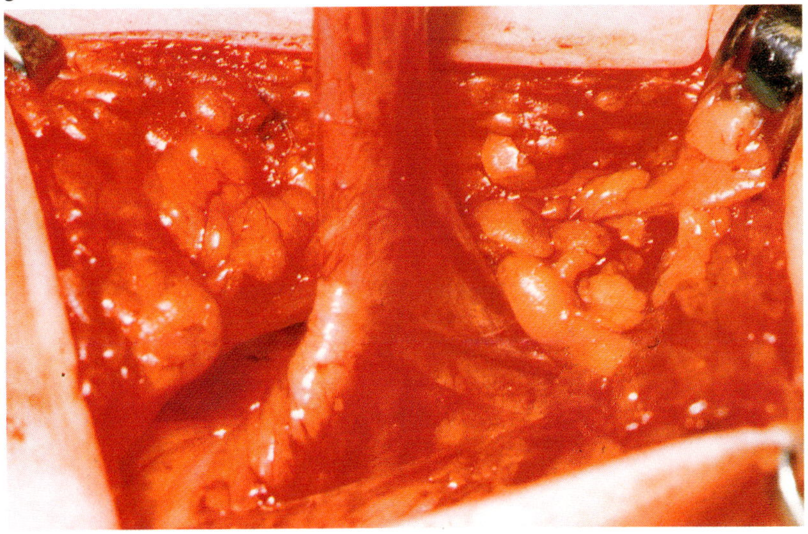

6

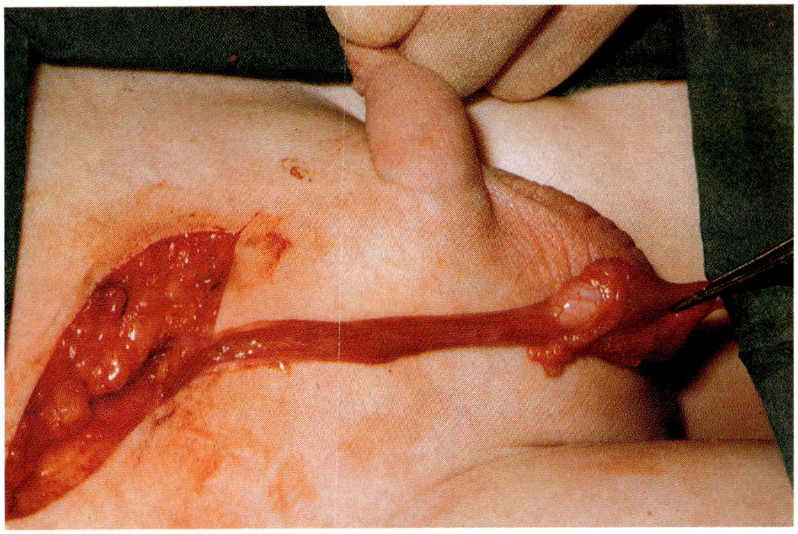

5 The tissue tethering the cord is well shown in close-up. This tissue will need to be divided and the cord mobilised down to and beyond the deep inguinal ring.

6 Full mobilisation can be measured externally when the testis can be seen to lie easily at the level of the scrotum.

7 In preparation for fixing the testis in the scrotum this is made prominent by inserting the forefinger down into it.

8 A transverse incision, along the line of the vessels, is made through the skin held aside by skin hooks.

9 This is deepened down to the dartos muscle which is incised into the scrotum.

7

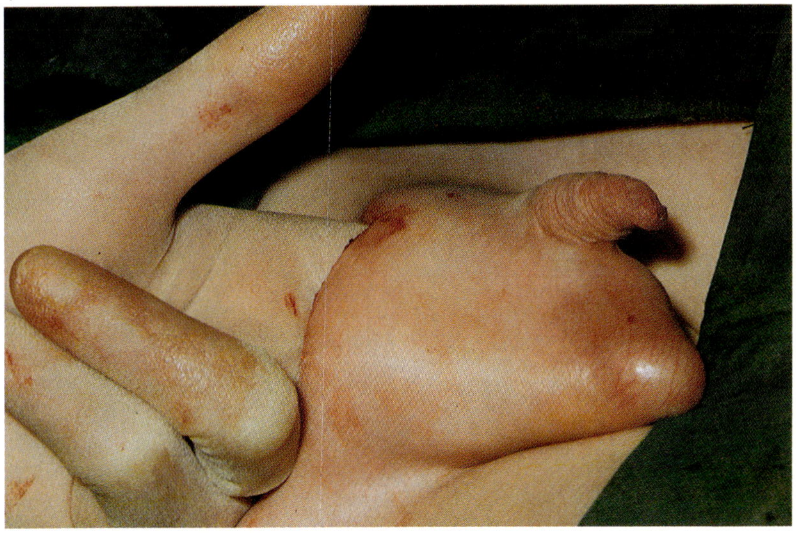

8

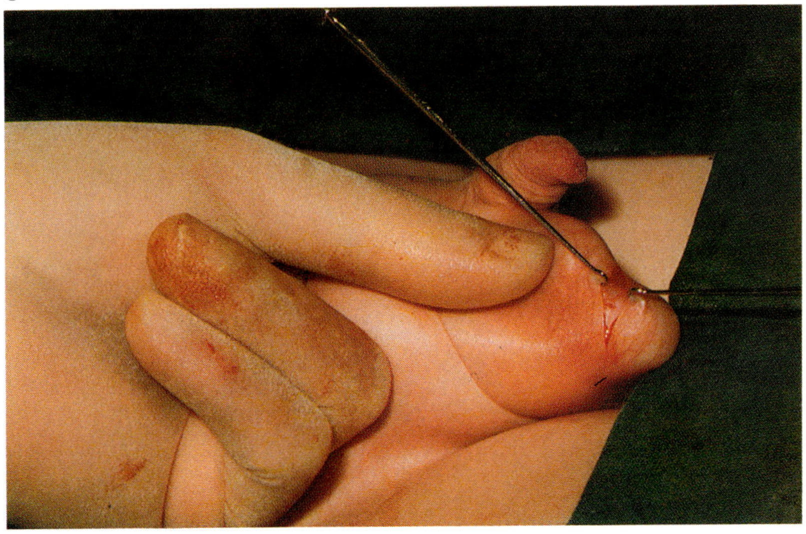

9

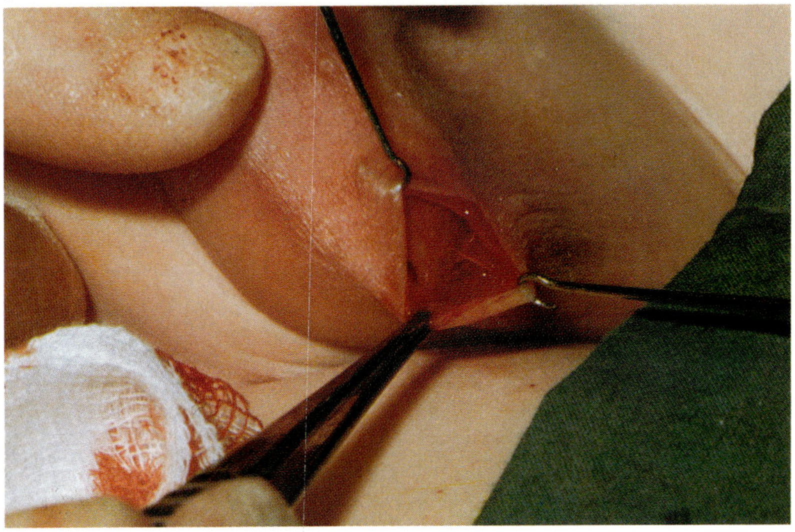

10

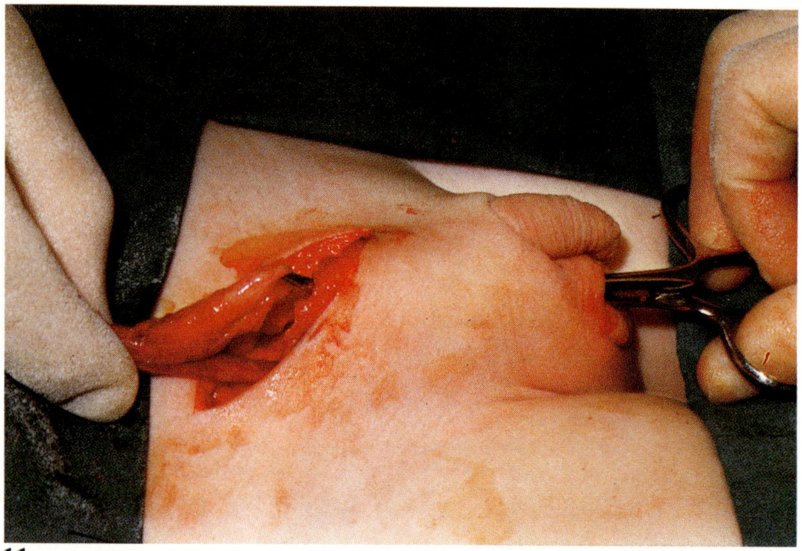

11

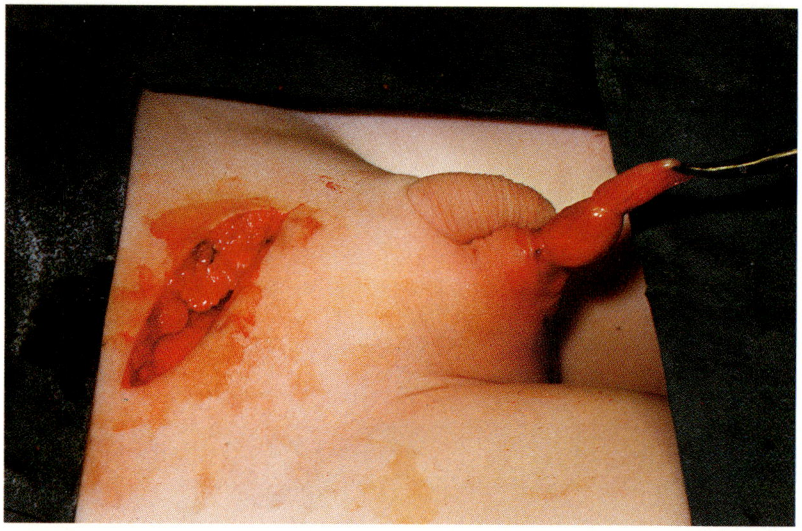

12

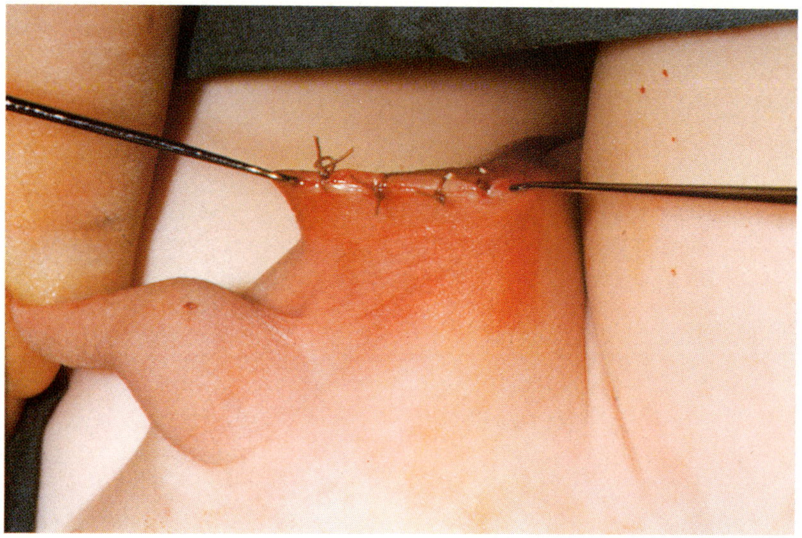

10 The testicular soft tissue is grasped and the testis is pulled down gently.

11 The testis now lies in a pouch between the dartos and the skin. The opening in the dartos is visible beyond the tie.

12 The skin is closed simply with catgut and the inguinal region with Prolene.

13 The completed operation. Note in this case the operation was simple but where the testis lies in the inguinal canal it may not be possible and it may be necessary to make a higher oblique incision in the iliac fossa to approach the spermatic vessel and vas deferens from above and mobilise further. **This is not, in such circumstances, a minor operation.**

13

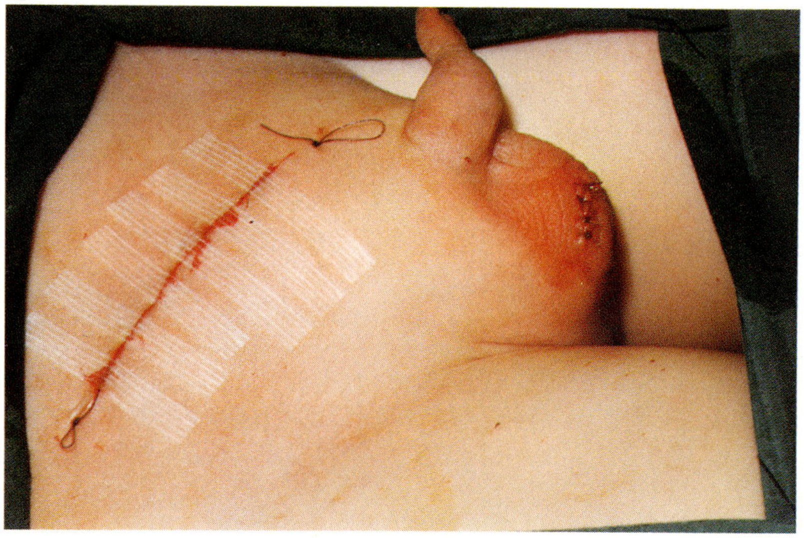

Excision of cyst of epididymis

Cysts of epididymis are usually easily diagnosed but occasionally mistakes are made where a solid tumour, for example of the upper pole of a testis, may be mistaken for a cyst.

1

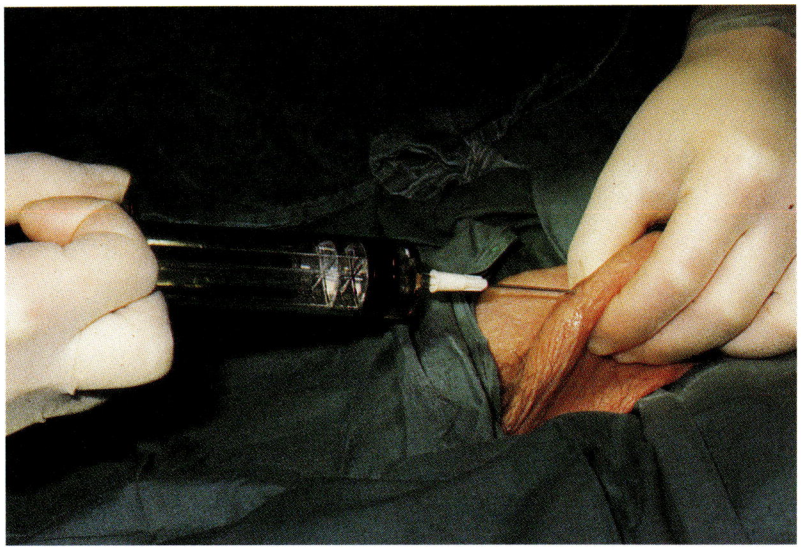

1 Aspiration may be a first step, as here, where clear fluid is aspirated. Usually general anaesthesia is used but it is possible to use local anaesthesia with block of the genitofemoral nerve, as well as local tissues.

2

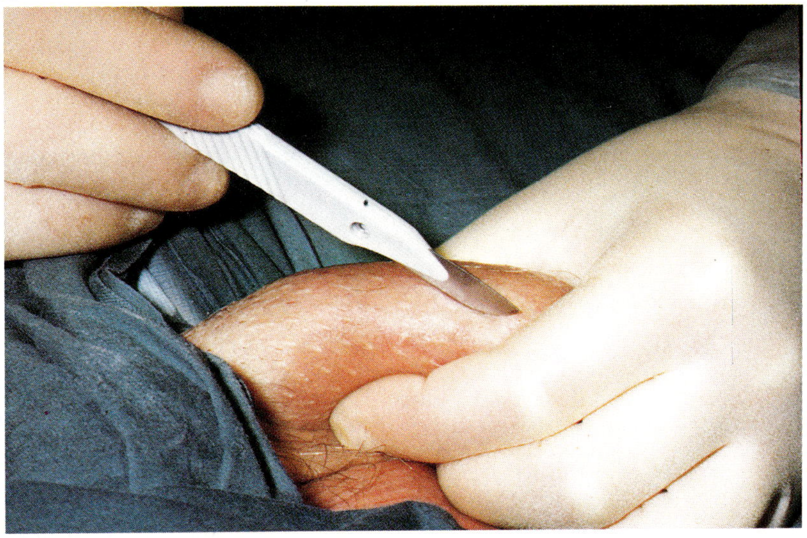

2 The cyst is held in one hand and a transverse incision made over it.

3

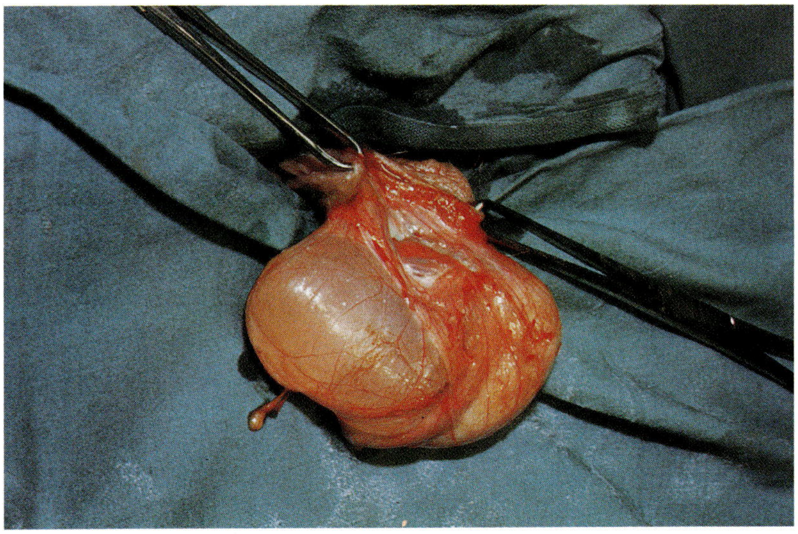

3 The testis is delivered through the opening in the scrotum. The cyst is clearly visible.

4 The cyst is enucleated very carefully by dividing the attachments. Bleeding needs careful control by diathermy or ligation. **Damage to the epididymis can compromise fertility.**

4

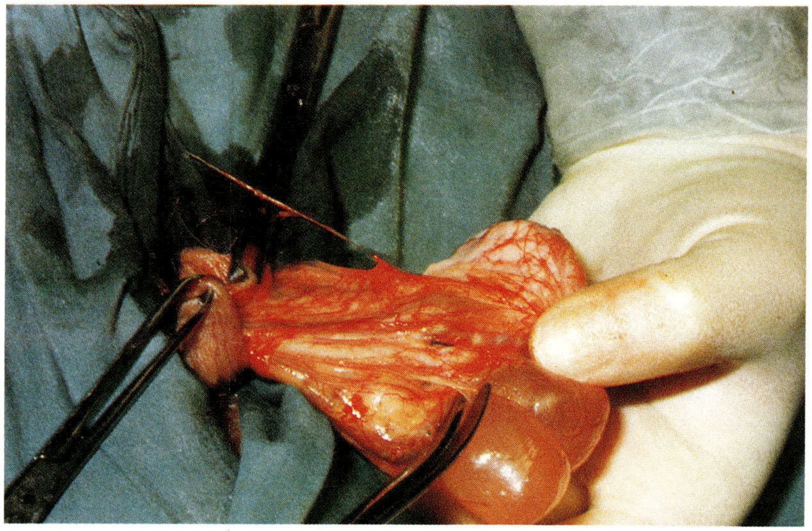

5 As the main cyst is being removed, a further small cyst is seen and should also be dissected out.

5

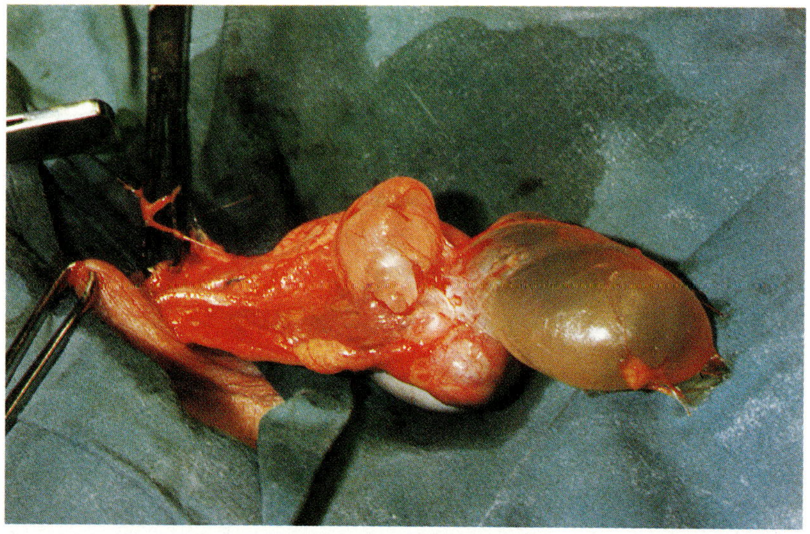

6 A clean excision has taken place leaving the caput epididymis testis clean.

7 The scrotum is sutured with catgut in two layers – one continuous, the outer one interrupted. Providing the dissection is satisfactory a drain is not required. A firm scrotal support will help to prevent haematoma.

6

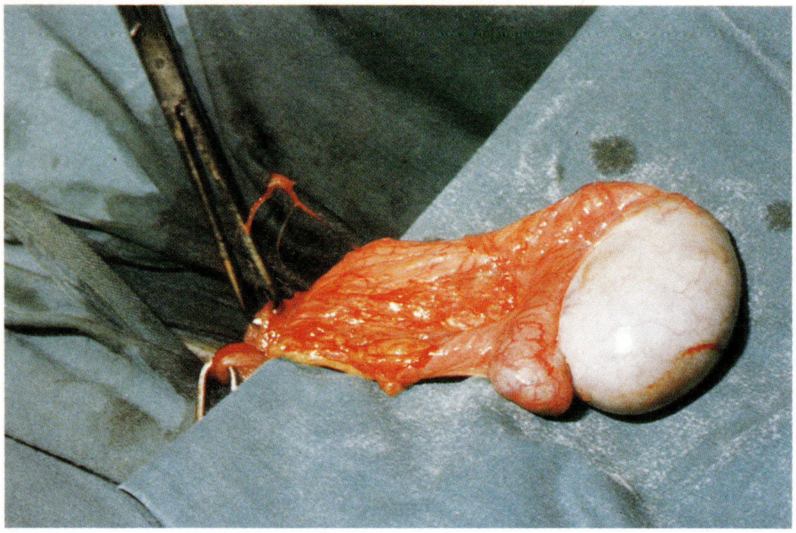

7

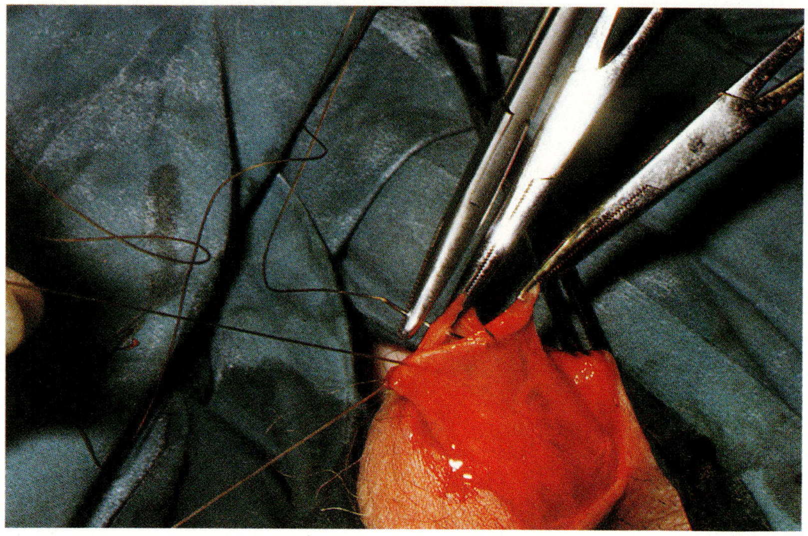

Lord's operation for hydrocele

Hydrocele is a common complaint where fluid accumulates inside the tunica vaginalis testis. It may be treated by: repeated aspiration; aspiration and injection of a sclerosing agent into the space; Jaboulay's operation where the excess of the sac is excised and the remnant stitched together behind the testis; finally the simpler Lord's operation detailed here.

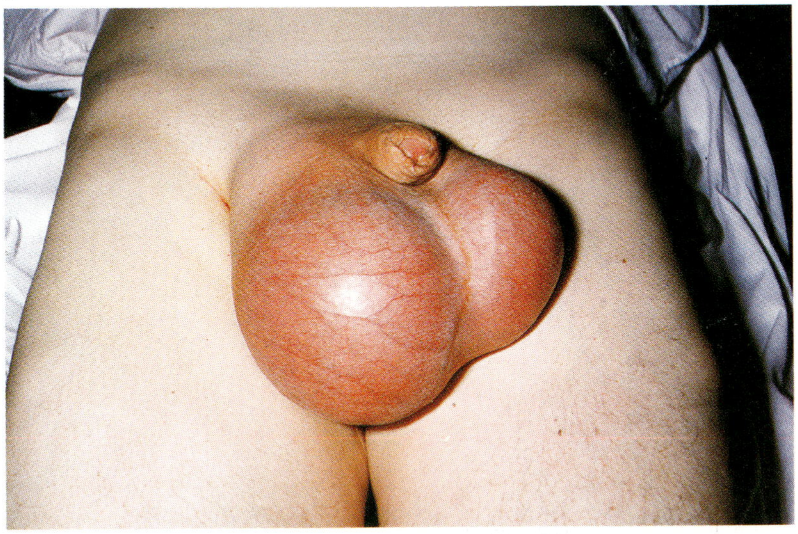

1 Bilateral hydroceles are obvious with the right one greater than the left. These may be dealt with in two operations or both done at the same time.

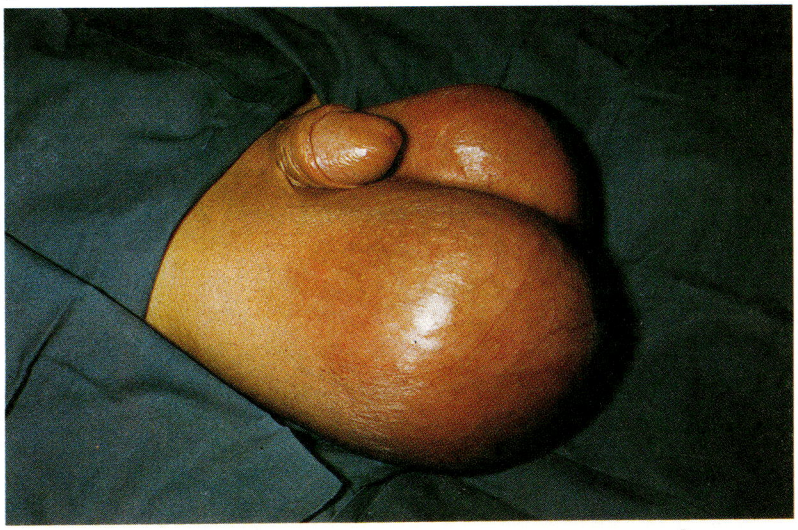

2 After shaving, the scrotal area is carefully cleansed with antiseptic solution.

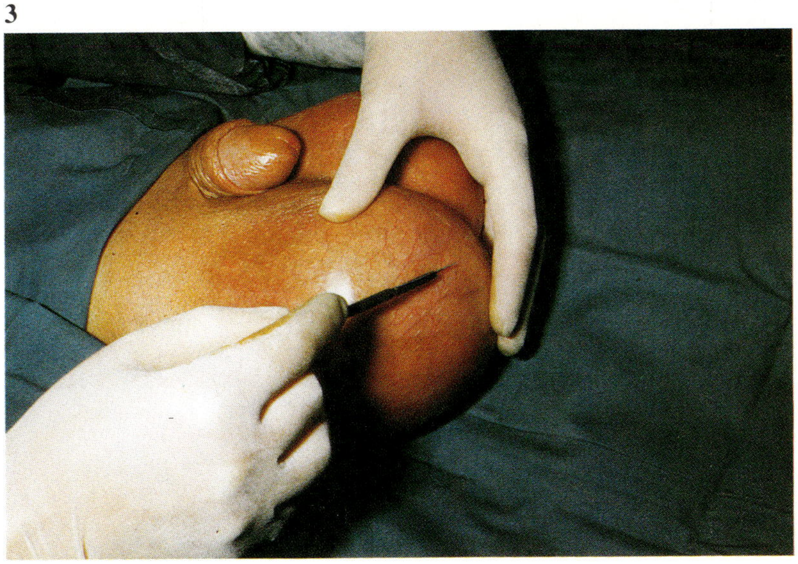

3 A transverse incision is made in the anterior surface which is held taut. The incision goes through the skin and dartos down to the tunica vaginalis.

4

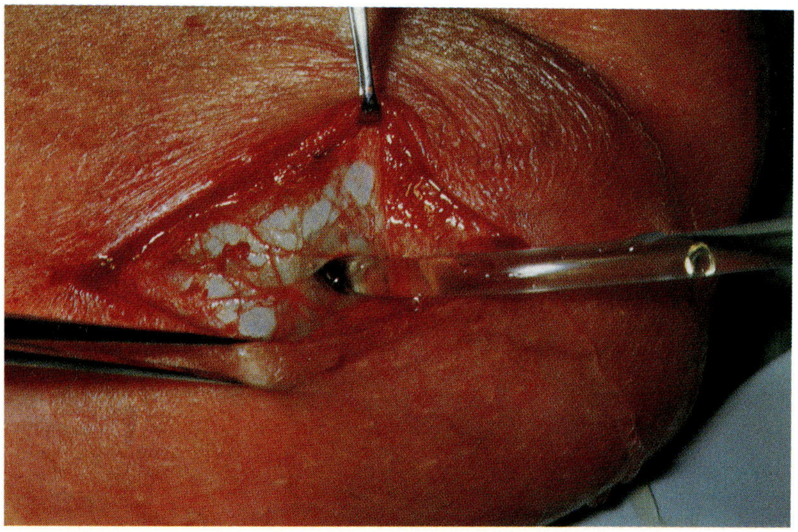

5

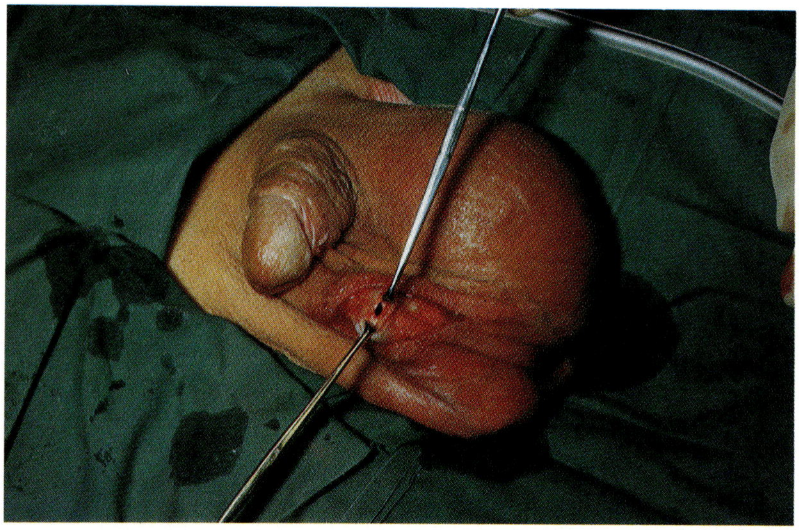

6

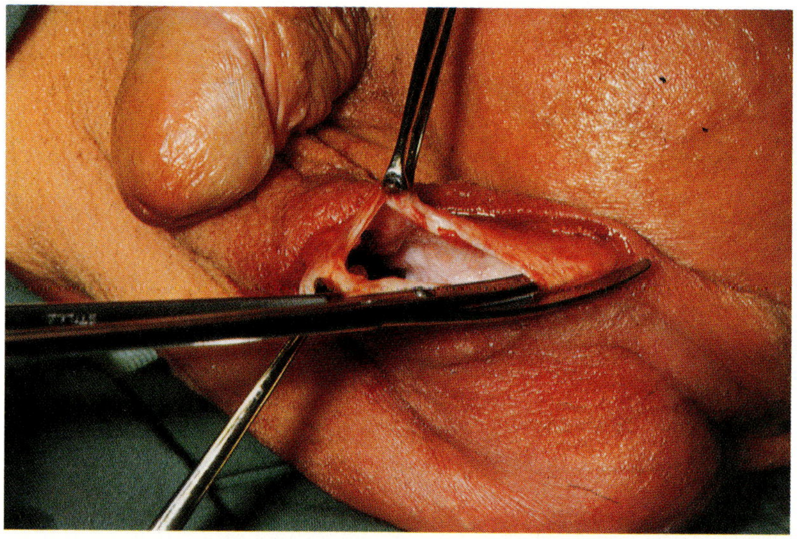

4 The tunica is exposed, a small incision is made into it and the fluid removed by sucker.

5 The opening of the tunica is grasped by forceps and may be enlarged by inserting the index finger first of one hand and then the other. This dislocation avoids bleeding.

6 Alternatively, as here, it may be opened by scissors with care to coagulate or tie any bleeding vessels.

7 The testis is extended through the hole and the tunica is then everted.

8 Full eversion is present with no bleeding from the edge of the tunica.

7

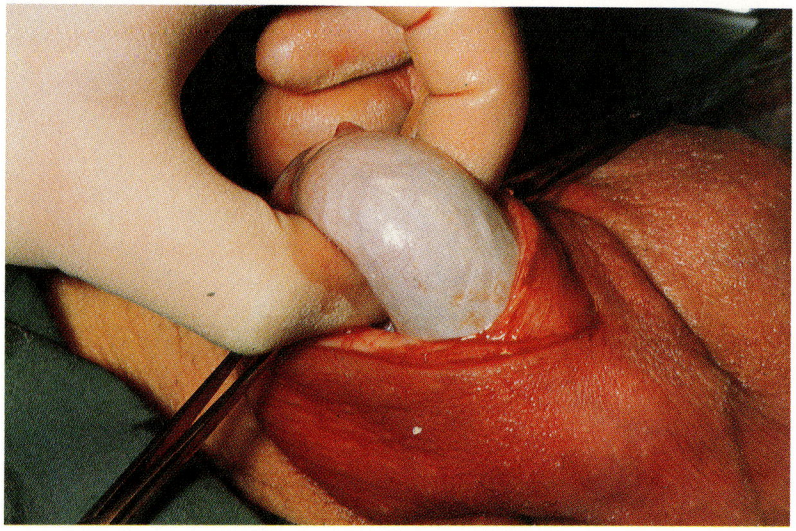

8

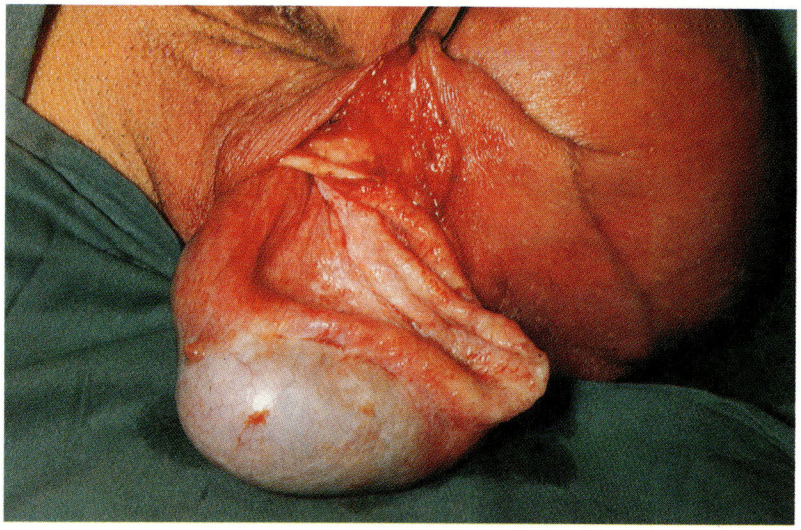

9

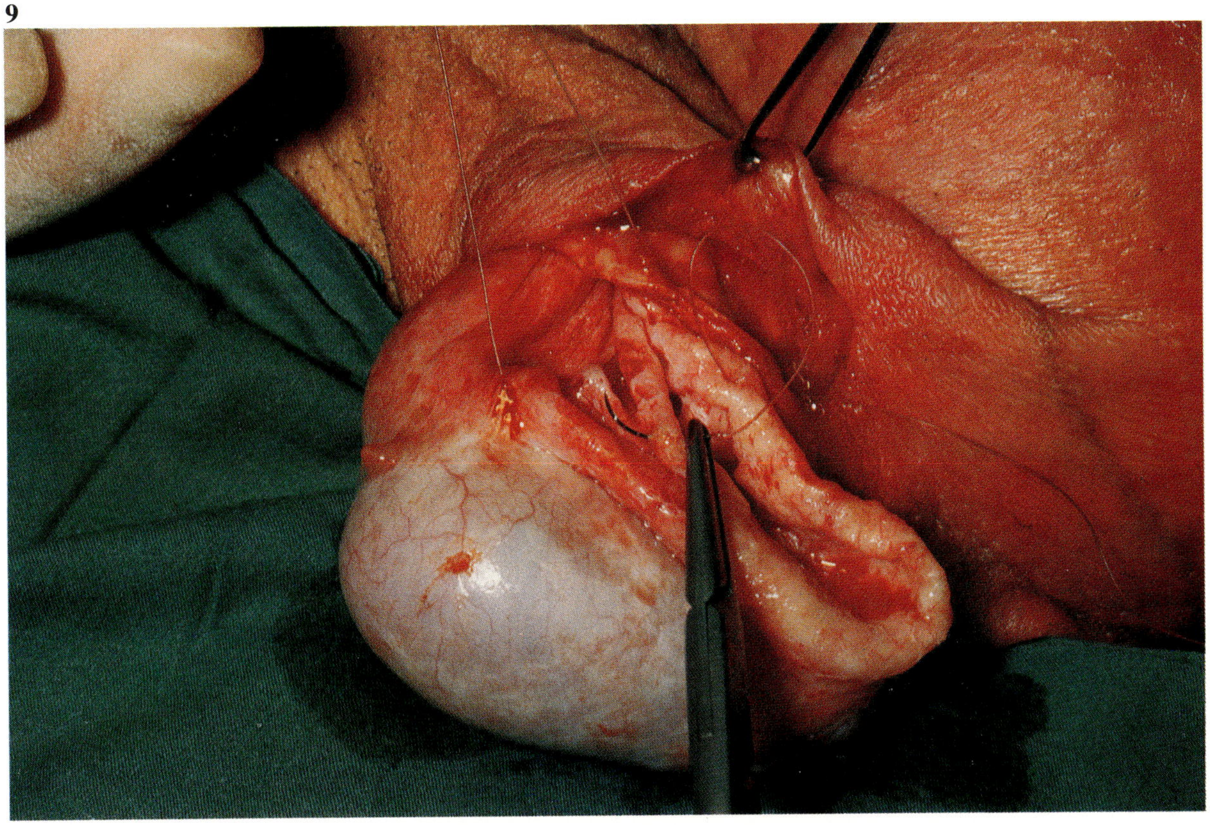

9 Catgut sutures are then inserted just through the free edge of the tunica then through the inner lining picking up the tunica in 1 cm bites and finally through the junction of the tunica with the testicle.

10

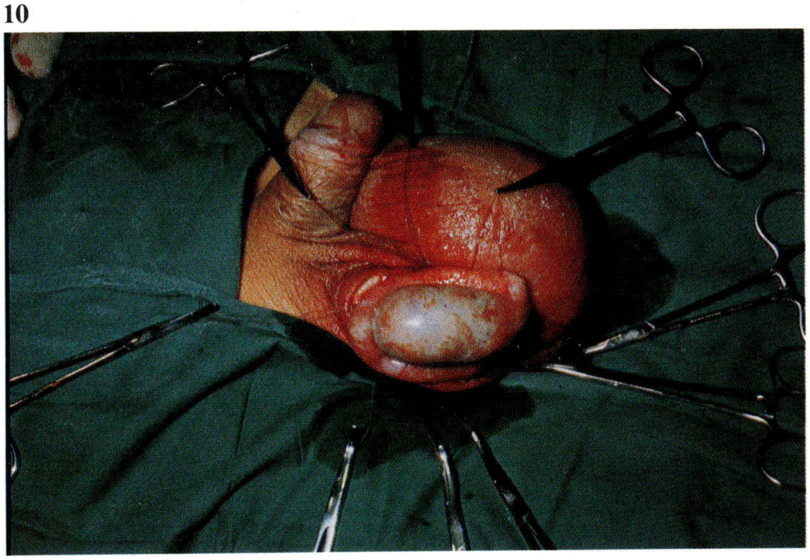

10 About 9-12 stitches are inserted circumferentially and tied, thus plicating the tunica and, as it were, gathering it up as a collar round the testicle.

11

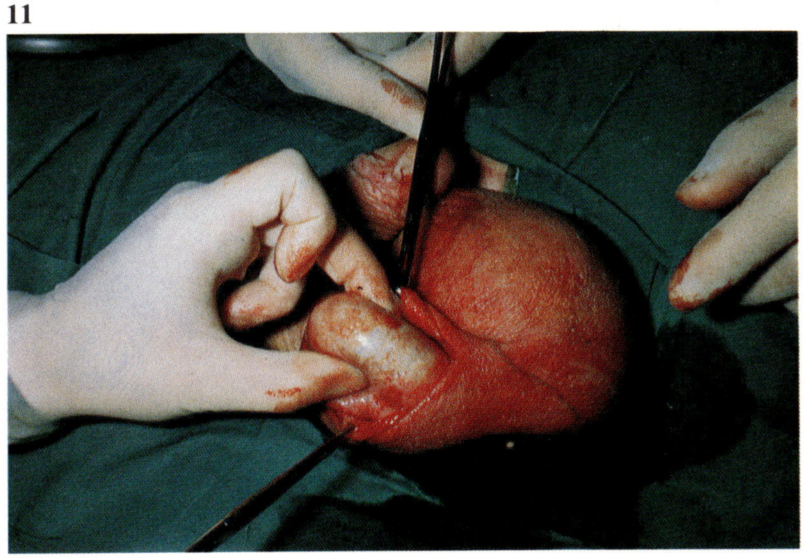

11 The testicle is now pushed back into the scrotum, stretching the latter to allow it to do so.

12 The dartos is now sutured with a running catgut stitch.

12

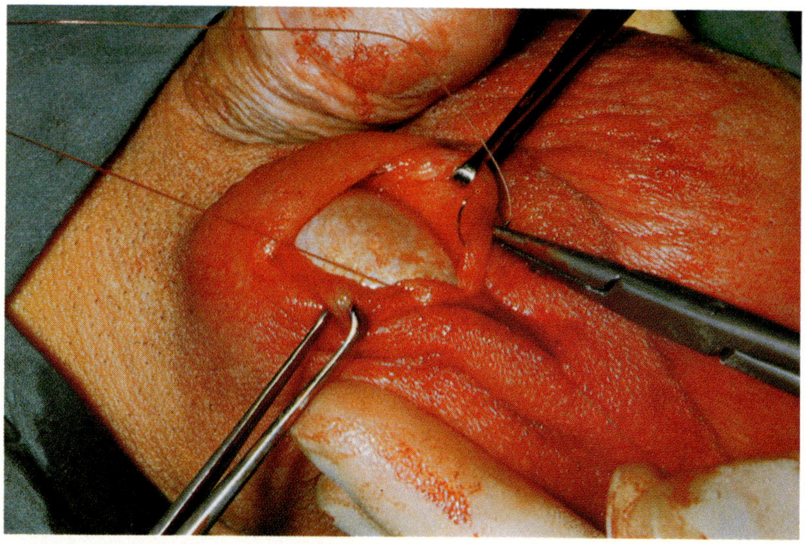

13

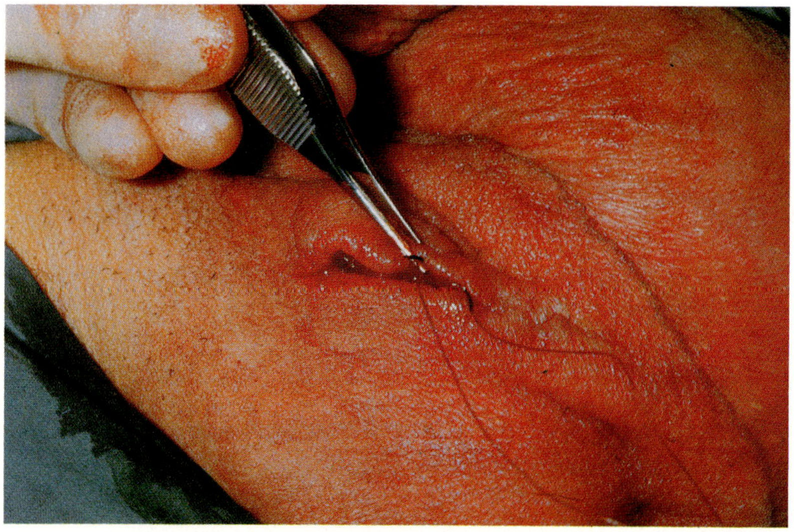

13 The scrotum is closed with subcutaneous catgut without drainage.

14

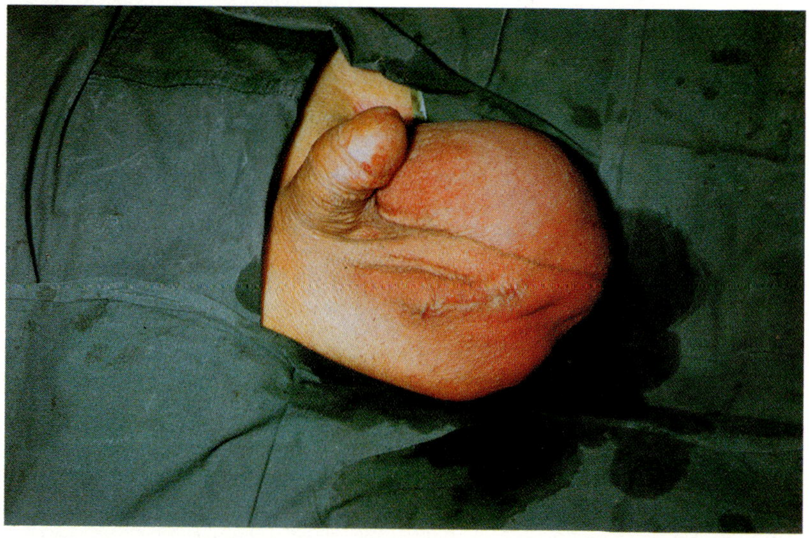

14 Final result of closure. If both hydroceles are done at the same time a transverse incision is made on both sides.

Repair of a baby's inguinal hernia

This is a relatively simple operation but should be carried out with delicacy of touch as the contents of the spermatic cord, in particular the vas deferens, can be damaged by rough handling. A complete knowledge of the anatomy of this area is essential.
Do not use diathermy because of the probability of spreading damage to delicate structures.

1 Typical appearance of a right inguinal hernia in an infant.

2 Two points are identified: the anterior superior iliac spine and the pubic tubercle. The incision is in the medial half of a line between the two points.

3 The skin incision is made.

4 The edges of the incision are retracted by tissue forceps or by skin hooks and dissection deepened to the superficial fascia.

1

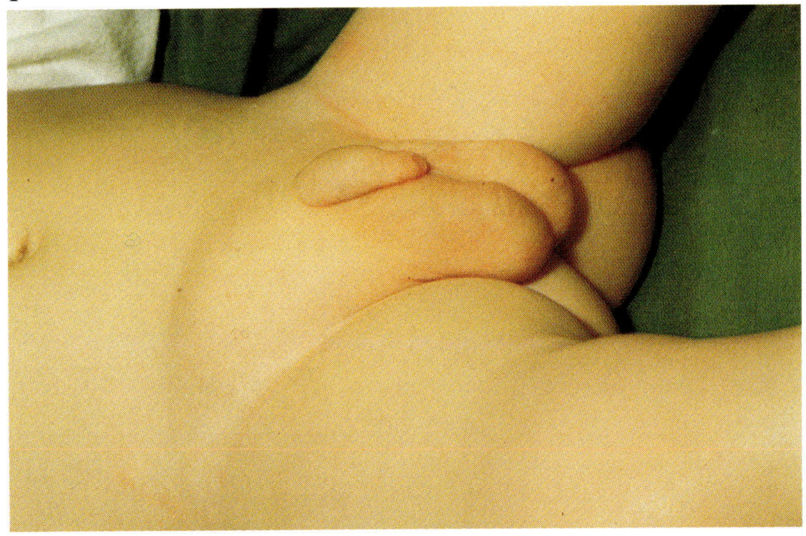

2

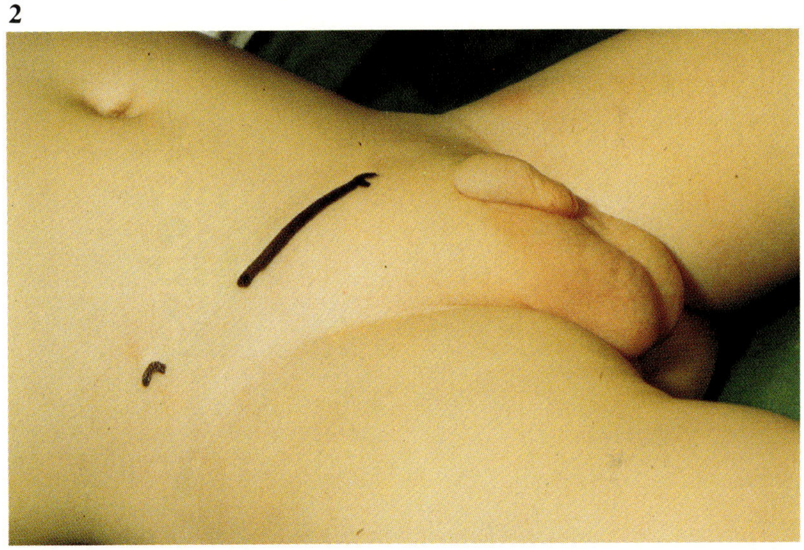

3

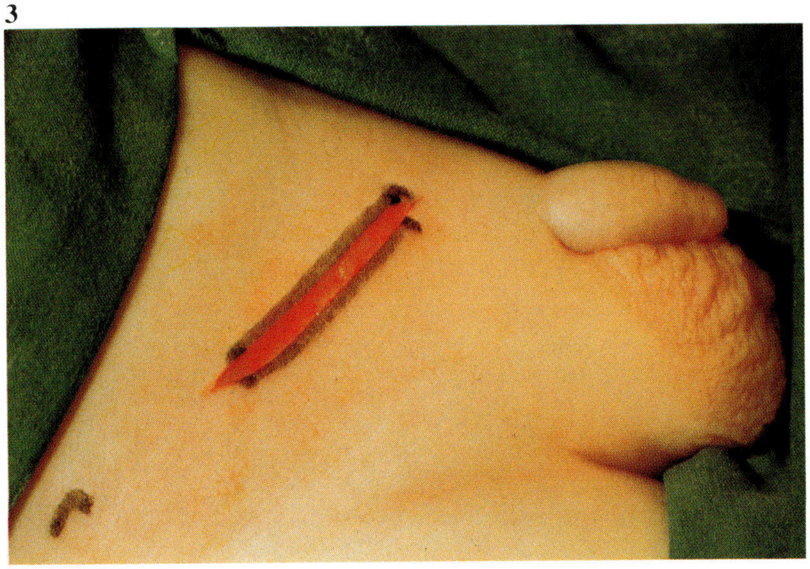

4

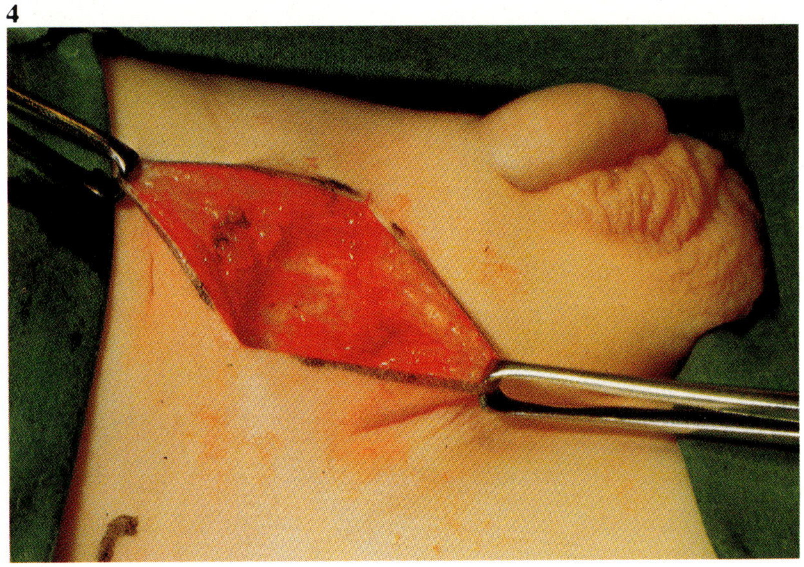

5

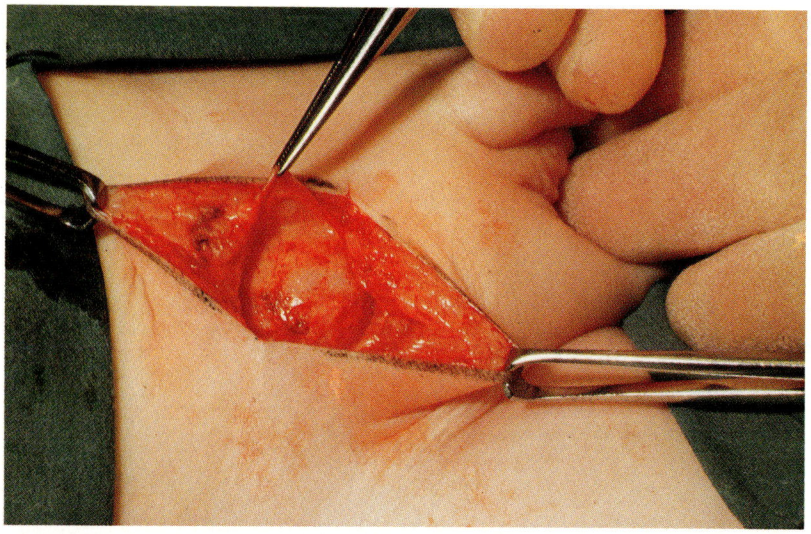

6

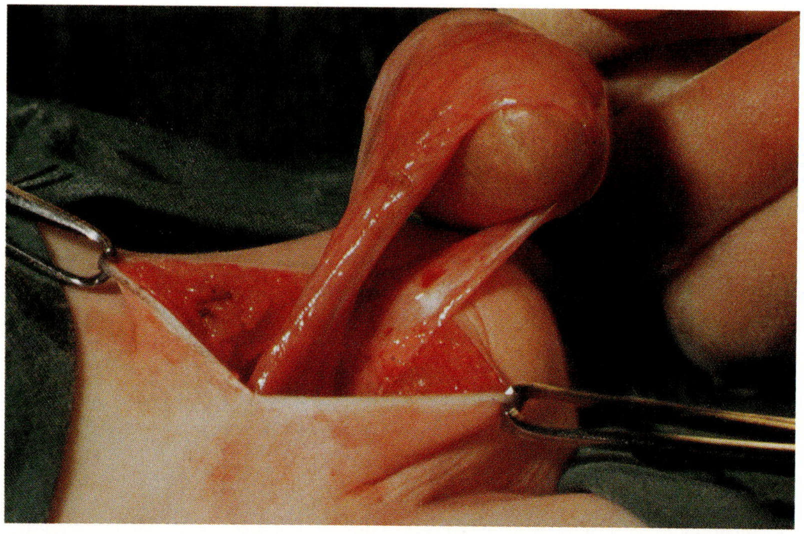

7

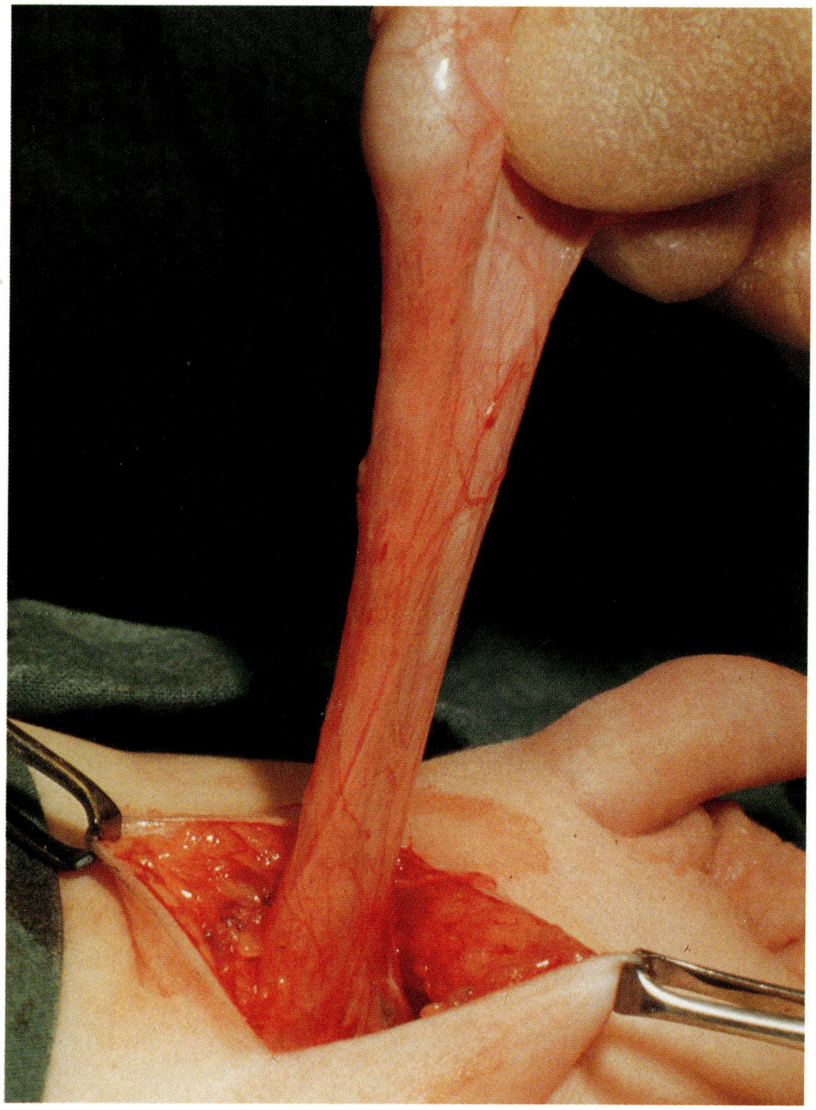

8

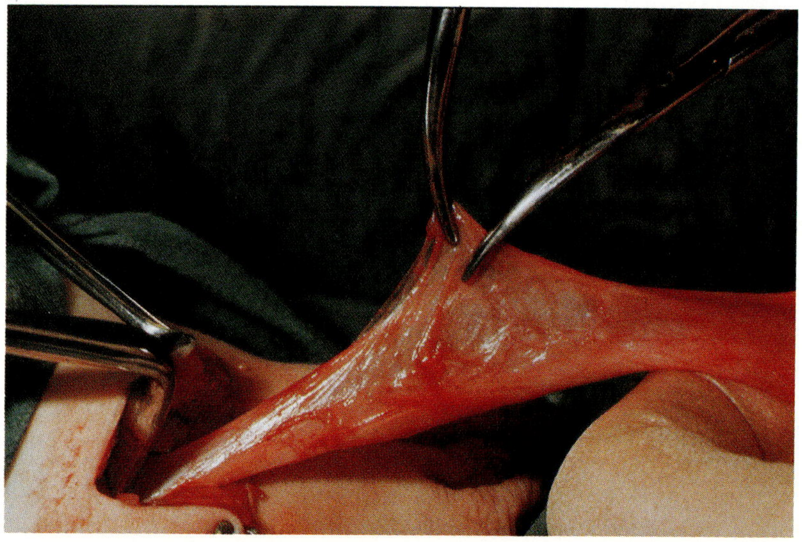

9

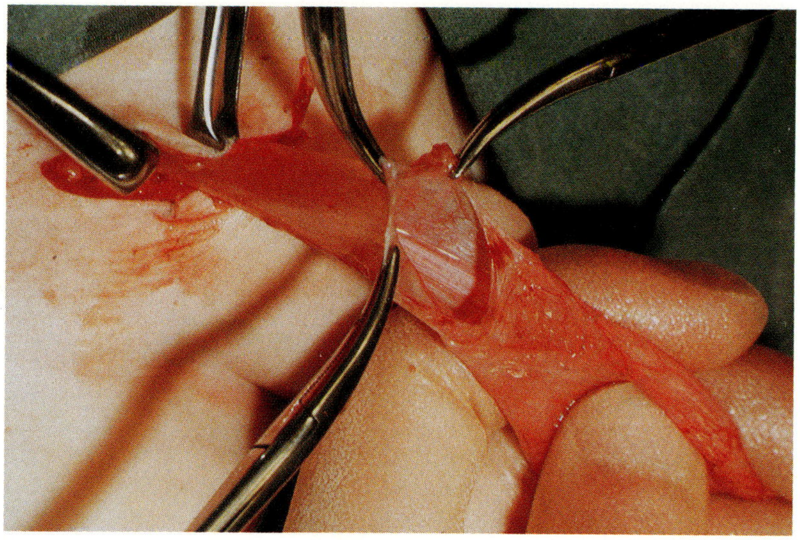

10

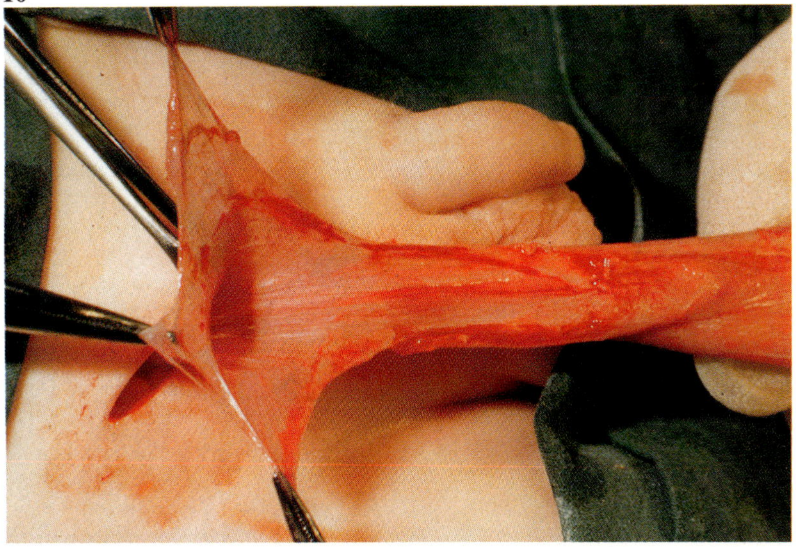

11

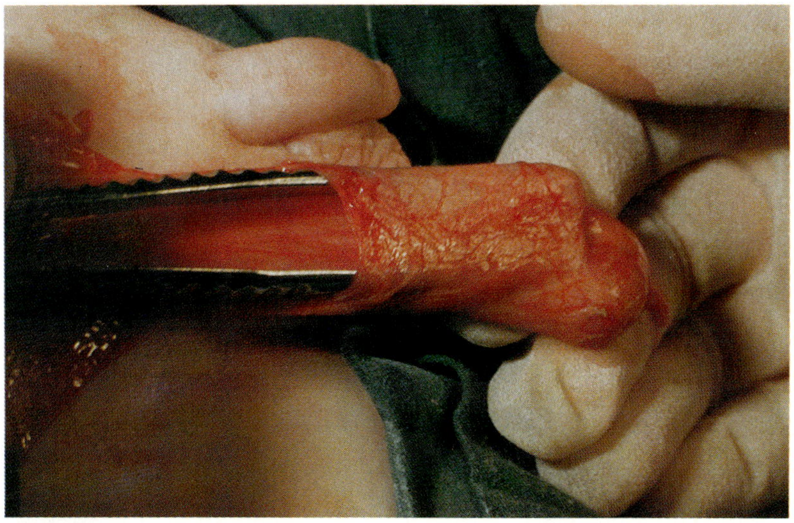

12

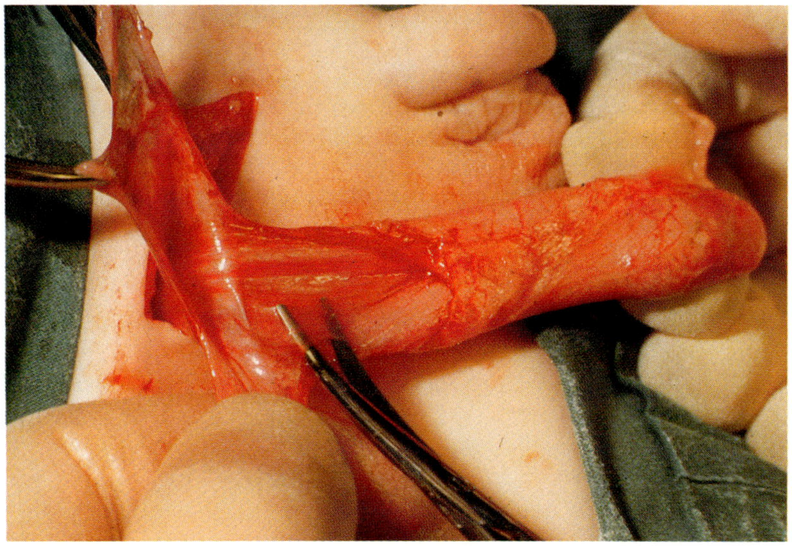

5 The superficial fascia is incised to expose the hernial bulge.

6 The spermatic cord is dissected out gently and held up.

7 The testis slips out easily from the scrotum and is now demonstrated.

8 The coverings of the cord are now dissected out carefully.

9 The processus vaginalis has been opened and the spermatic vessels and vas deferens lie behind.

10 The processus vaginalis is being dissected proximally to the deep inguinal ring.

11 The processus extends distally to the testis in this case.

12 The posterior wall of the processus vaginalis is being separated with care from the posterior structure. The vas deferens is visible. This dissection should be done with great care.

13

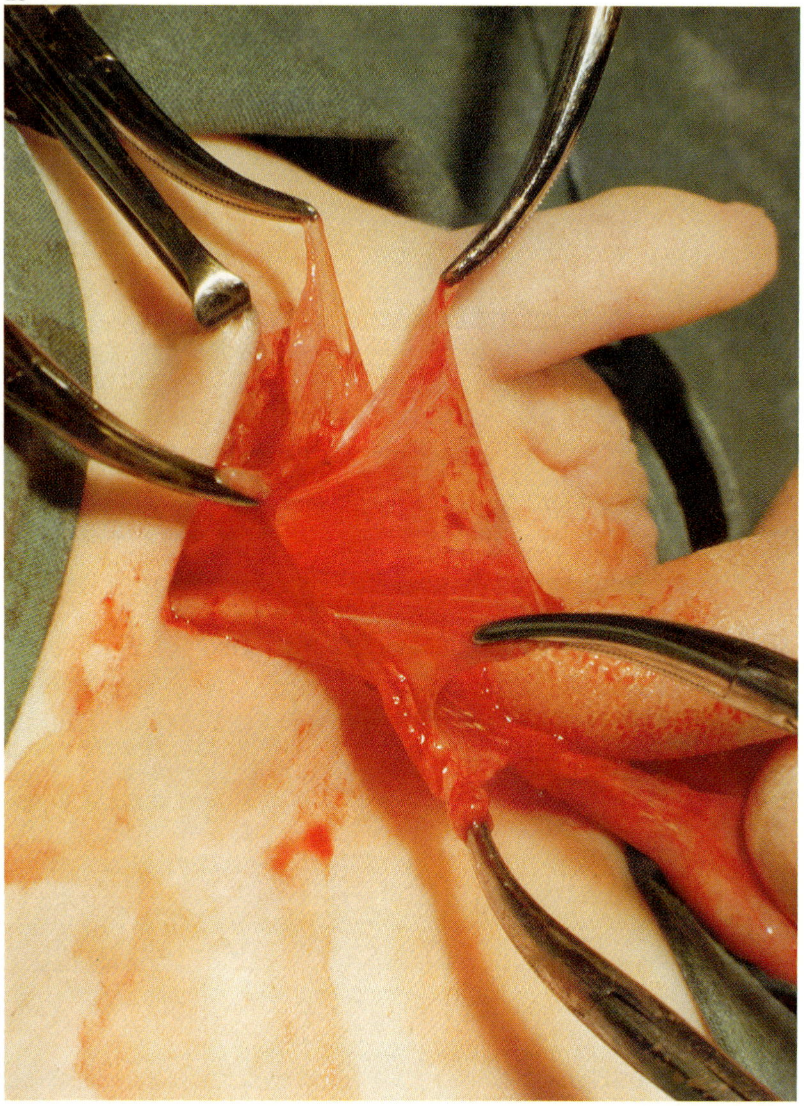

14

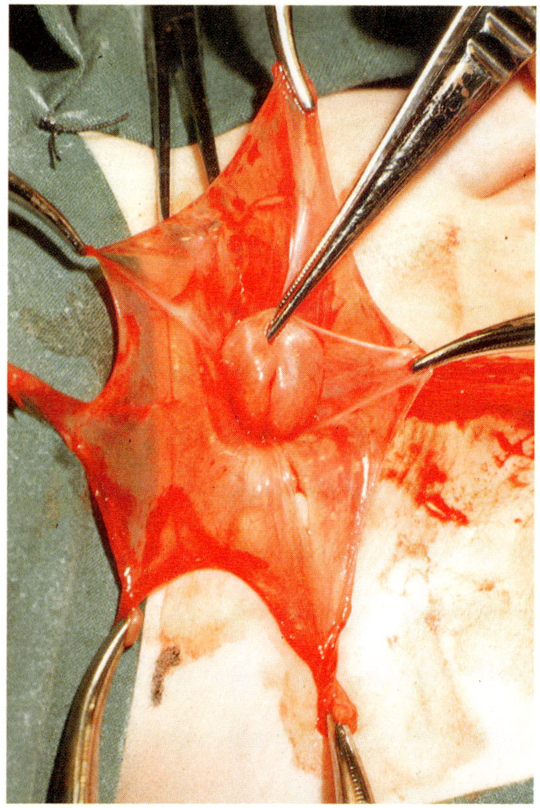

15

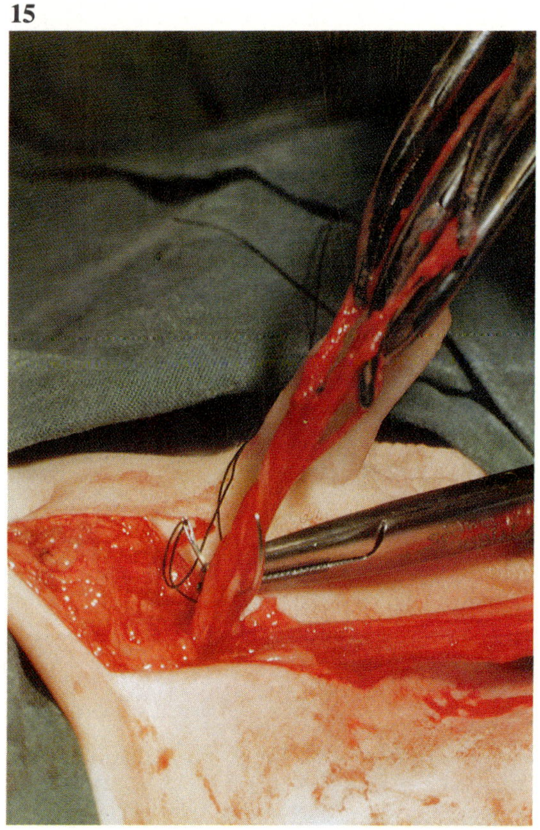

13 The proximal processus is being raised from the other contents of the cord.

14 Dissection has been continued down to the deep inguinal ring. A portion of bowel is visible.

15 The proximal processus is being twisted round to exclude any bowel in it and a catgut suture is placed through the neck of the processus.

16

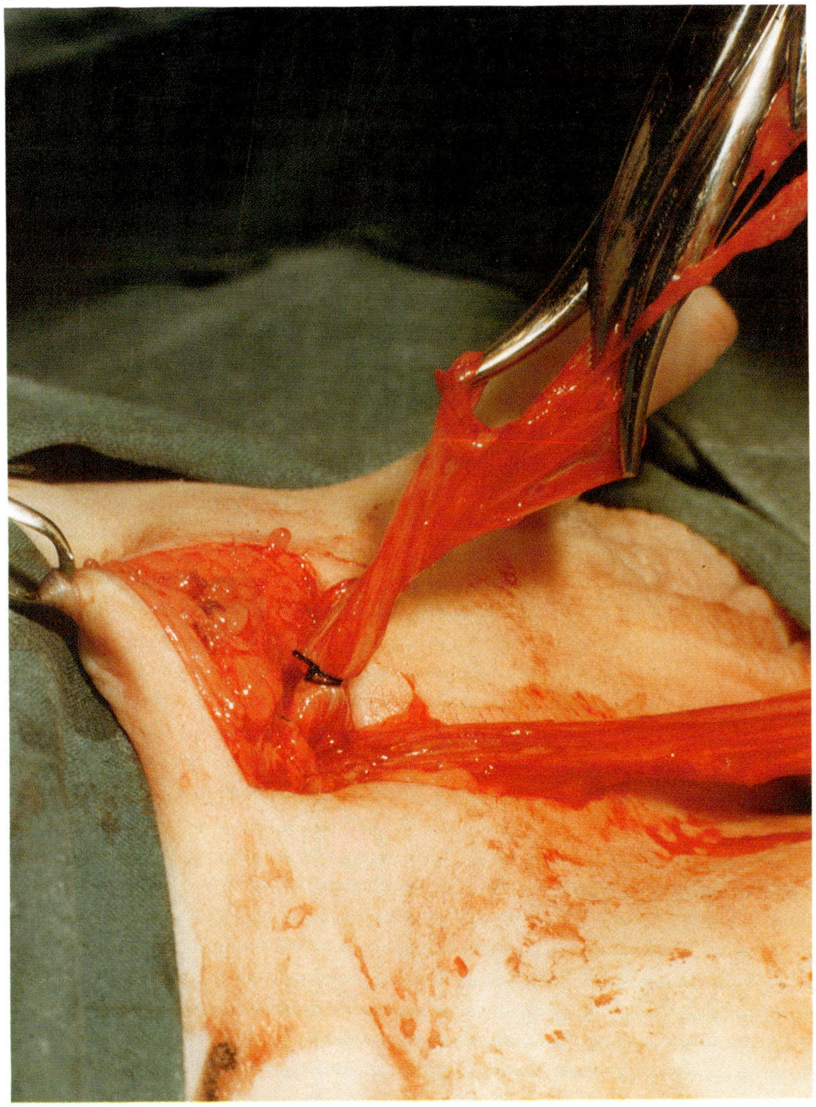

16 Suture ligation is complete. The excess processus is now cut distal to the suture which retracts inwards.

17

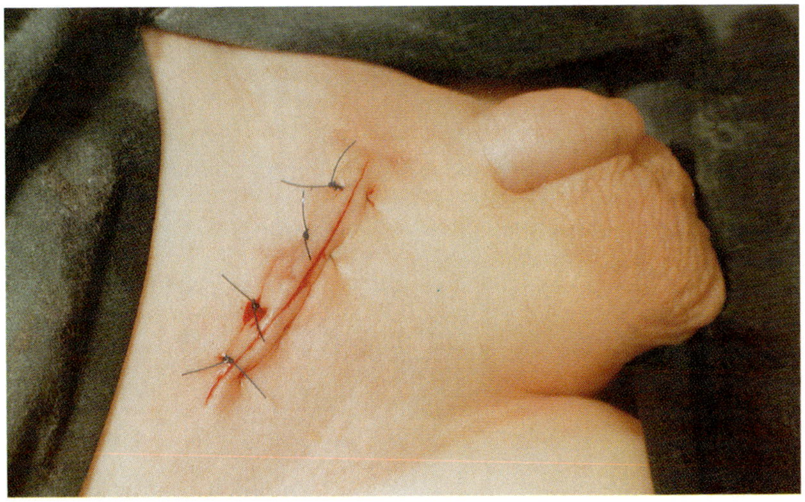

17 The testis is replaced in the scrotum and the wound closed with interrupted Prolene.

Epigastric hernia

An epigastric hernia is a protrusion of extraperitoneal fat through a defect in the linea alba. Why the defect is there is not really certain. **The hernia can present as a swelling or may be painful and, indeed, the fat swelling may become gangrenous.**

1

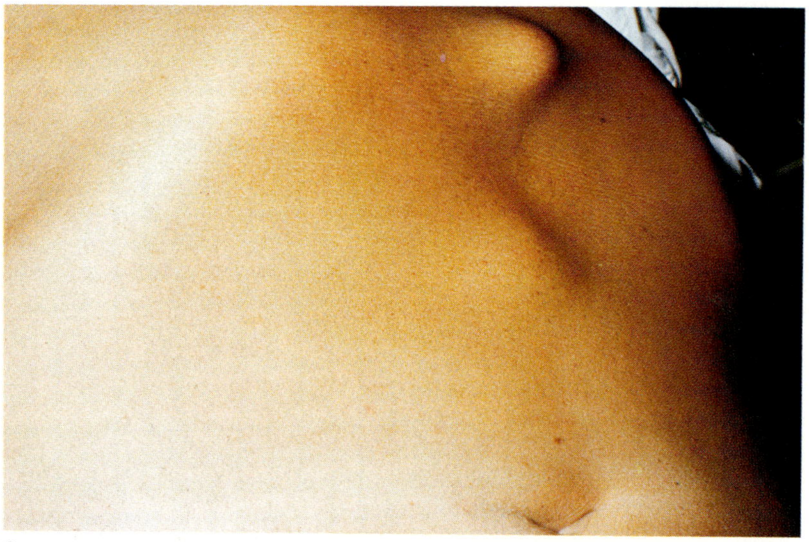

1 Characteristic picture of the swelling between the prominent xiphisternum and the umbilicus.

2

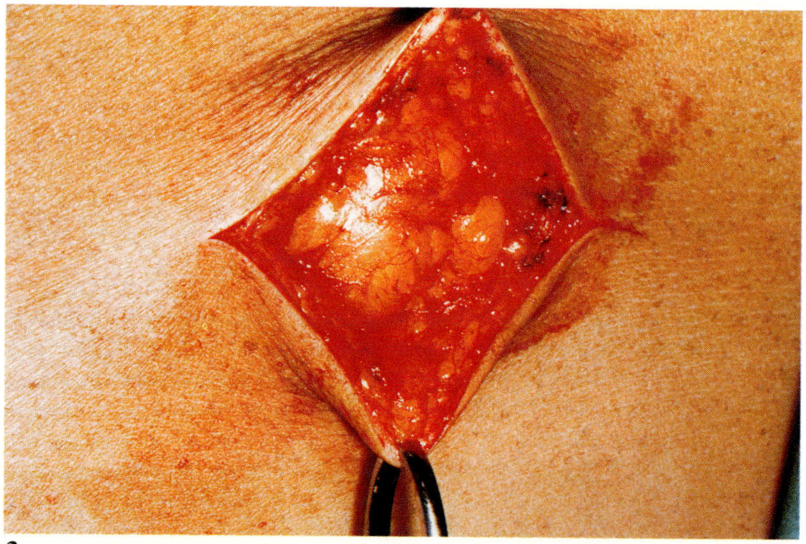

2 The incision may be vertical in the line of the linea alba or, as in this case, transverse over the swelling. General anaesthetic is usual but local anaesthesia can be used.

3

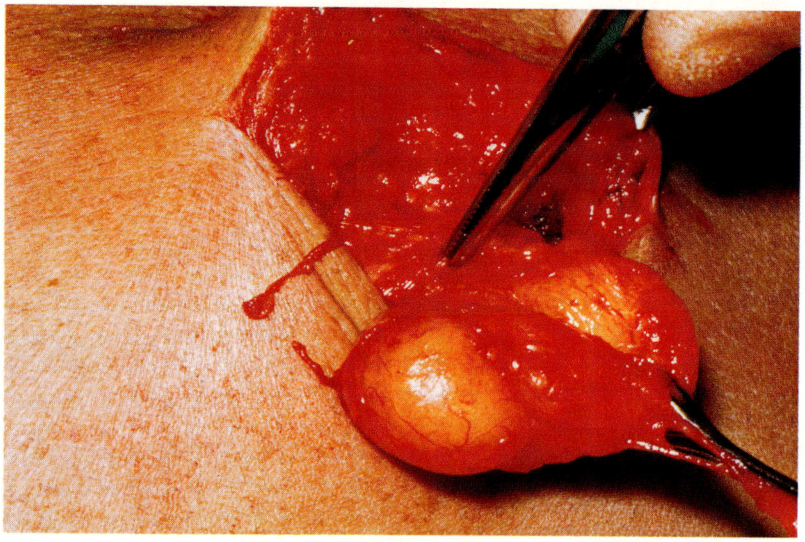

3 The fatty mass is dissected down to the neck which protrudes through the hole in the linea alba.

4

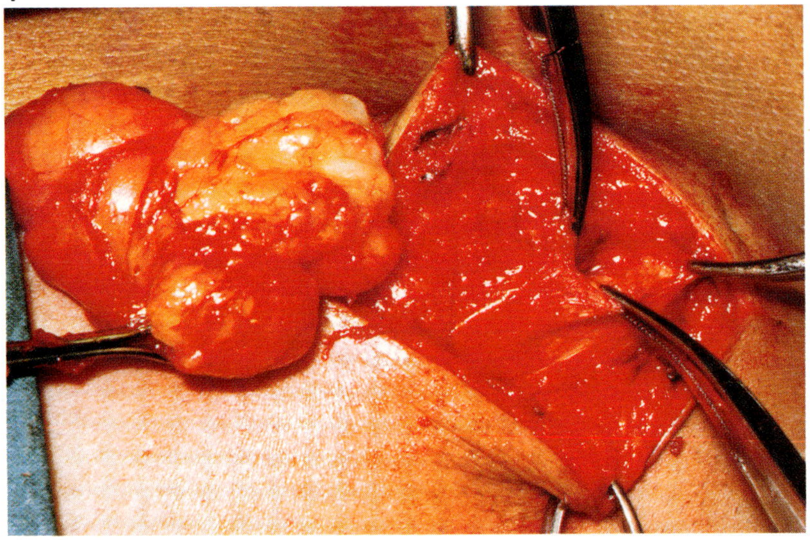

5

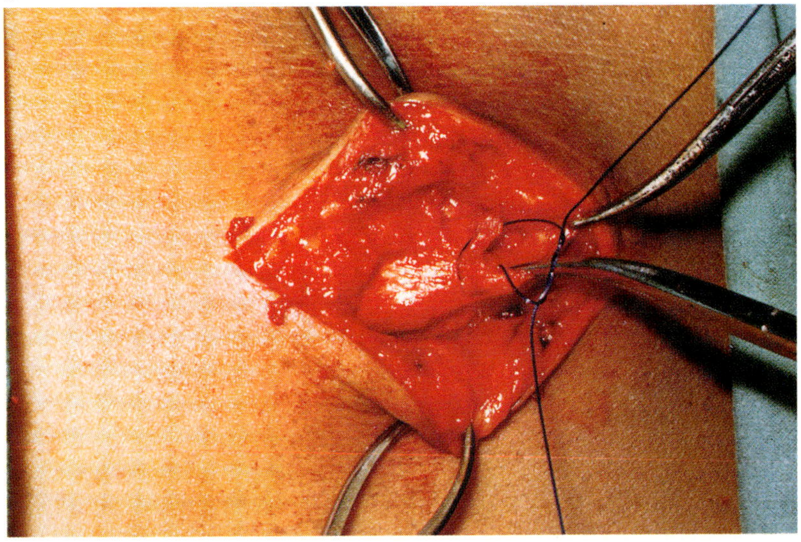

6

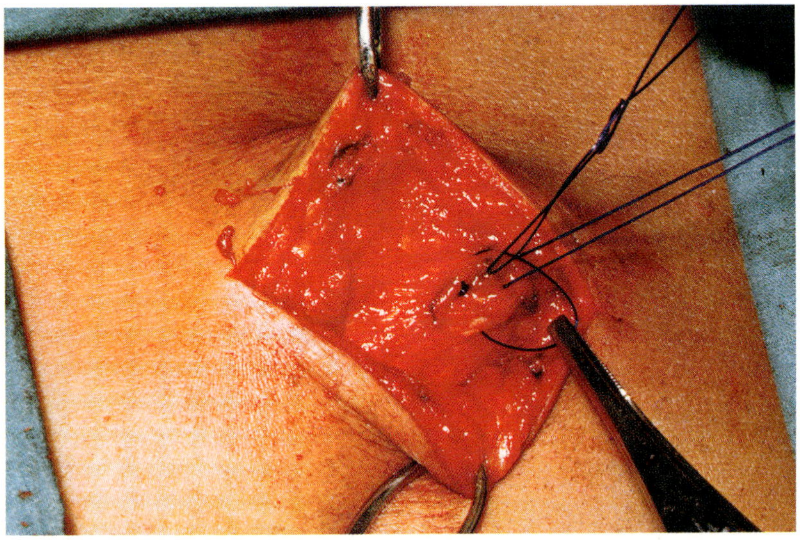

4 With removal of the mass the defect in the linea is clearly exposed.

5 The hole may be closed by simple stitches of non-absorbable material, in this case Prolene. The margins are being inverted with a buried Prolene knot.

6 These sutures are all that is required in this case.

7 The closure is satisfactory and can be tested by asking the patient to cough if the procedure is carried out under local anaesthetic.

8 The sutured area is now being reinforced by a further layer of Prolene sutures.

7

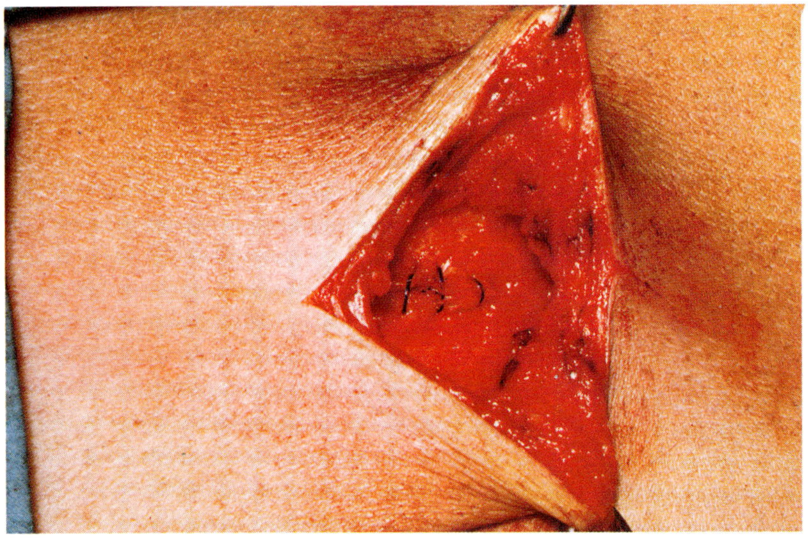

8

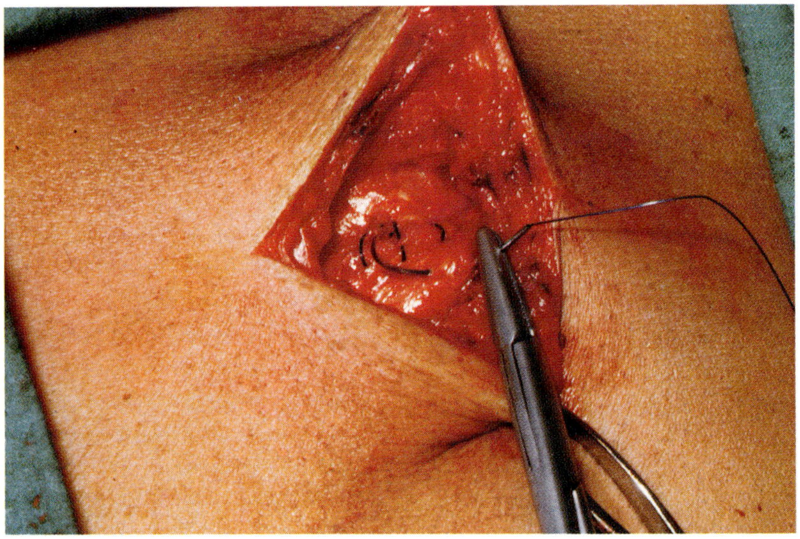

9

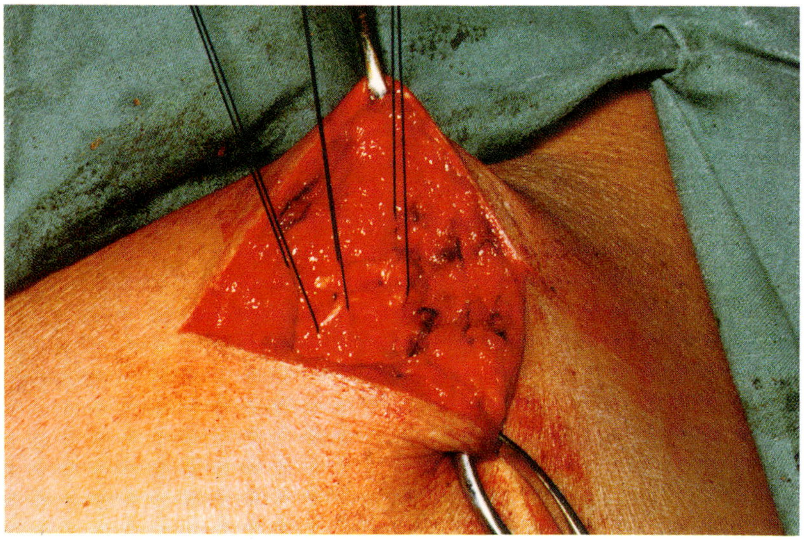

10

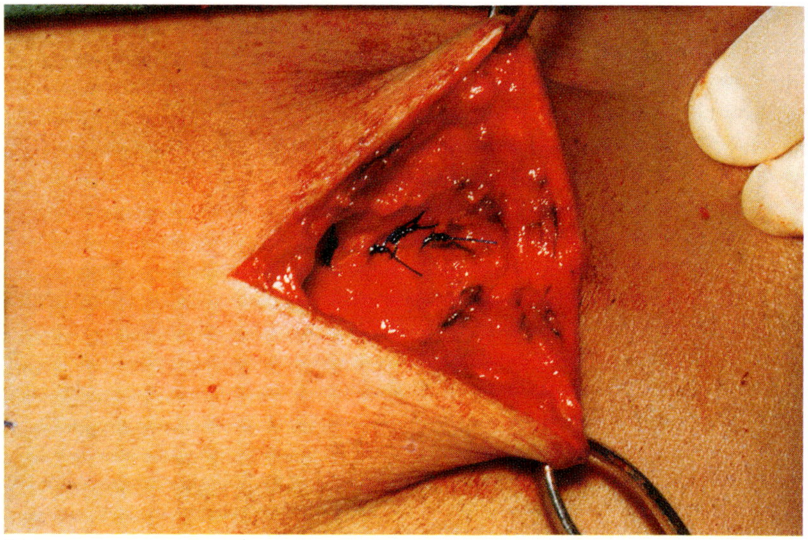

11

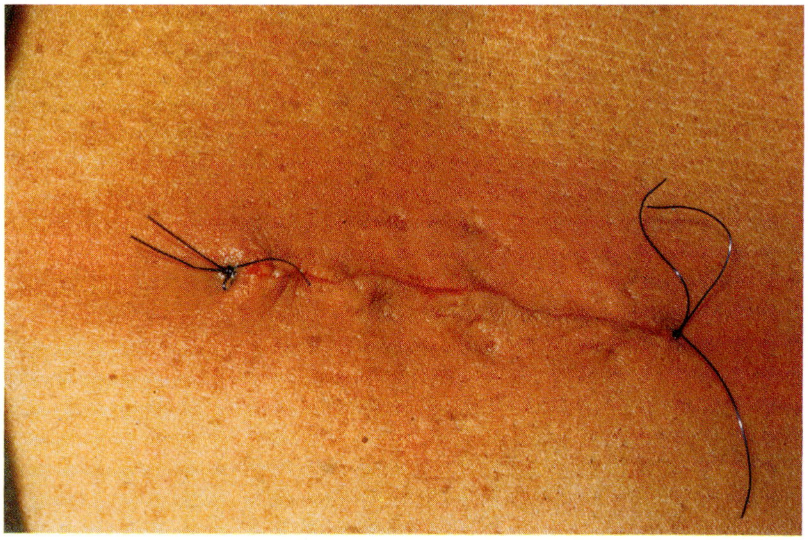

9 The third suture is now ready for tying down.

10 The repair is now completed.

11 The skin is closed with a continuous subcutaneous Prolene stitch.

Repair of direct inguinal hernia

1

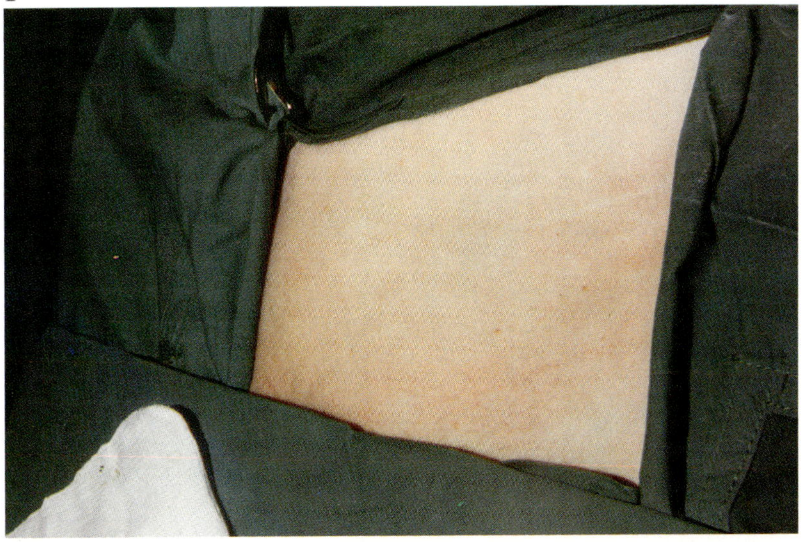

1 This patient had a recurrent direct inguinal hernia. The scar is just visible. As the hernia is in an area of possible infection, care must be taken to clean the area and isolate it well.

2

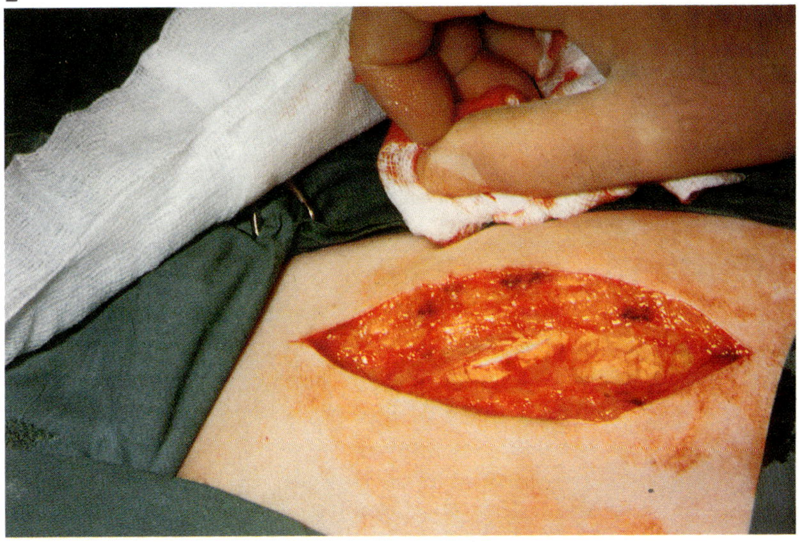

2 Incisions vary from the oblique one starting above the pubic tubercle, where the opening of the external ring is, extending obliquely upwards and laterally, as shown here, to a more transverse incision in a skin crease.

3

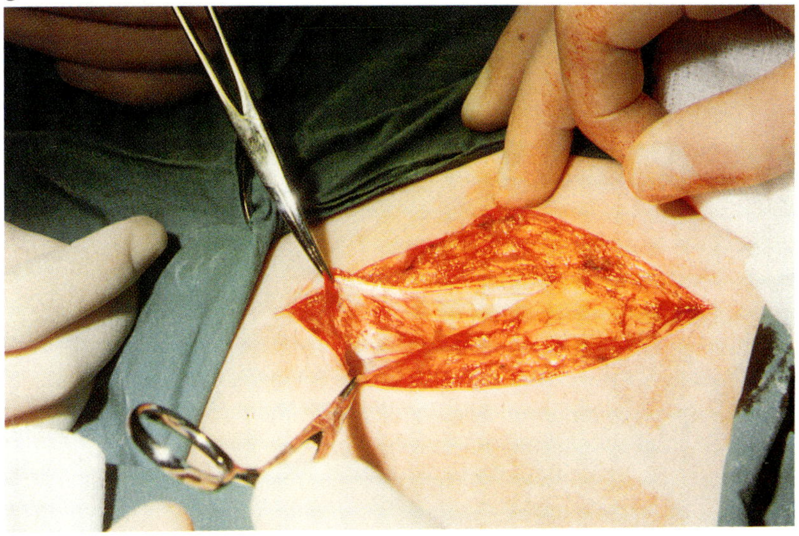

3 The external oblique is opened along the line of the inguinal canal.

4

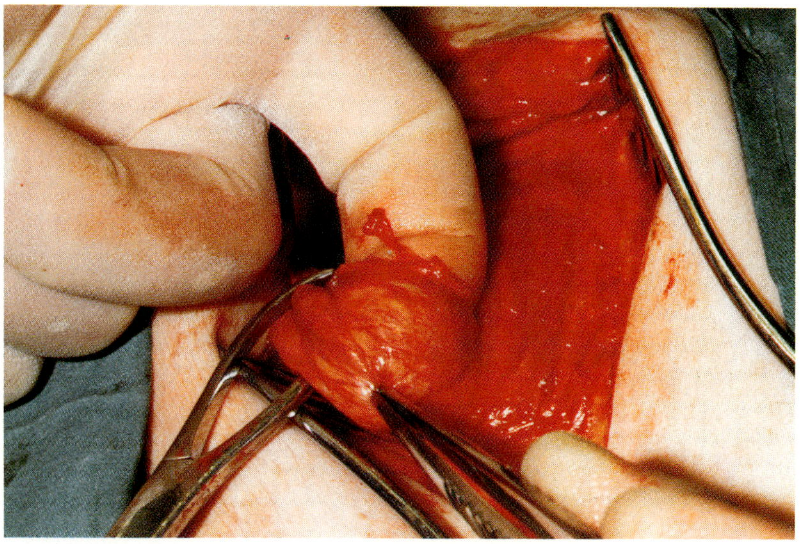

5

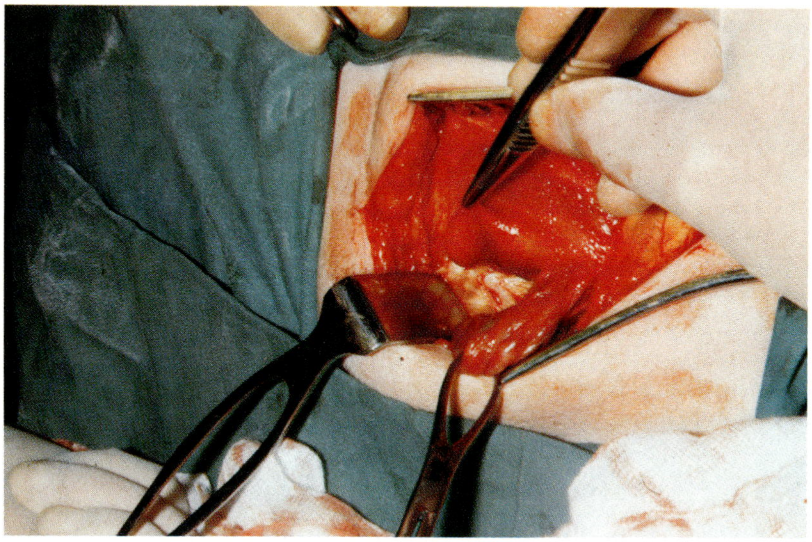

6

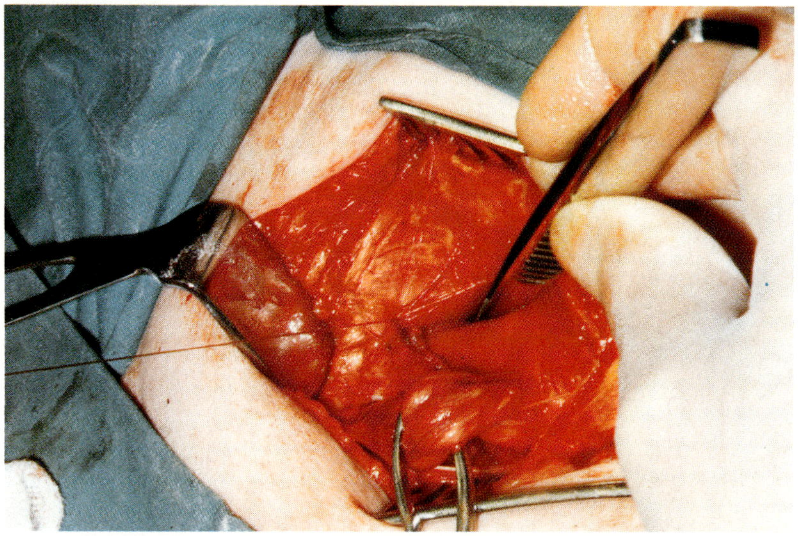

7

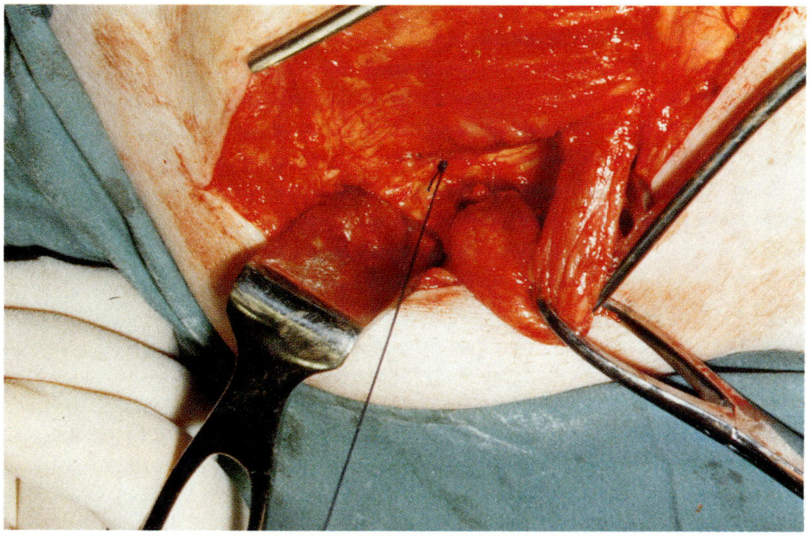

8

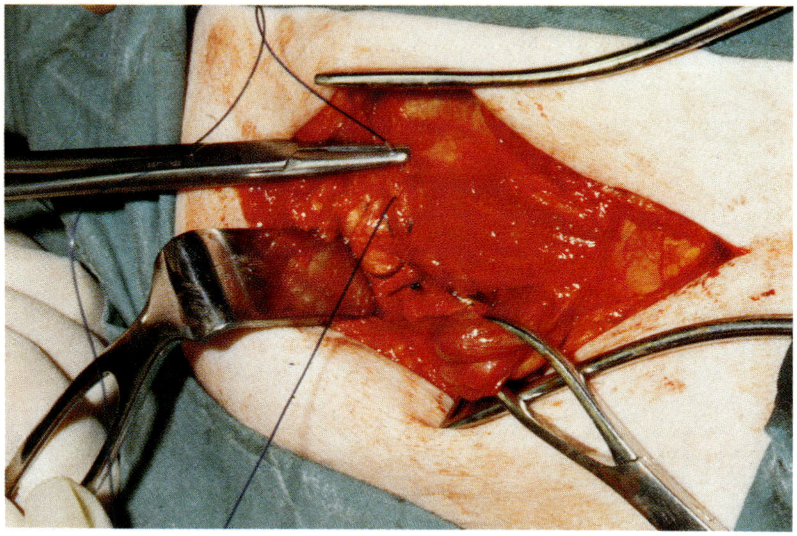

9

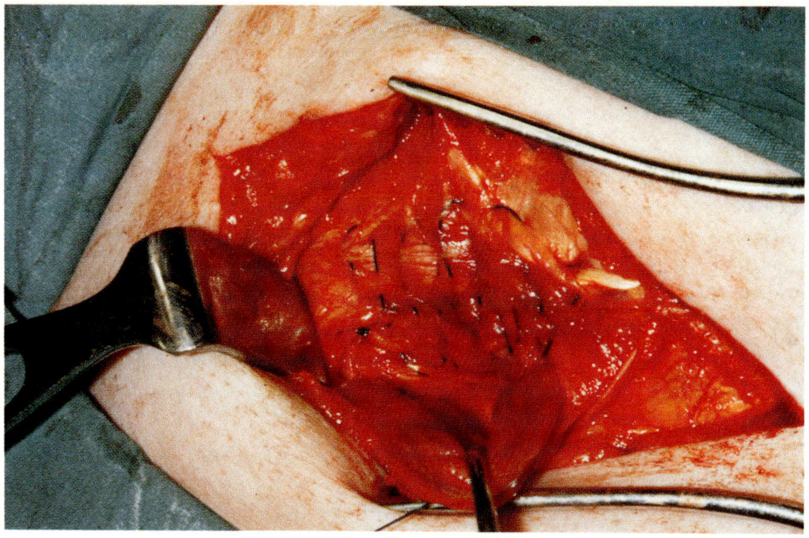

4 The spermatic cord is isolated and the tissues are separated, looking for a possible indirect sac.

5 With the cord drawn downwards the inguinal ligament is seen and above it, held up in the dissecting forceps, is the sac of a direct hernia.

6 The sac has been invaginated by the forceps and the transversalis fascia is being sutured by a continuous catgut suture.

7 The first stitch looking down from above the wound is being inserted between the medial end of the conjoint tendon and the pubic tubercle and is firmly tied. This is the really important stitch which must be deep into the tissues on the tubercle. If it gives way the hernia will recur. A non-absorbable suture such as Prolene O or silk is used.

8 Looking from below, the Prolene suture is continued as a darn passing in and out of the conjoint tendon above and through the inguinal ligament.

9 The completed darn is shown.

10 The external oblique is now being closed with No.0 Prolene. Care is taken not to narrow the external ring too much. It should allow the tip of the little finger to enter it.

11 The lateral closure of the external oblique is nearing completion.

12 Closure of skin is a matter of choice using Prolene as interrupted mattress sutures or as a continuous subcuticular suture which is more cosmetic.

10

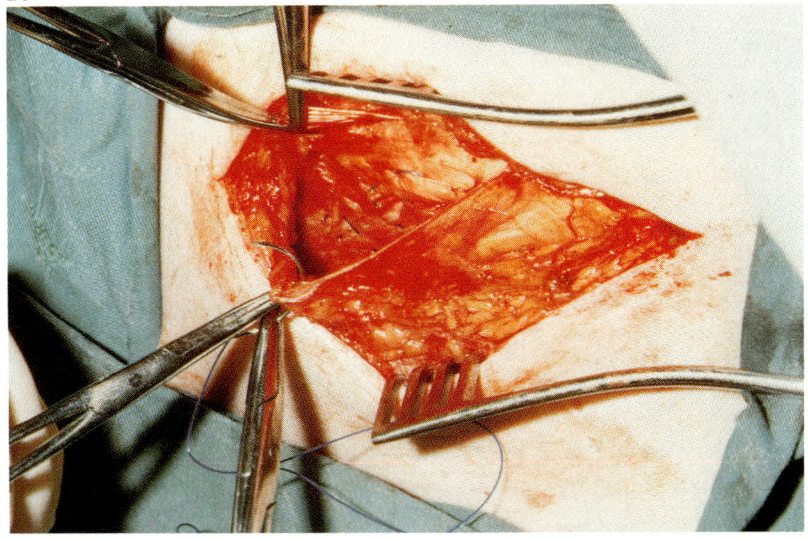

11

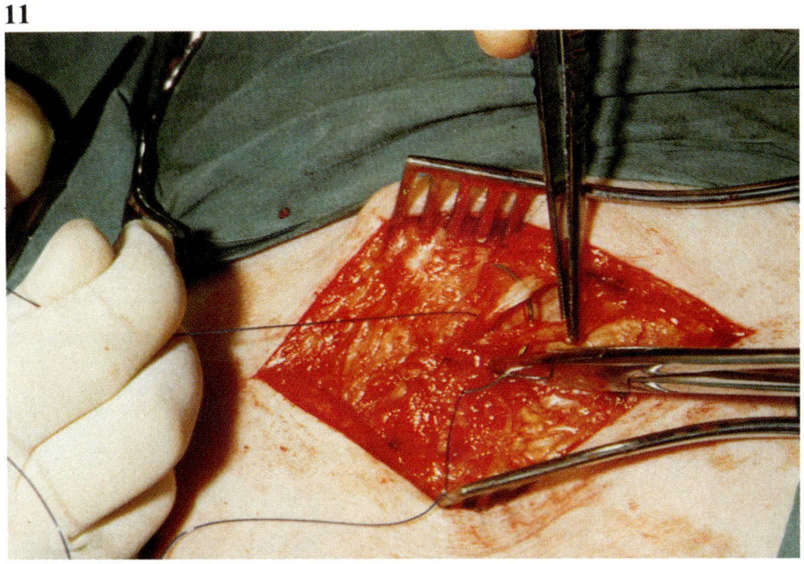

12

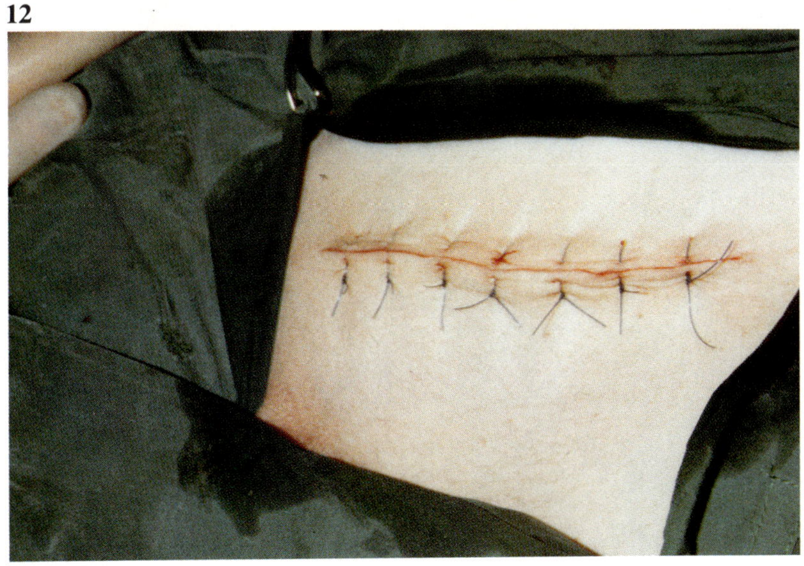

Inguinal hernia repair under local anaesthesia

There are occasions when general anaesthetic is not possible in repair of hernias and spinal anaesthetics. In these cases local anaesthesia may be preferable.

There are three nerves which must be blocked in addition to local skin infiltration. These are:

1] Iliohypogastric which lies between the external and internal oblique muscles, passing across these muscles above the inguinal canal area.

2] Ilioinguinal which runs below the iliohypogastric nerve and emerges through the superficial inguinal ring.

3] Genitofemoral nerve which has two branches: the genital which follows the spermatic cord to supply the cremaster muscle and skin of the scrotum and the femoral branch which lies alongside the external iliac artery passing to the skin of the femoral triangle.
Lignocaine 0.5 per cent with adrenaline is satisfactory to block the nerves using a 30-35 ml syringe and a 23 gauge needle.

The areas marked by X indicate sites for injections of local anaesthesia. The anterior-superior iliac spine is indicated laterally. 2 cm medially is the injection area for the ilioinguinal and iliohypogastric nerves. The next two crosses indicate upper and lower areas of infiltration anaesthesia and the medial cross the opening of the external ring above the pubic tubercle.

1

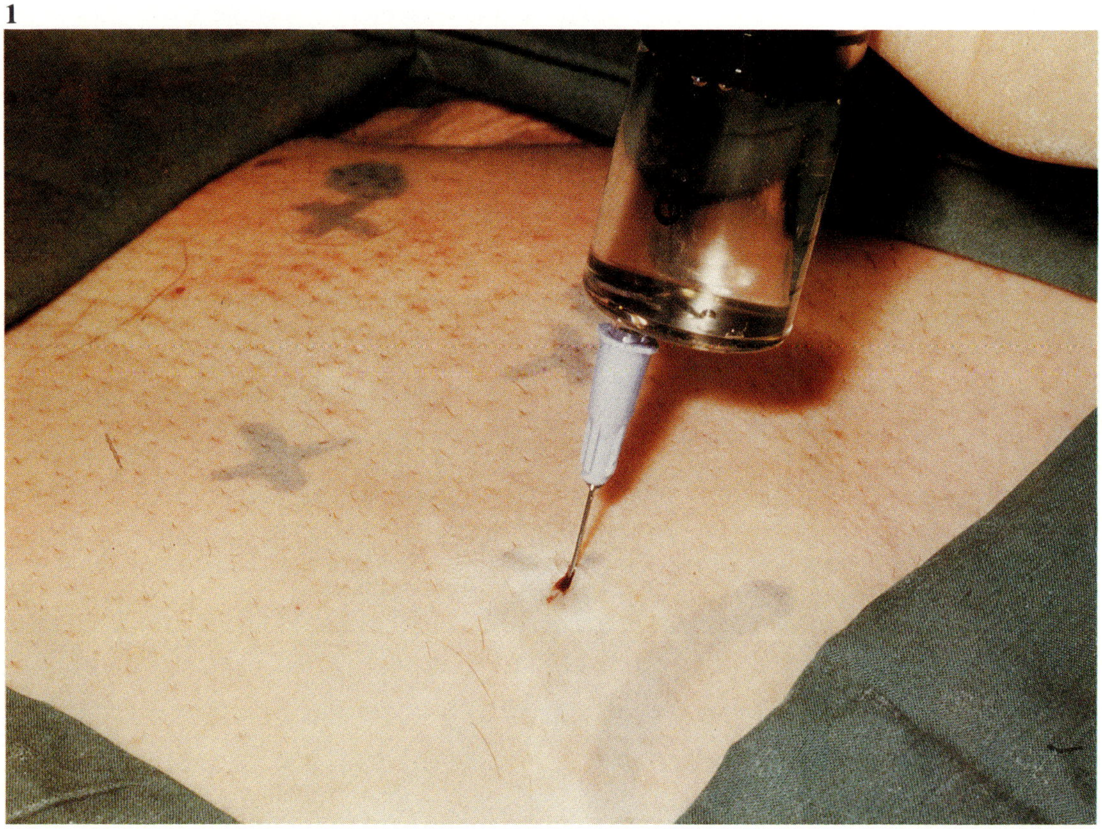

1 The first injection is made at a point of 2 cm medial to the anterior superior iliac spine. Through a skin weal about 10 ml is injected just deep to the external oblique aponeuroses. This blocks the ilioinguinal and iliohypogastric nerves. The penetration of the aponeuroses can be felt by a distinct 'give' as the needle passes through.

2

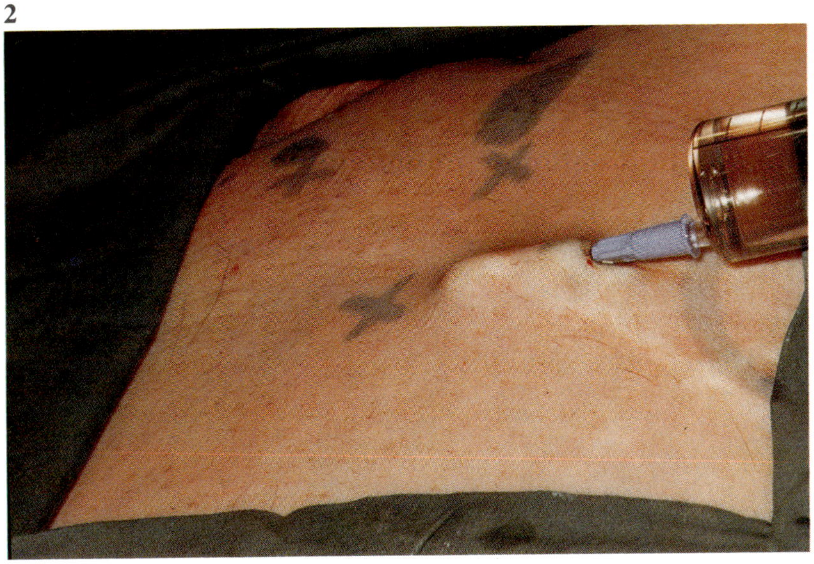

3

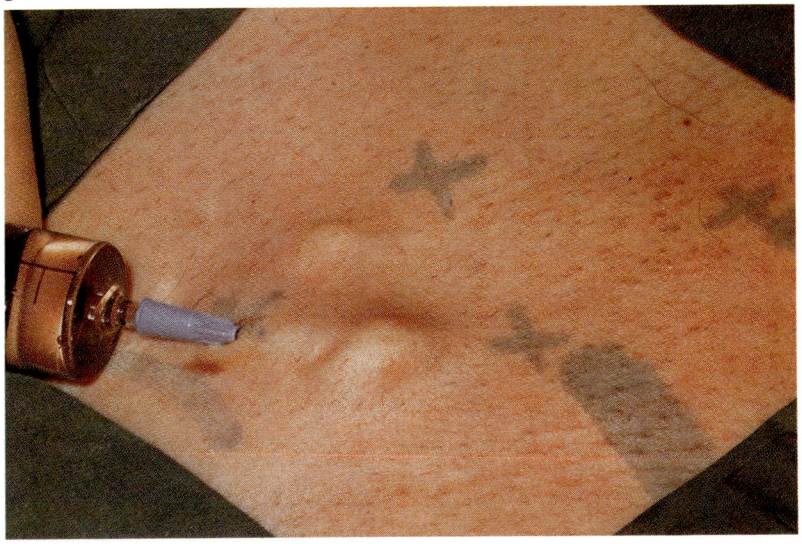

4

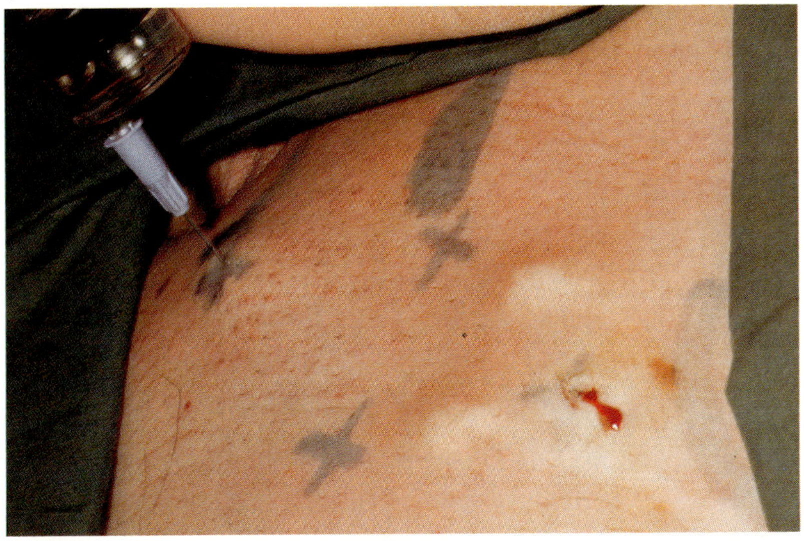

2 At the same injection further anaesthetic is injected subcutaneously 2.5 cm in a fan-wise direction towards the cross marking. The upper about 2.5 cm above the mid inguinal point.

3 Another 10 ml injection is made to the lower mark 2.5 cm below the mid inguinal point. The place of the femoral artery is noted by the wide mark.

4 A further injection is made just lateral to the pubic tubercle and about 5 ml is infiltrated around the bone itself.

5 The injection gradually deepens down to the bone. A further injection of 10 ml is made subcutaneously superolaterally. No attempt should be made to infiltrate the spermatic cord at this point because of the risk of producing a haematoma by damaging the venous plexus.

6 When the ilioinguinal canal is now opened the ilioinguinal nerve is sought and infiltrated with 2-3 ml of anaesthetic.

5

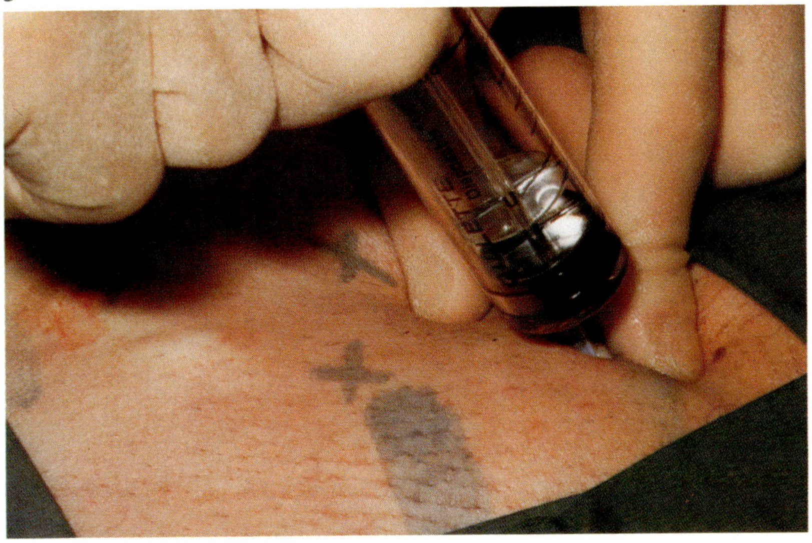

6

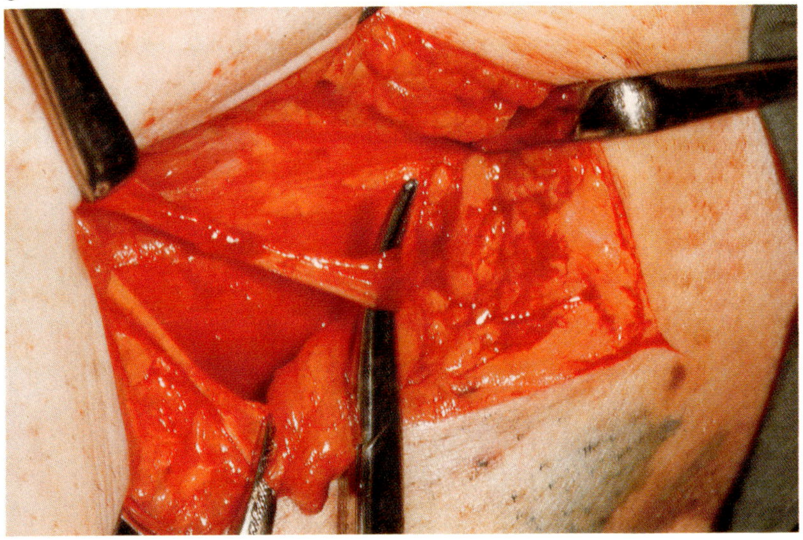

7

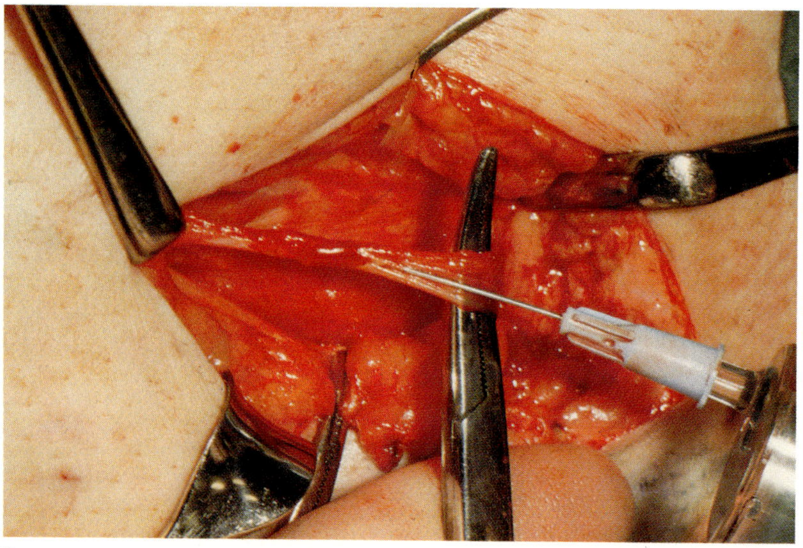

8

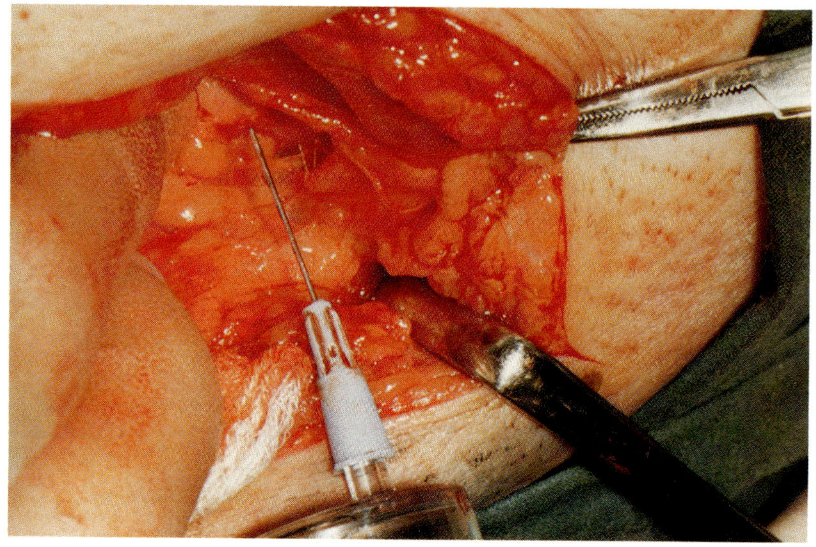

9

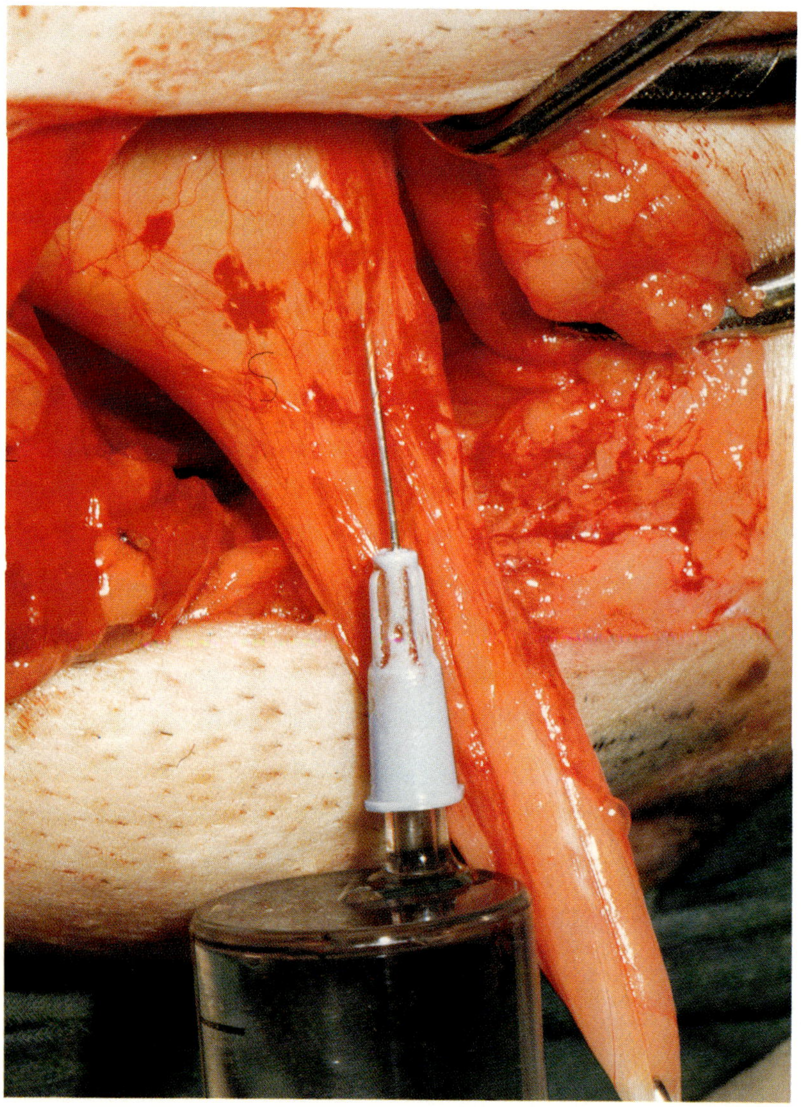

7 The injection of the ilioinguinal nerve is shown.

8 The genital branch of the genitofemoral nerve is found behind the spermatic cord and is blocked directly.

9 This patient had a direct hernia and the neck of the sac is blocked after the epigastric vessels have been displayed.

10 Further injection of the peritoneum alongside the spermatic cord. The peritoneal sac is elongated by traction. The spermatic cord is on the left of the picture.

10

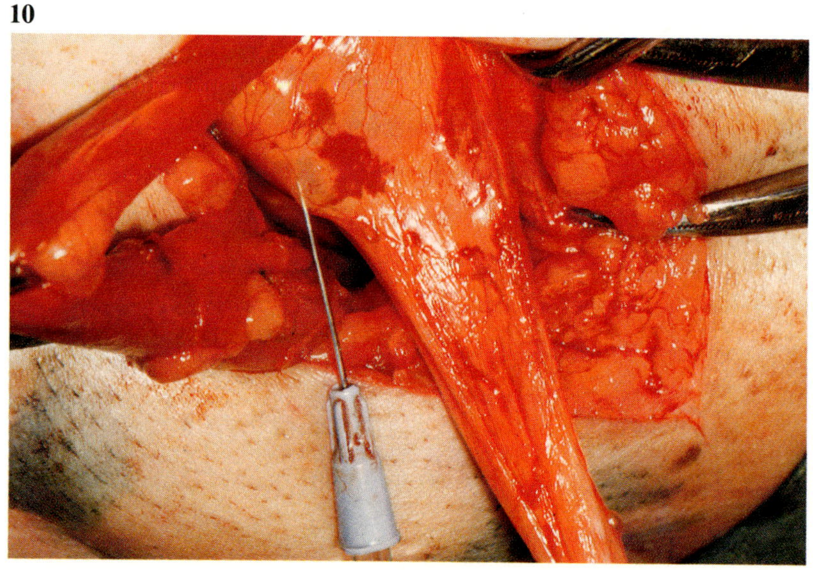

11

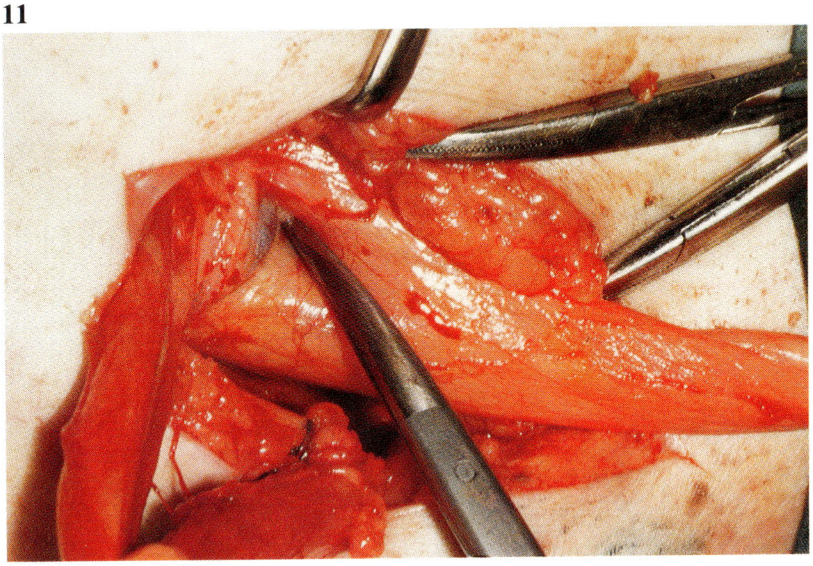

12

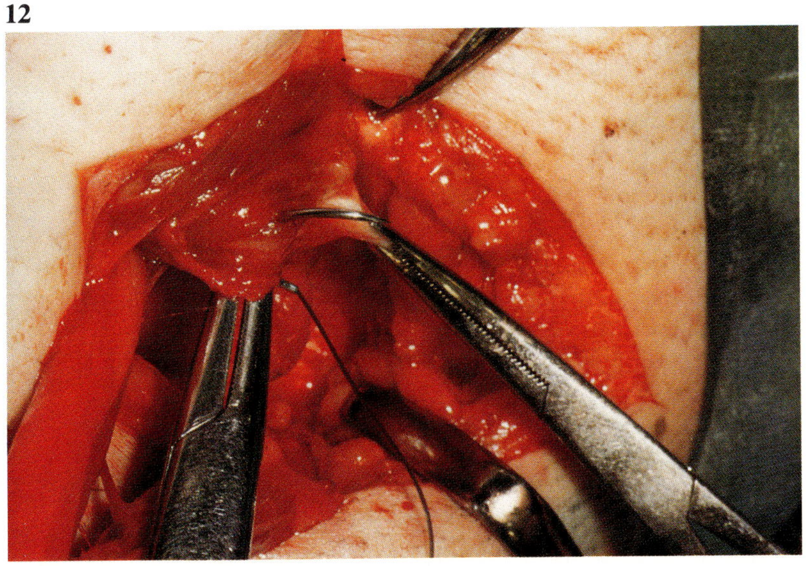

13

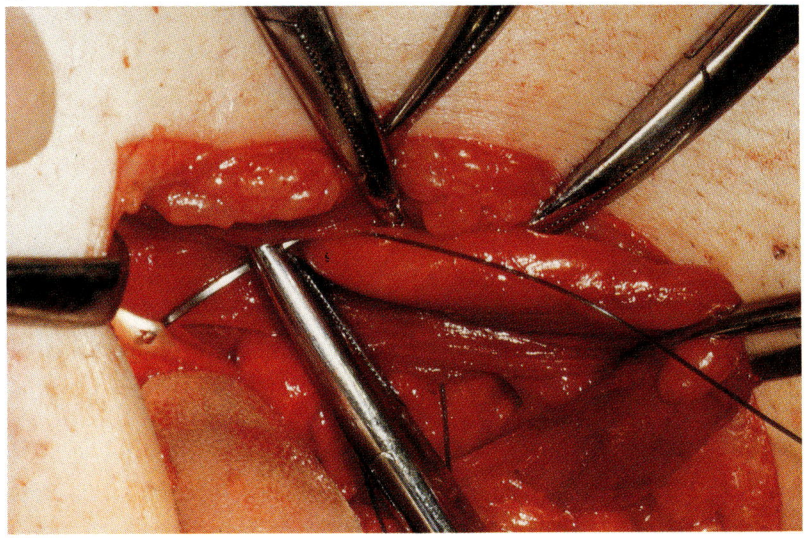

11 The hernial sac was quite long and, when held in forceps, became elongated. The forceps at the base of the sac demonstrate the inferior epigastric vessels.

12 Although the direct sac is not usually removed it was in this case and the neck sutured.

13 The repair of the inguinal canal is done using a Prolene darn.

Appendicectomy

1 The standard incision is made one third above and two thirds below McBurney's point which is at the junction of the lateral and middle thirds of a line between the umbilicus and the anterior iliac spine. Often a curvilin bar incision is made in line with the skin-crease in the area.

1

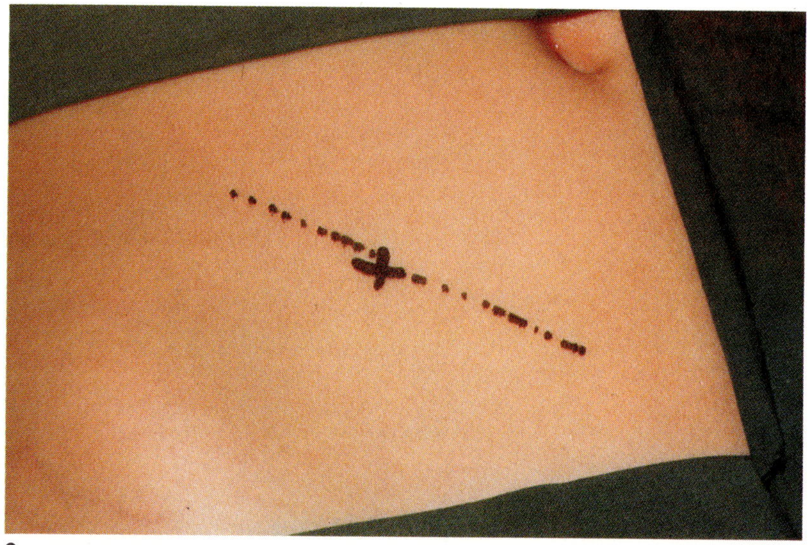

2 The external oblique aponeurosis is incised in the line of the skin incision.

2

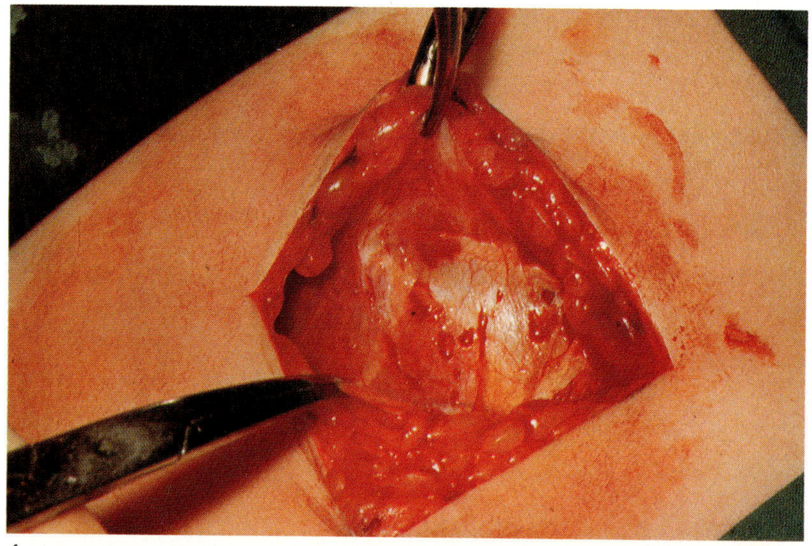

3 The internal oblique and transversus muscles are split in the line of their fibres to expose the peritoneum. This is carefully picked up in haemostats with care not to include the underlying bowel in the forceps.

4 The appendix may be readily accessible and can be easily picked out or it may lie in the pelvis or, as in this case, be retrocaeal as is found in about 33 per cent of these cases.

3

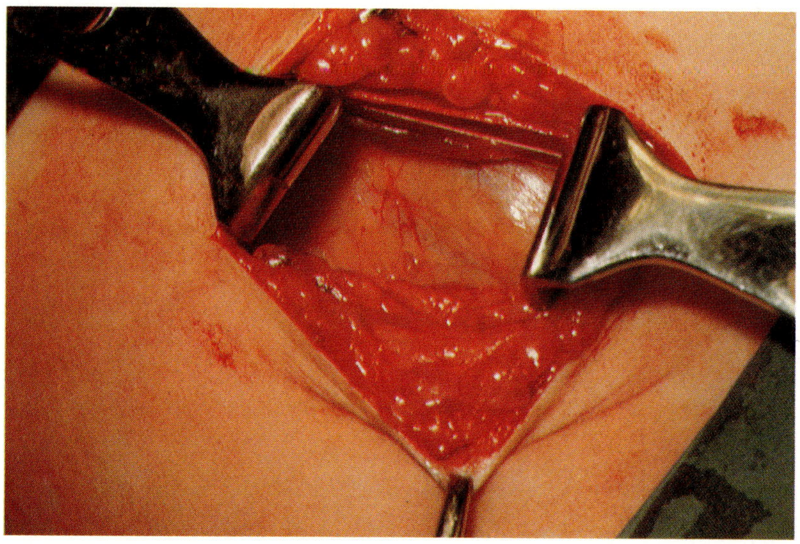

4

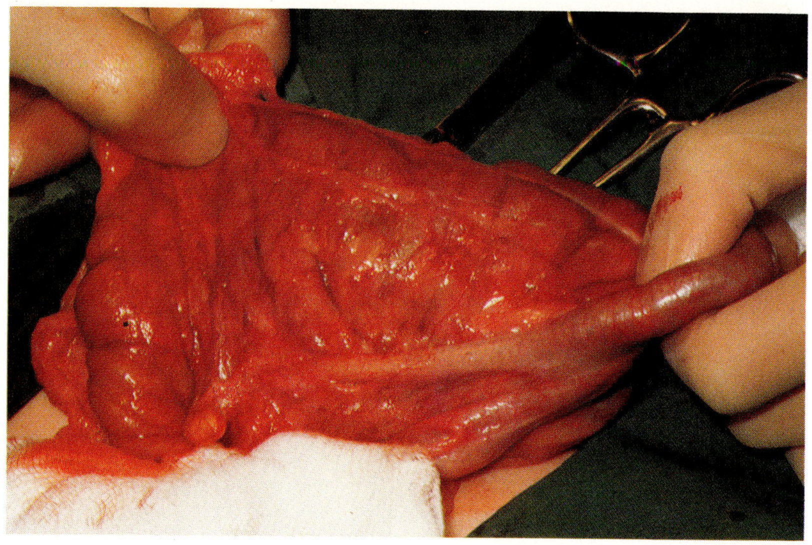

5

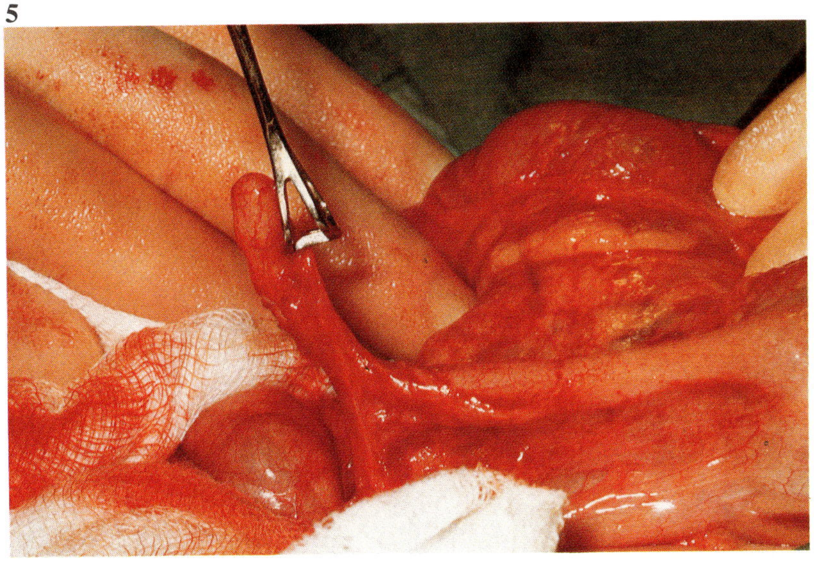

5 The tissue at the tip of the appendix is grasped in atraumatic tissue forceps. Before this can be done it may be necessary to mobilise the caecum by incising the tissues on its lateral side.

6

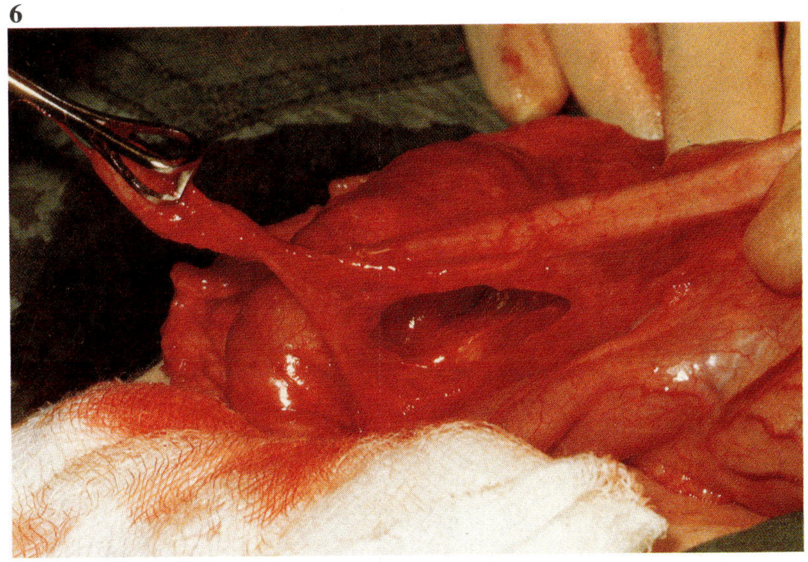

6 The mesoappendix is gradually mobilised and the appendicular artery which often runs or branches in the free edge is caught and tied.

7

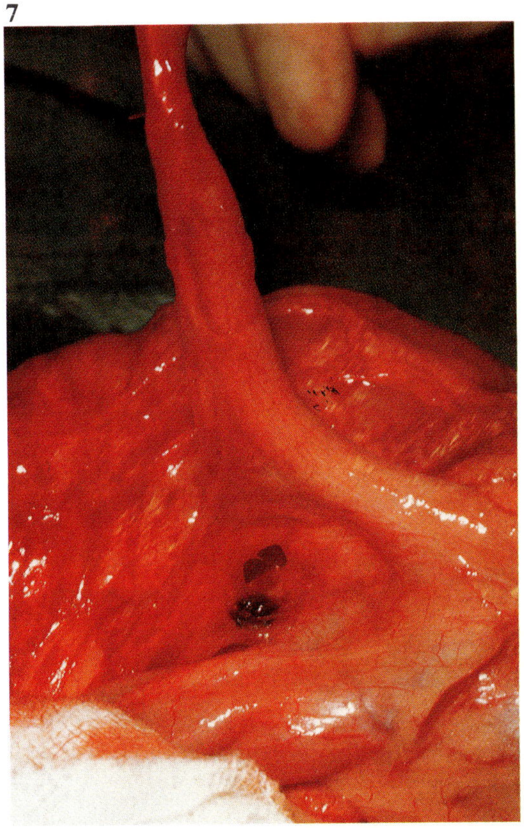

7 Smaller vessels towards the base of the appendix are also tied or, if very small, coagulated with diathermy.

8

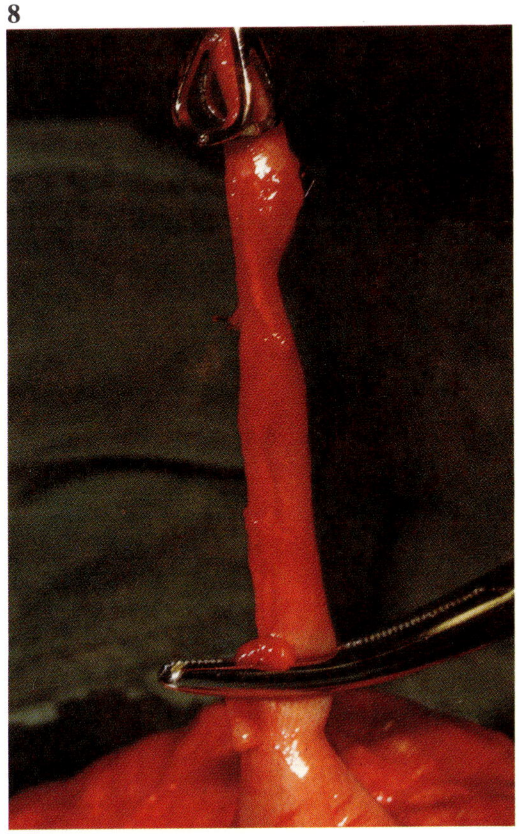

8 The fully mobilised appendix is clamped at its base.

9

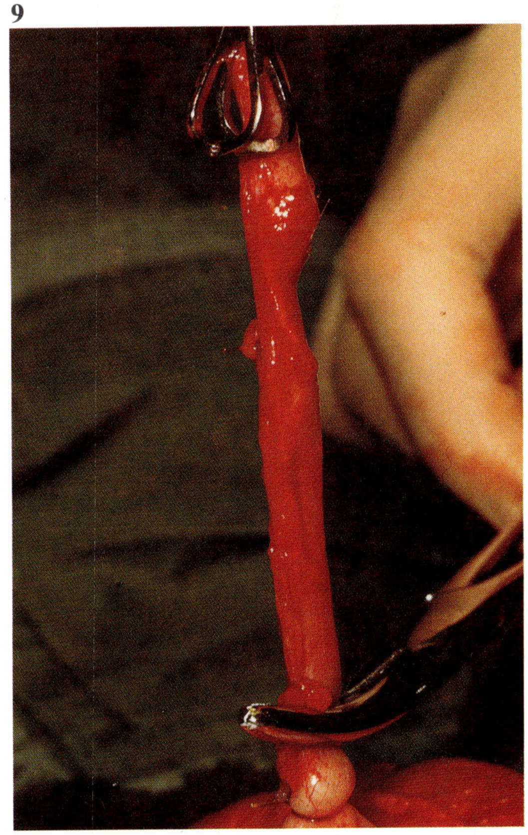

9 A catgut ligature is tied proximally or the clamp can be released and the catgut tied over the clamped area. The forceps are reapplied distal to the tie.

10

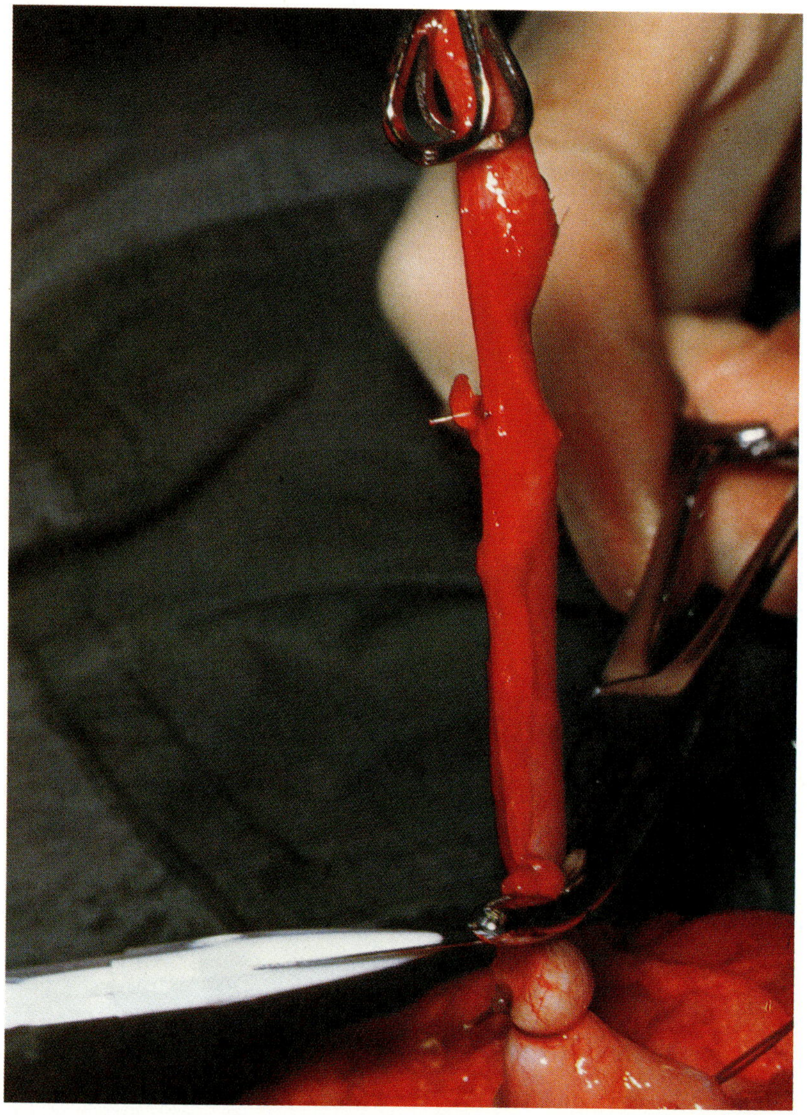

11

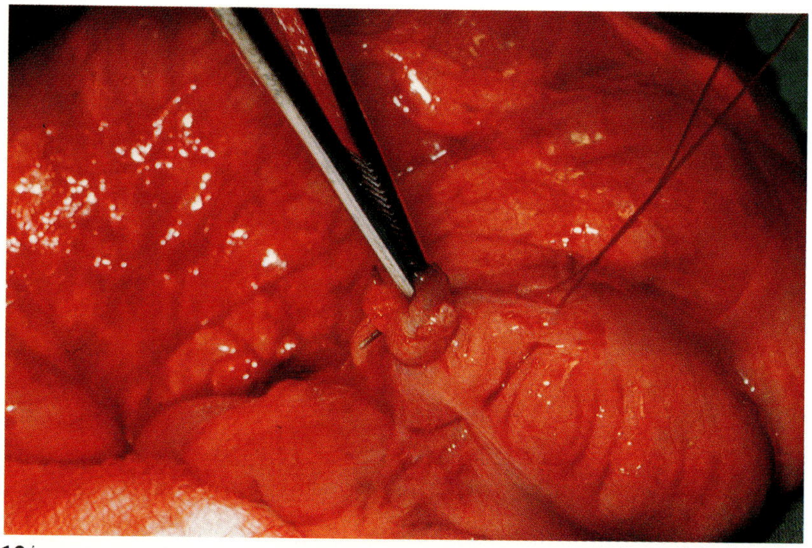

12

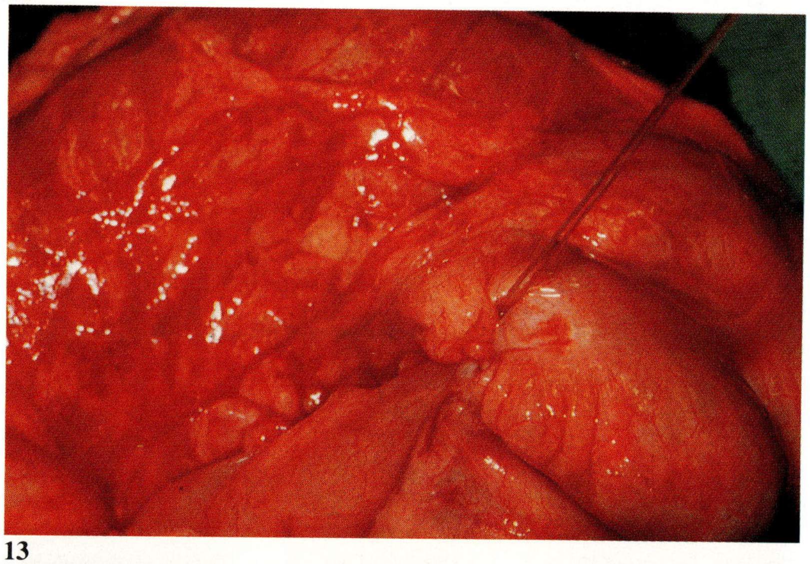

13

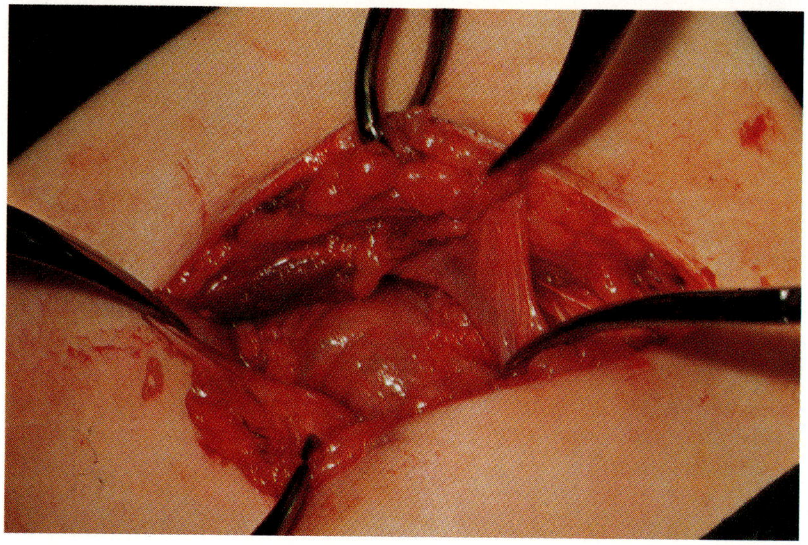

10 A purse string suture of 2/0 chromic catgut is inserted into the caecum encircling the base of the appendix about a half to three-quarters of an inch from its base.

11 The appendix has been divided and is now being invaginated through the catgut purse-string.

12 The purse string suture is tied securely. It is wise if there is not too much inflammation to look at the last 2-3 feet of the small bowel to exclude a Meckel's diverticulum. If it is long and narrow a wedge excision of it may be done. If wide and short, its presence should be stated in the operation notes. **Much depends on the amount of inflammation in the appendix and the possible hazards of extending the operation.**

13 Closure of peritoneum is simply effected by a 2/0 catgut suture, again avoid picking up the bowel in the stitch.

14

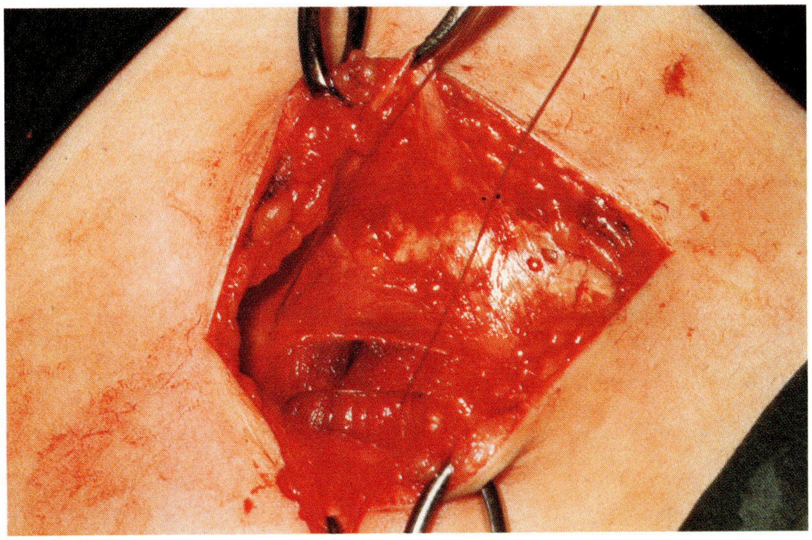

15

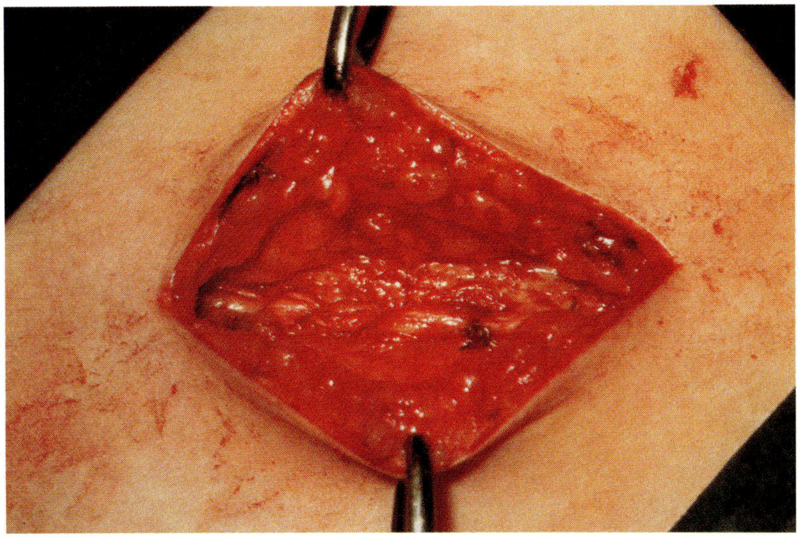

16

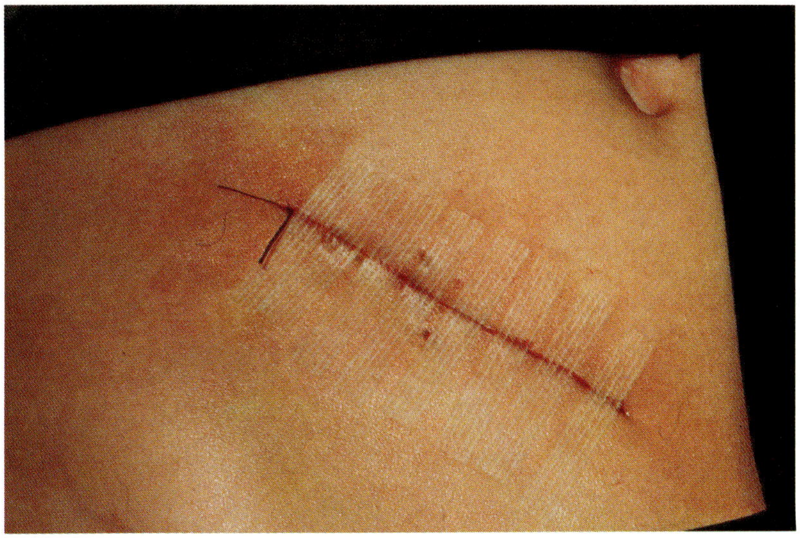

14 The transverse and internal oblique muscles are brought together loosely with interrupted catgut sutures.

15 The external oblique layer is closed with running catgut stitch.

16 The skin may be sutured with continuous or interrupted Prolene or, as here, a subcutaneous Vicril suture with steristrips to reinforce it and close the skin neatly.

If there is marked inflammation and possible or actual soilage, it is reasonable to close the peritoneum and muscle and leave the wound open with a pack and re-suture later.

Fistula-in-ano

This usually follows an abscess in the ischiorectal area which has burst into the rectum and outwards to the skin. The fistulae may be high level, i.e. inner opening above the anorectal ring. This is the rare type and difficult to manage. The other type is the common one described here, the low level, i.e. the inner opening is below the rectal ring.

1

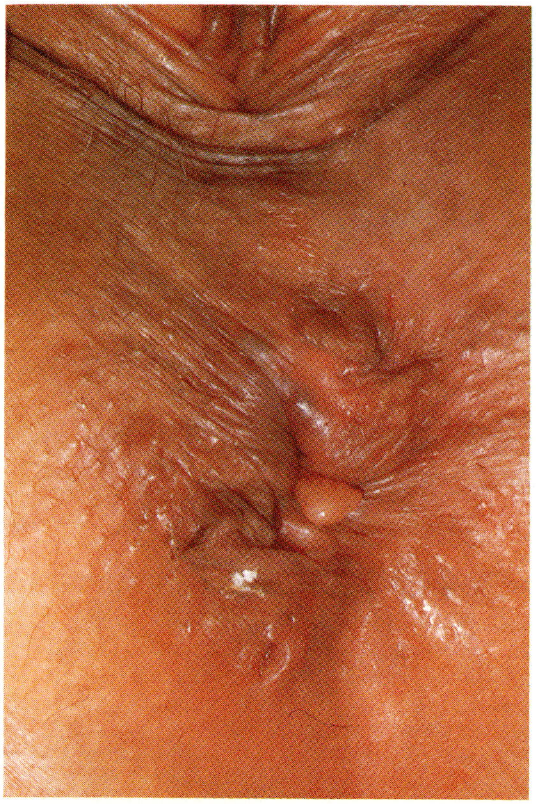

1 The outer opening is just visible at 7 o'clock as an individual oval area.

2

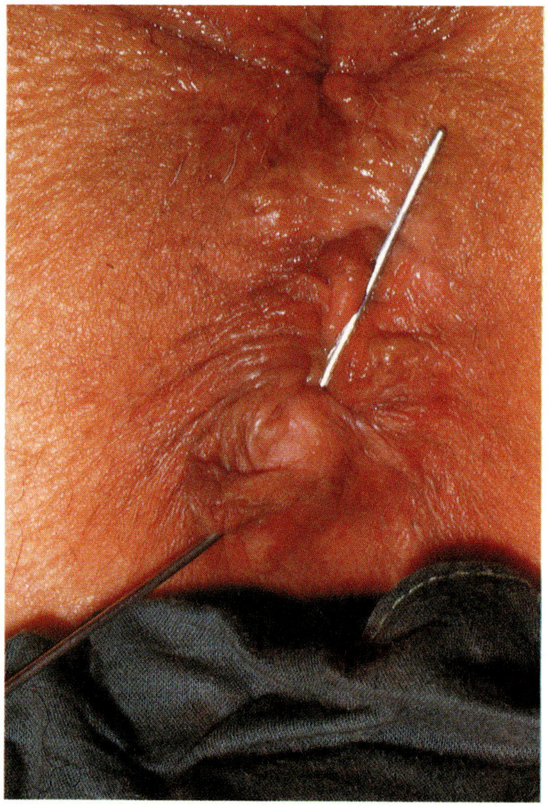

2 A probe is inserted through it and appears through the anal canal. If the probe transverses the sphincter mechanism, then senior opinion should be sought at once.

3

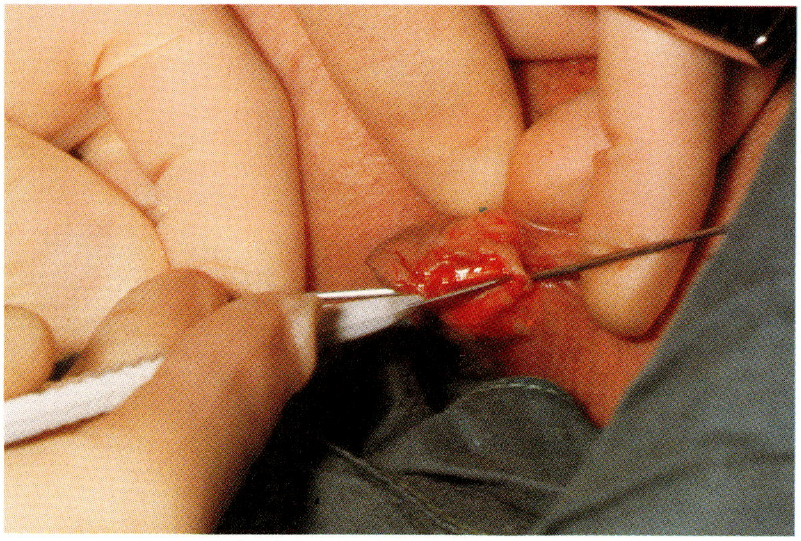

3 The canal outlined by the probe is cut open.

4

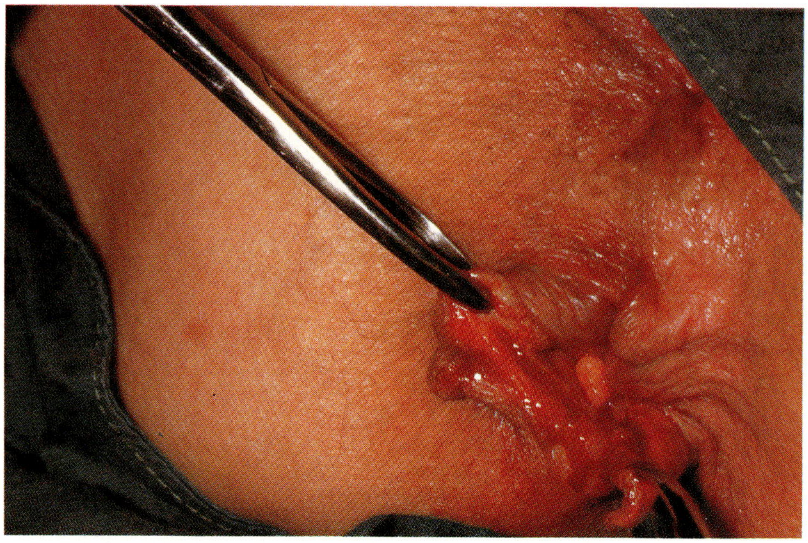

4 The area of the opened fistula is demonstrated.

Haemorrhoidectomy

There are numerous ways of dealing with haemorrhoids: injection, rubber bands, cryotherapy, etc. It is important before resorting to surgery to make sure that the patient has had proper dietary advice and is taking a high-fibre diet, and to make sure that there is no lesion higher up. The patient over the age of 40 years with *recent* haemorrhoids should have haemorrhoidectomy only after previous large bowel investigation, such as a double contrast barium enema and/or colonoscopy.

1

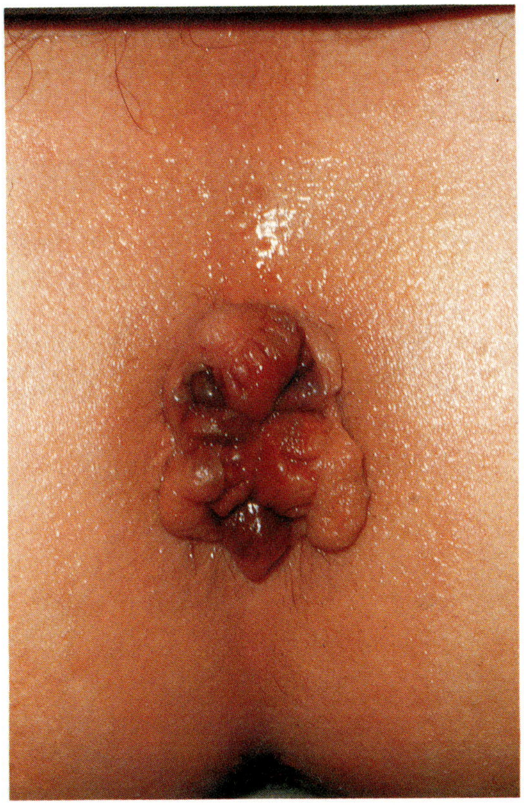

1 Patient is in lithotomy with prominent piles. The patient may be in lithotomy position which I prefer or may be done on his side or in the jack-knife position. General anaesthesia or spinal anaesthetic is satisfactory.

2

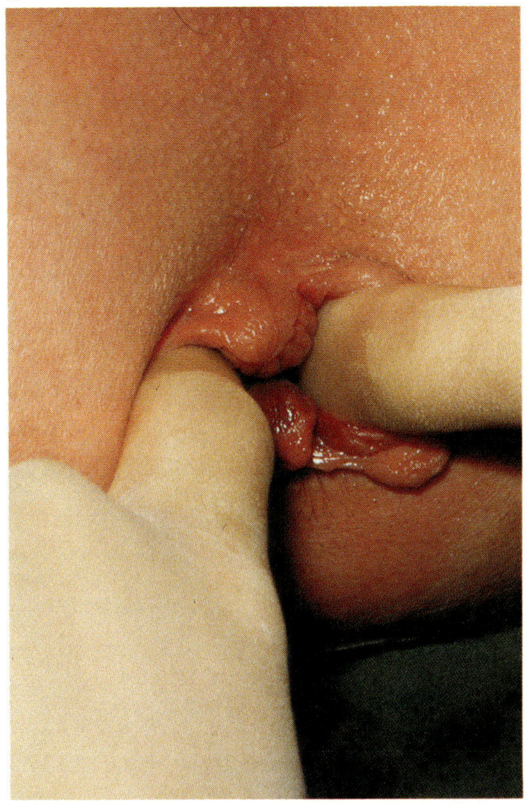

2 The anus is gradually dilated to stretch the sphincter. This makes operation easier and when fully dilated lessens incidence of postoperative anal spasm.

3

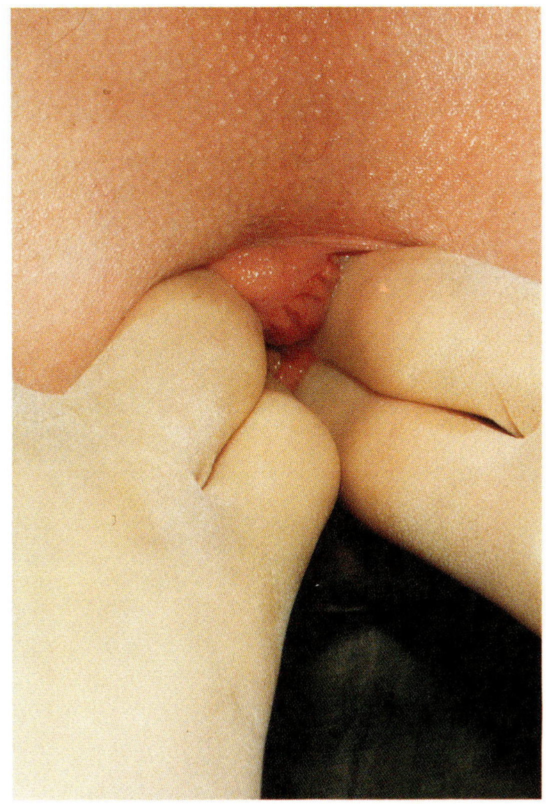

3 Further dilation to four fingers.

4

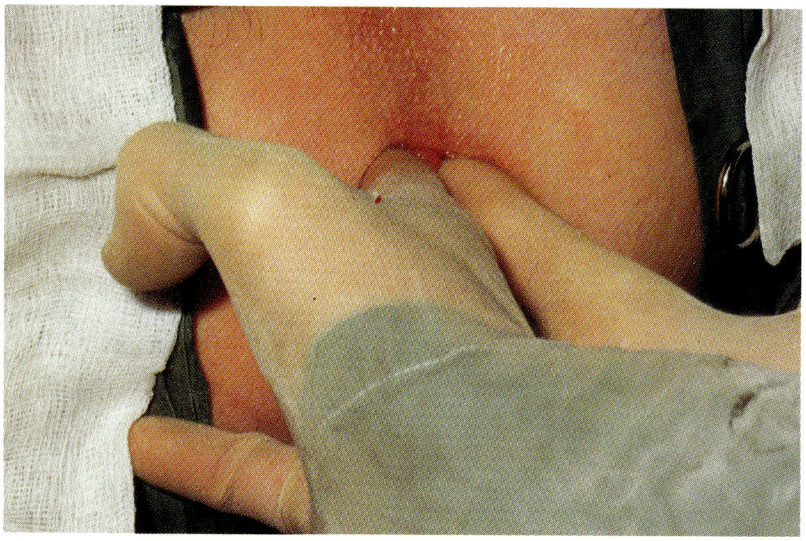

4 Full dilation accomplished.

5

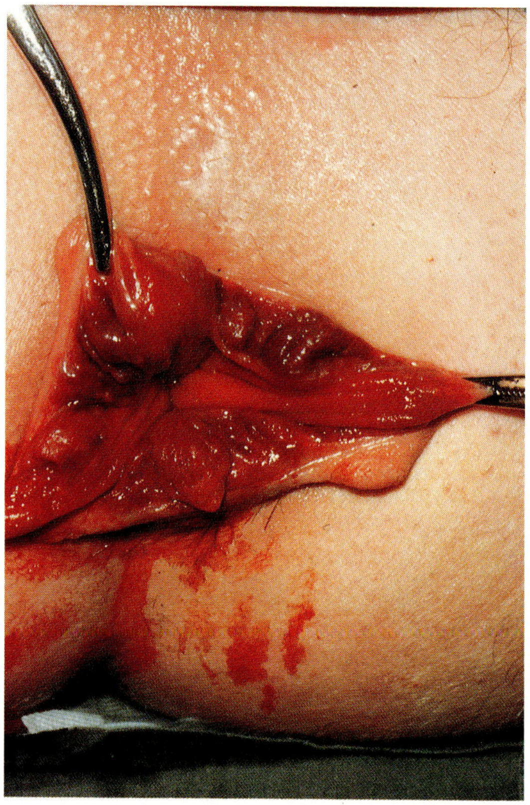

6

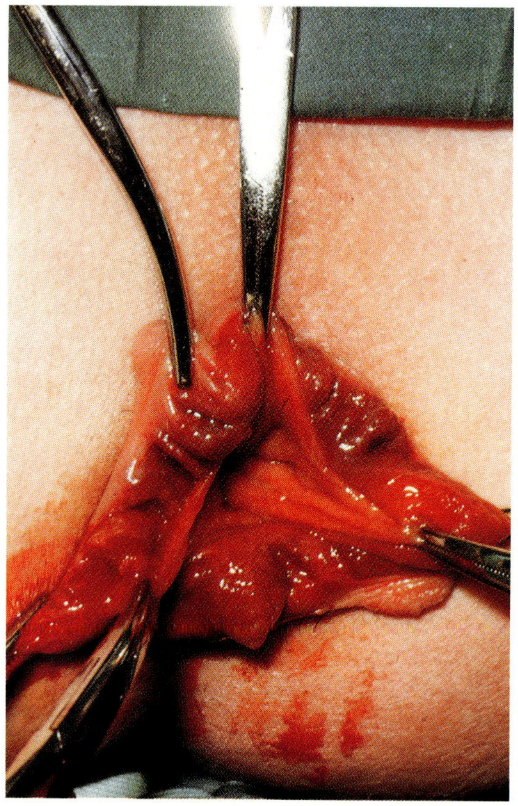

7

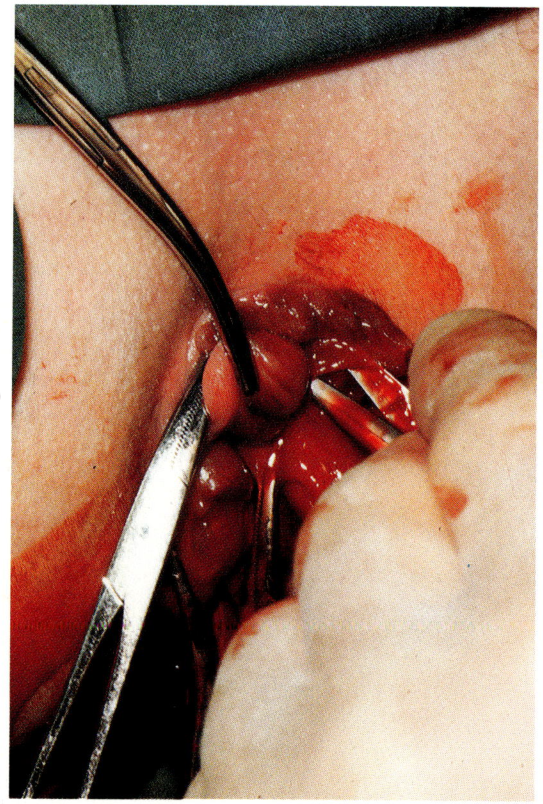

5 Forceps grasp the main haemorrhoids of 3, 7 and 11 o'clock. Secondary haemorrhoids are visible between these.

6 Further forceps grasp the haemorrhoids at the upper border of the pile and this makes prominent the junction between haemorrhoid and anal skin and normal rectal mucosa.

7 With tension on the inner forcep the junction between haemorrhoid and anal skin is incised with scissors and a submucosal resection is begun. Normally one starts at the 3 o'clock haemorrhoid then 7 o'clock and finally 11 o'clock to prevent the blood dripping down from the upper area and obscuring the lower field. Dissection can be facilitated by injecting 3 ml of 1 per cent lignocaine – adrenalin 1:200,000 solution subcutaneously at each of the three primary pile sites.

8

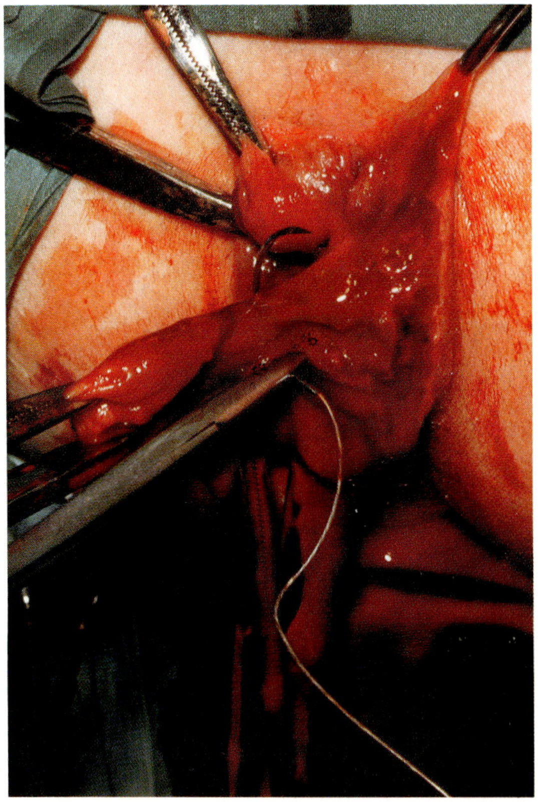

9

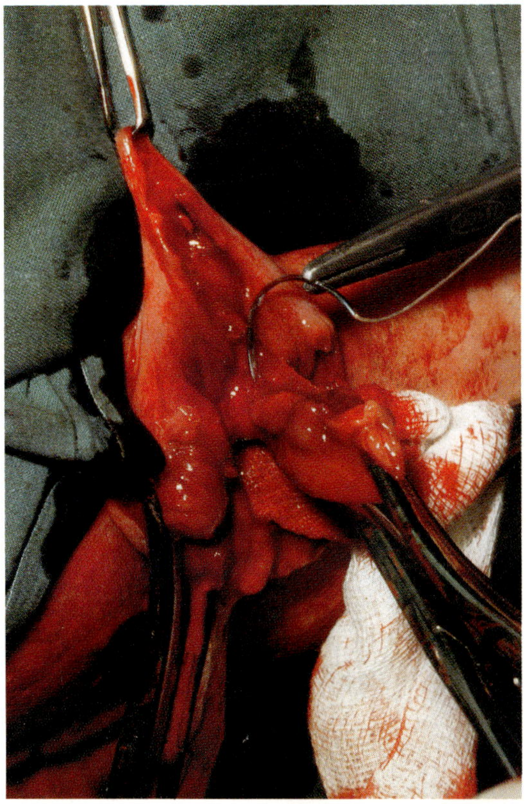

10

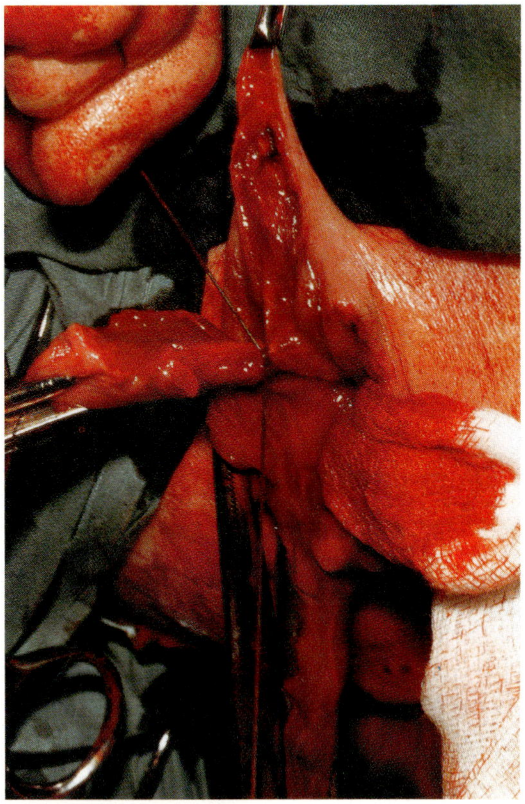

11

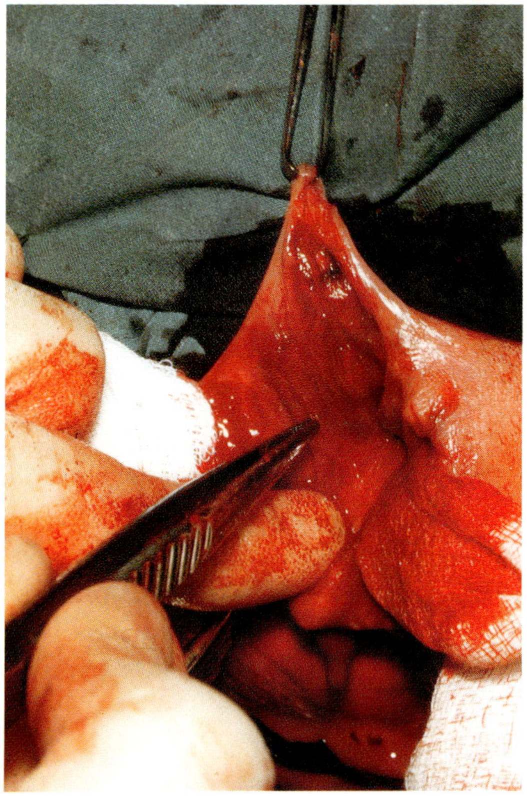

8 The right lateral or 3 o'clock haemorrhoid has been fully dissected and clamped; a catgut stitch is inserted through the base and tied. The haemorrhoid is then cut off.

9 The 11 o'clock haemorrhoid is now dealt with similarly (out of the order suggested above).

10 The 7 o'clock haemorrhoid is now sutured and cut off distally.

11 The clean area after removal is visualised and all bleeding points have been ligated. It is important to leave bridges of normal skin and muscle between the operative areas to prevent stenosis.

12

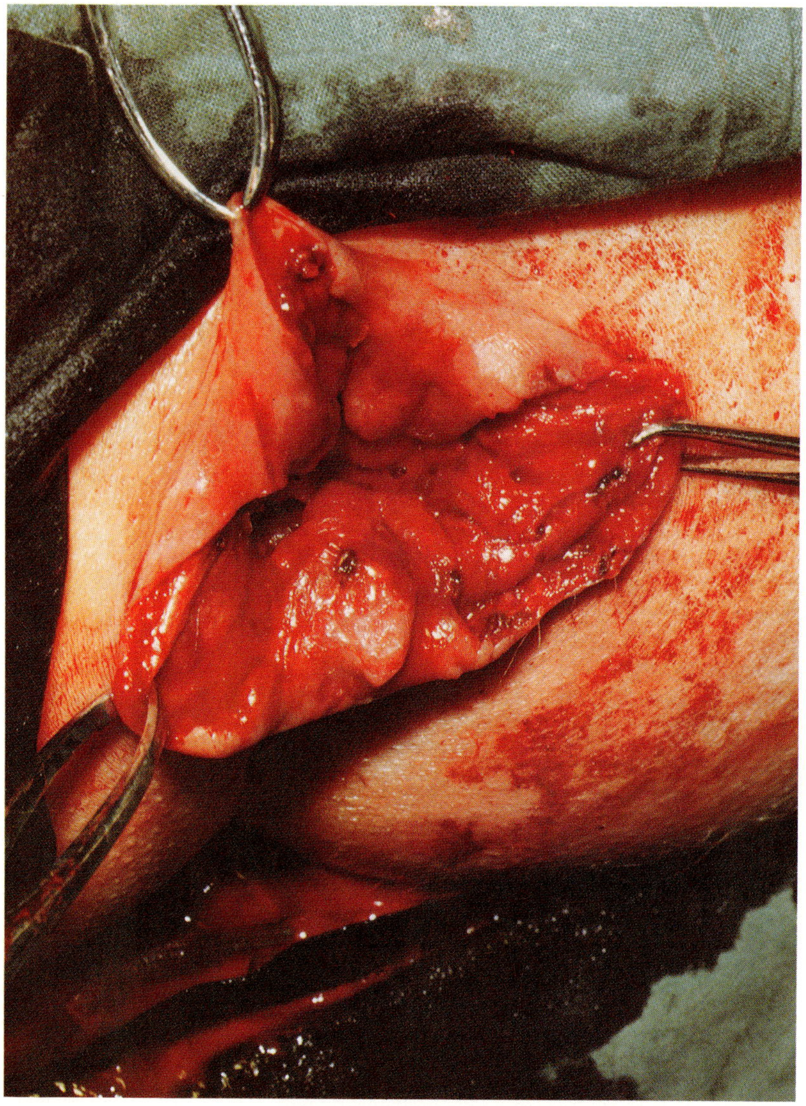

13

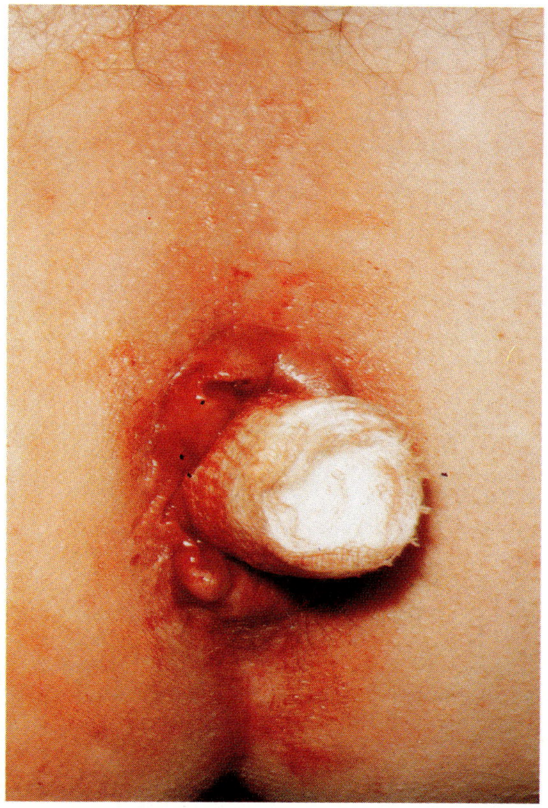

12 All three haemorrhoids have been excised and a relatively dry field is present. Note skin bridges between areas.

13 Some put a rolled piece of gauze into the anal canal as a tampon to reduce postoperative ooze. It should not be inserted far up the rectum and should be removed next day to limit anal spasm. I really prefer to tuck in the edge of 3 Vaseline gauze swabs which will come out easier in the bath next day.

Closure of a colostomy

Closure of a colostomy is a relatively simple procedure but failure to do it properly can result in peritonitis with death. The closure can be extraperitoneal, which avoids the risk of intraperitoneal leakage but may leave a hernia, or intraperitoneal, which prevents any stenosis at the area of closure but has risks of leakage. This risk can be avoided by proper preparation of the bowel prior to closure, i.e. low residue diet, enemas and by a meticulous suture technique.

1

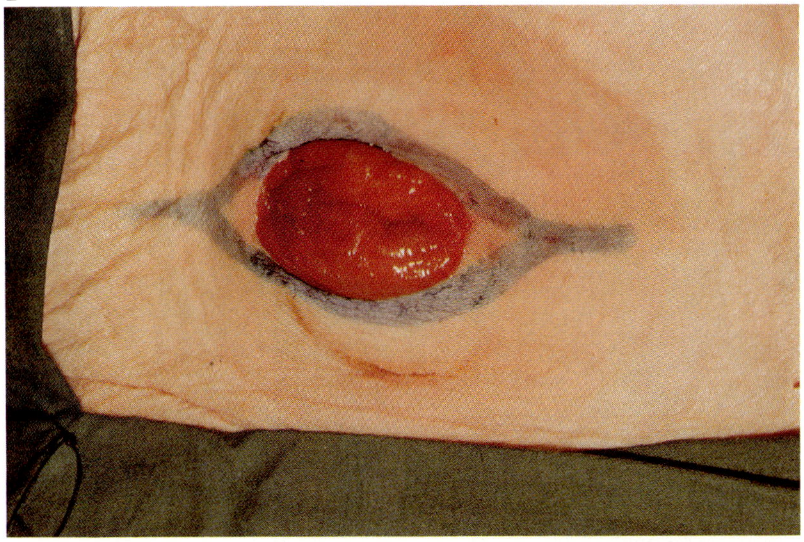

1 The skin incision round the opening of this transverse colostomy is outlined.

2

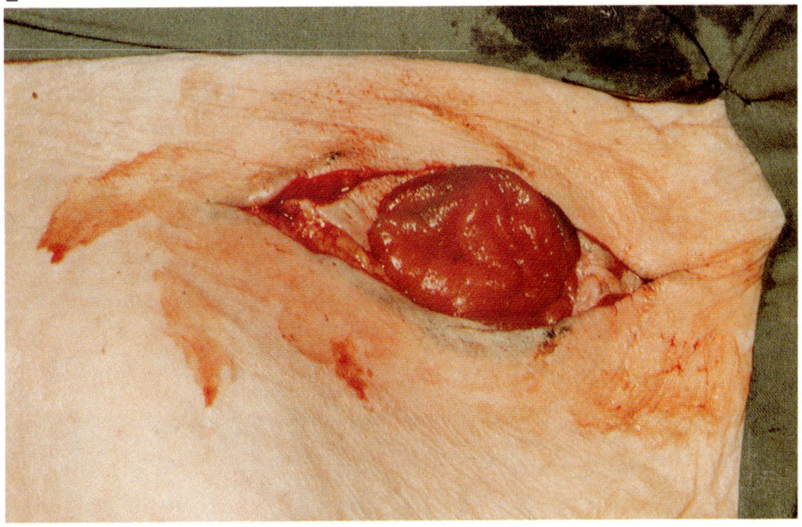

2 The skin incision is deepened leaving some skin attached all round the mucosa.

3

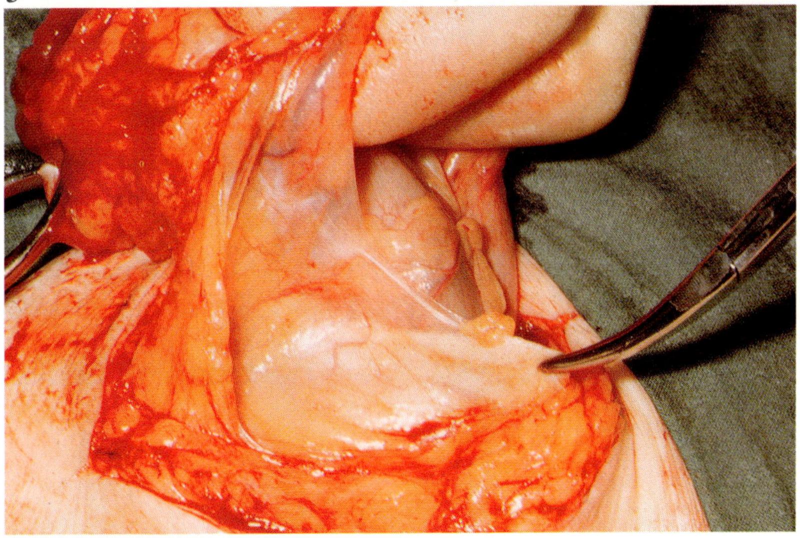

3 The peritoneum is opened up and the bowel isolated by division of adhesions.

4

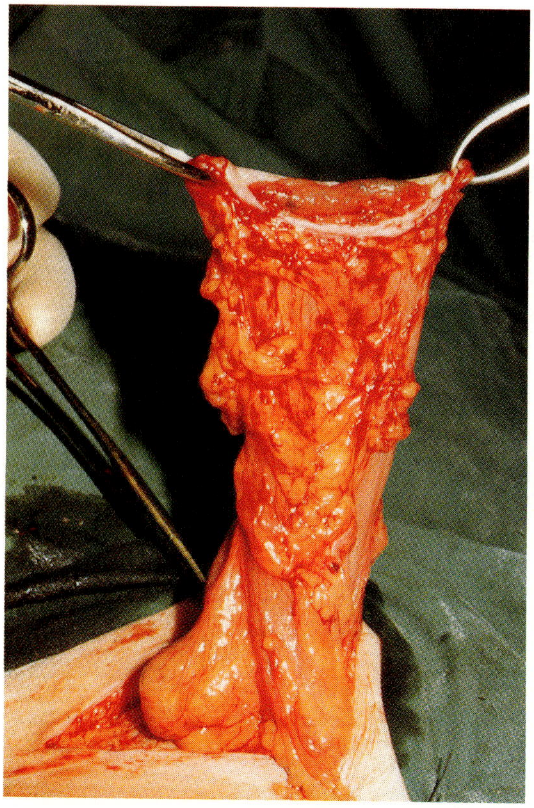

4 The bowel is held up ready to excise the skin attached to the mucosa and invaginate this.

5

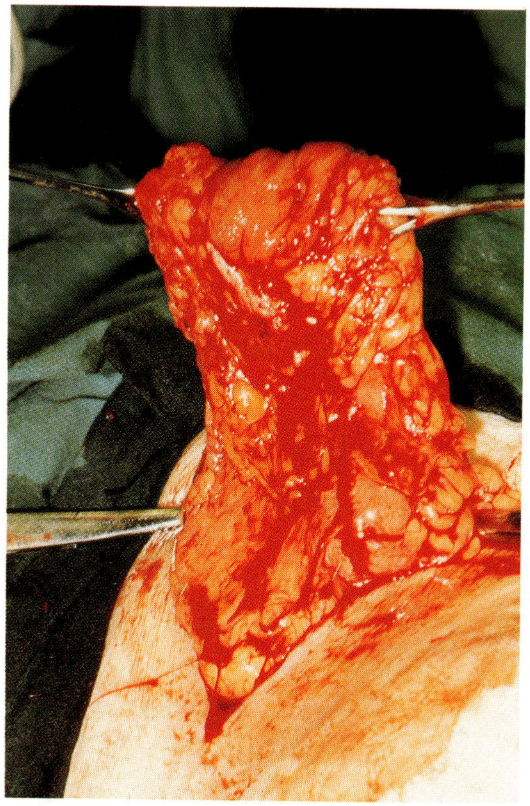

5 The skin has been dissected off. There is always some bleeding from the margin of the bowel when some fibrotic mucosa is also removed. The bleeding is easily stopped.

6

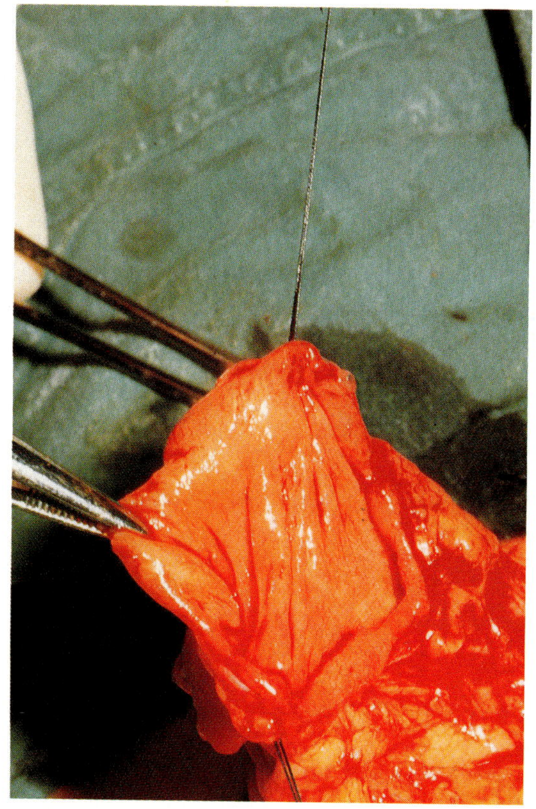

6 The bowel is closed in one layer or two, the latter being safer but should not produce narrowing. The mucosal layer was closed with continuous catgut.

7

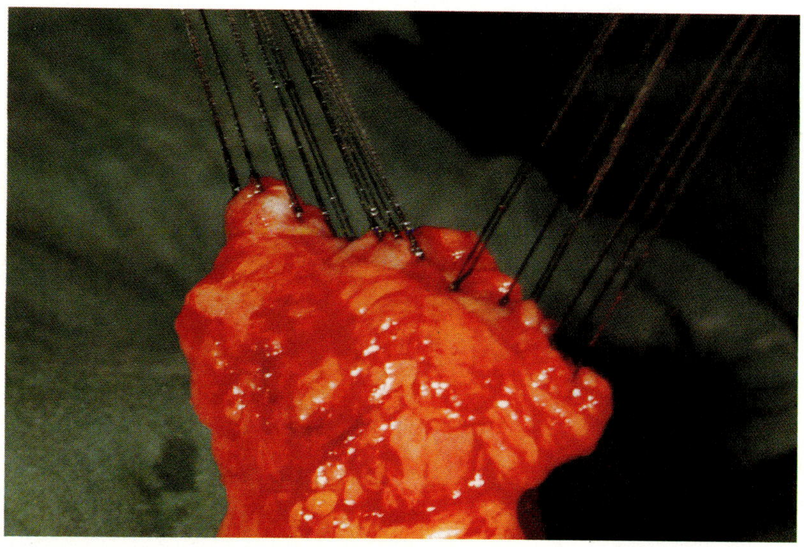

7 The seromuscular layer was closed with Neuralon.

8

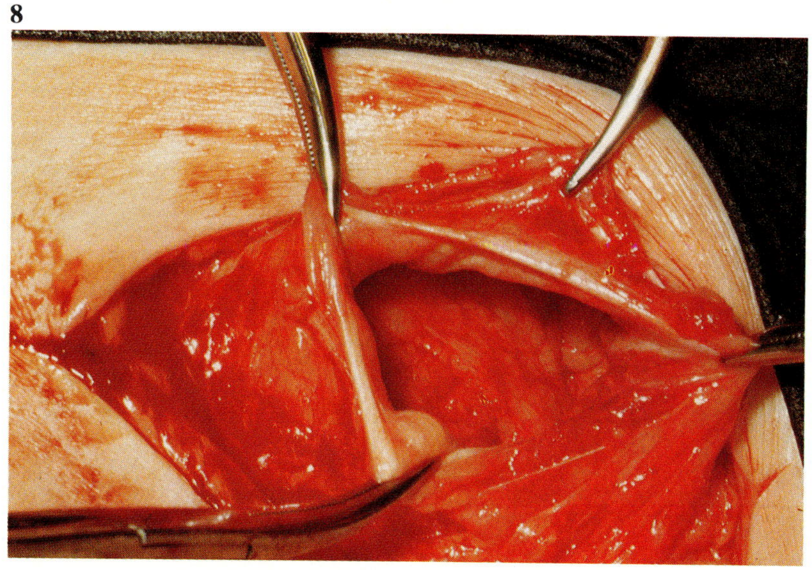

8 The bowel is placed back in the abdomen and the peritoneum is closed with catgut and the muscle with Prolene.

9 The skin is closed with Prolene leaving a drain in the subcutaneous tissues. Anal dilatation may be done at the end of the procedure, especially if a sigmoid colostomy is closed. It is thought to lessen pressure in the distal bowel.

9

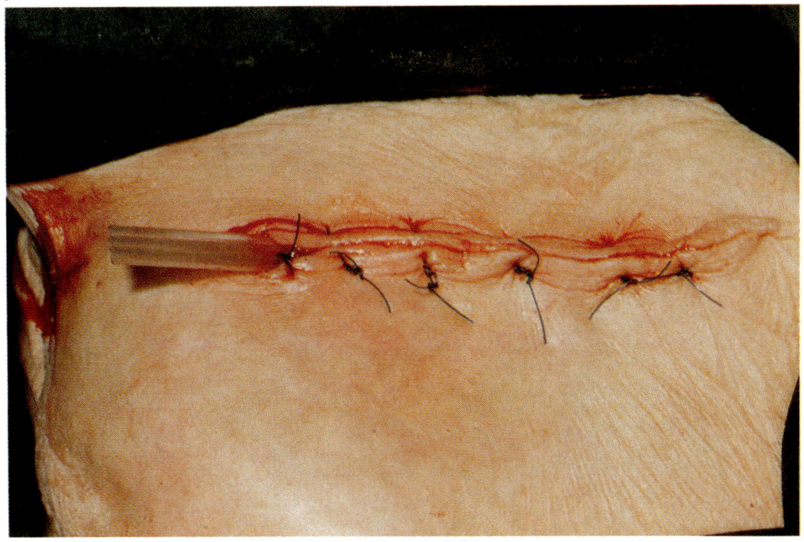

Pilonidal sinus

Pilonidal sinus is most common in the natal cleft, especially in black-haired hirsute men. The black hair is coarser and harder than the others and tends to penetrate the skin more easily.

1

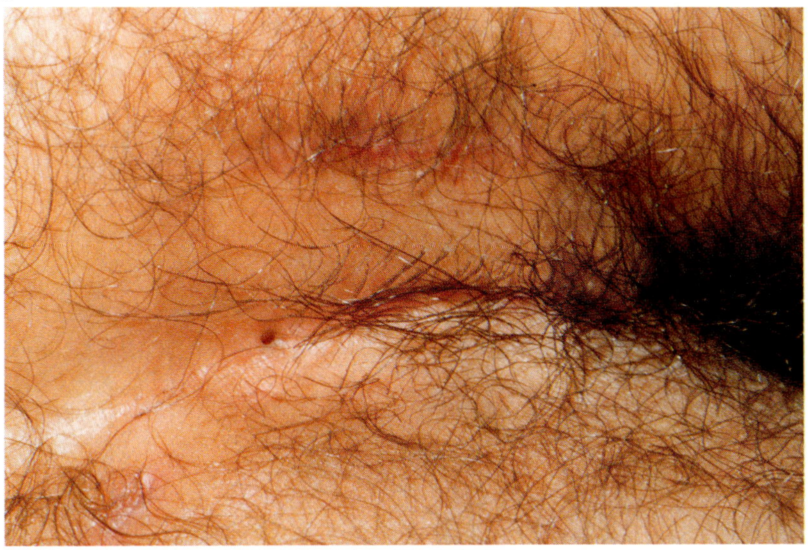

1 The sinus is apparent in the midline. Above is the scar of an incision of a previous abscess and in the lower left part of the picture is a further scar. There is a good appearance of the bending back of the black hair.

2

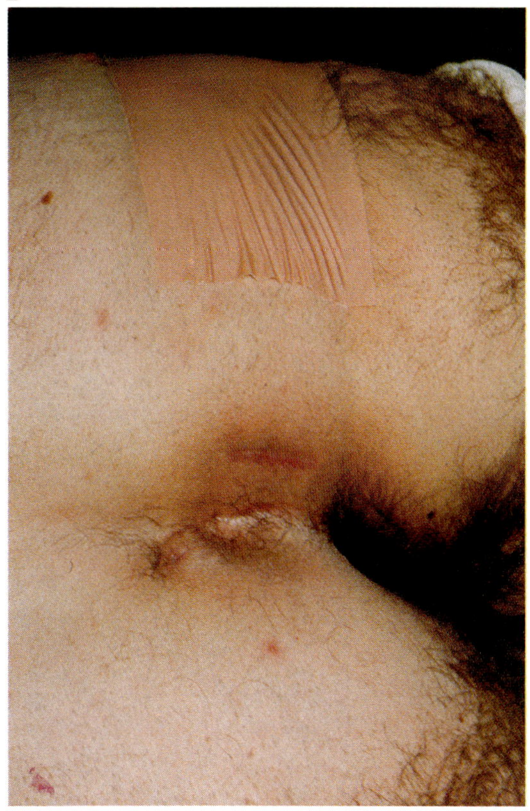

2 After shaving the skin for operation the scars are more visible. Note retraction of the left buttock by elastic adhesive opens up the area for excision.

3

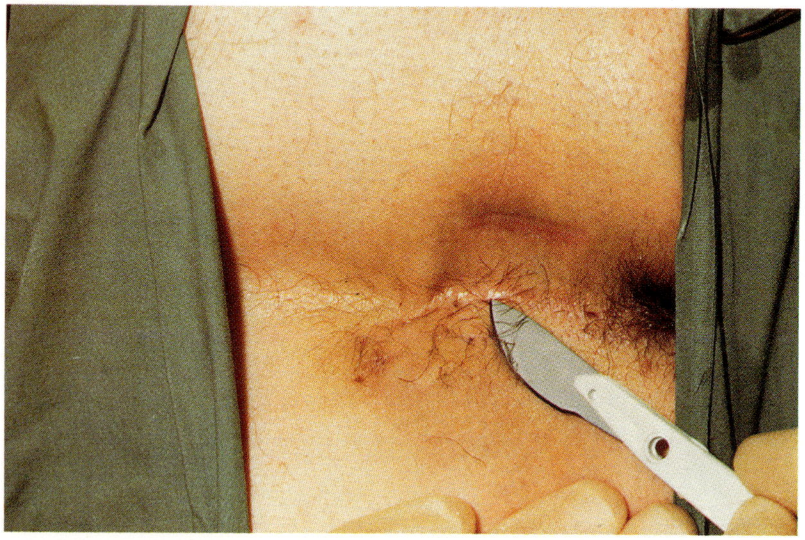

3 The remaining hairs are carefully excised by scalpel.

4

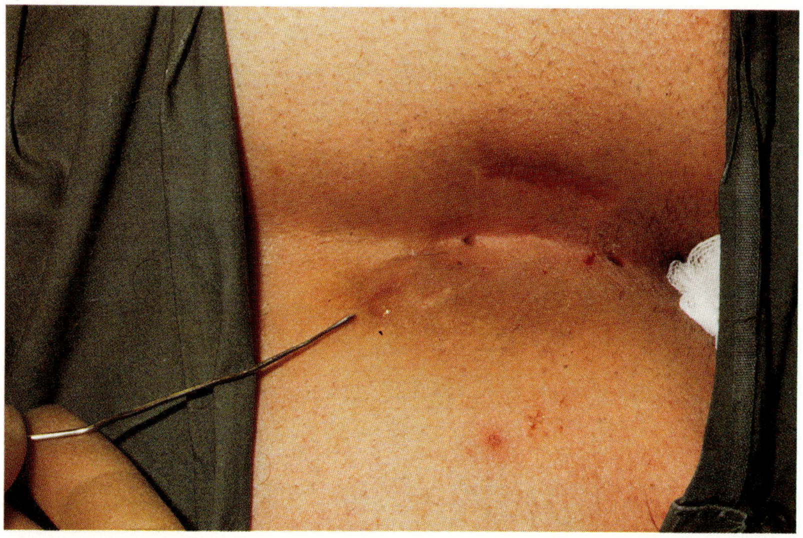

4 The sinuses are probed to get some idea of their extension and the amount of excision required.

5

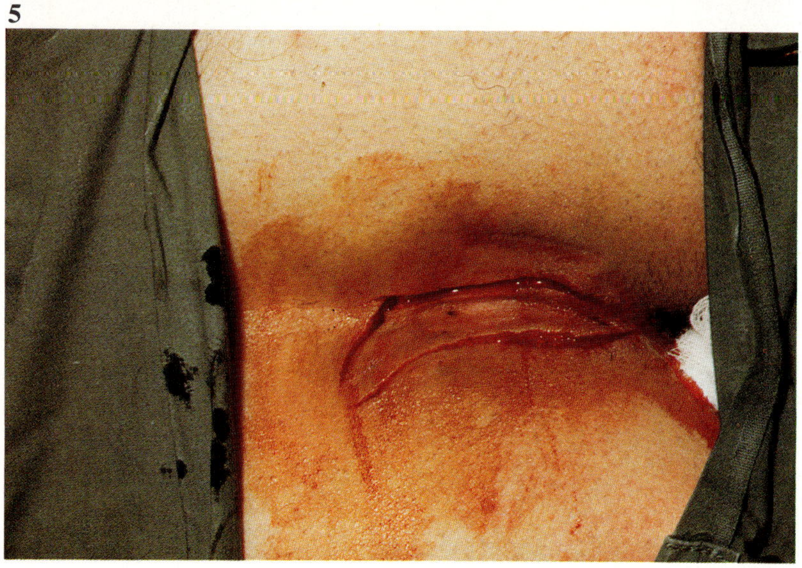

5 The area for excision is now determined.

6 On deepening the incision a buried hair is seen in the lower wound.

6

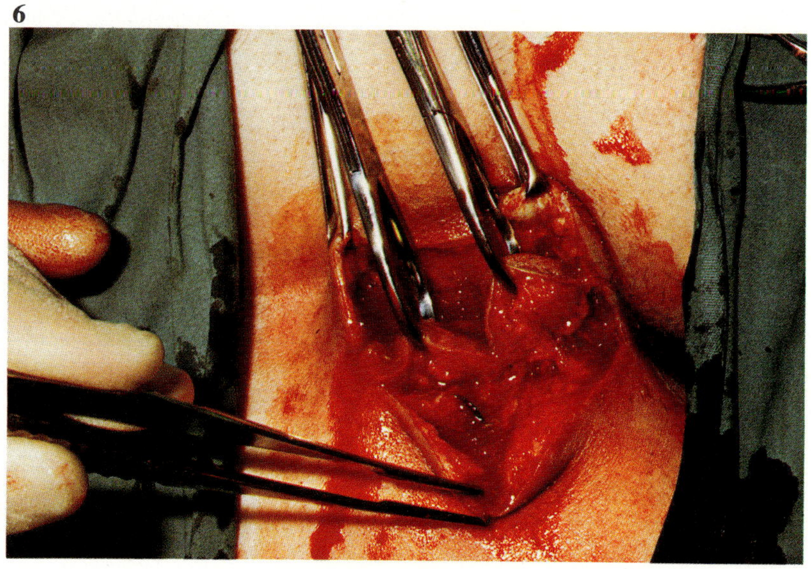

7 The upper wound is deepened down to sacral fascia.

7

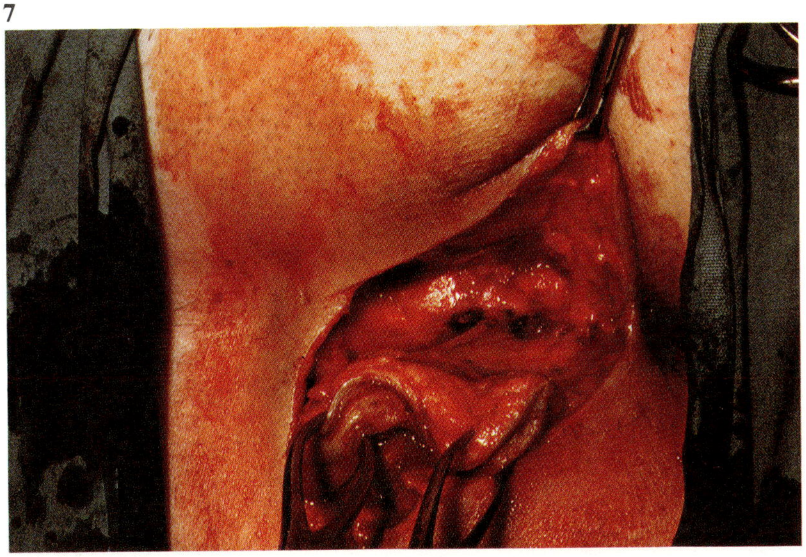

8 The lower wound encircles the remains of the previous abscess, now fibrotic.

8

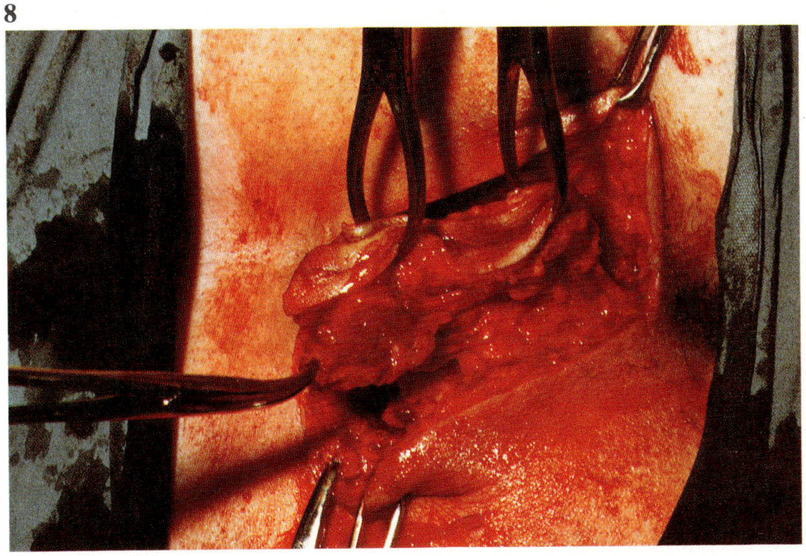

9 Total excision is now complete and bleeding areas sealed by diathermy.

10 The excised tissue is shown with the buried hair, which was crunched up in a 'nest'.

9

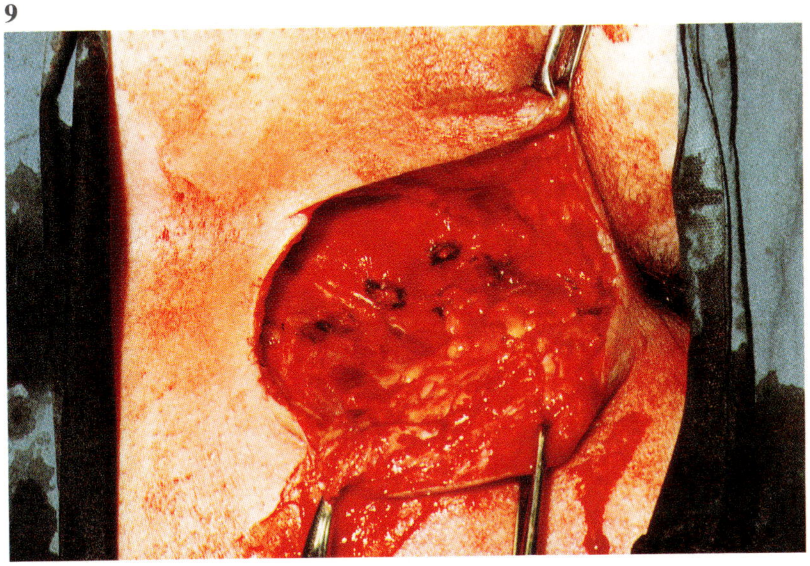

10

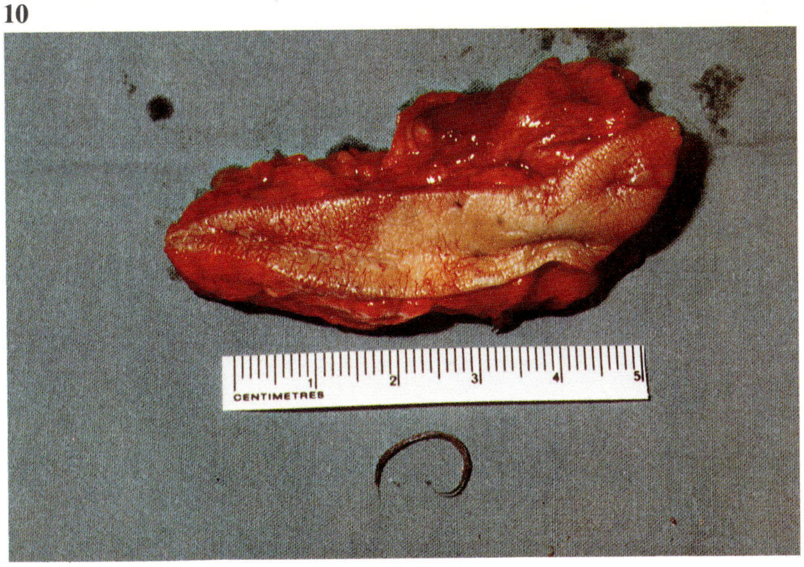

11

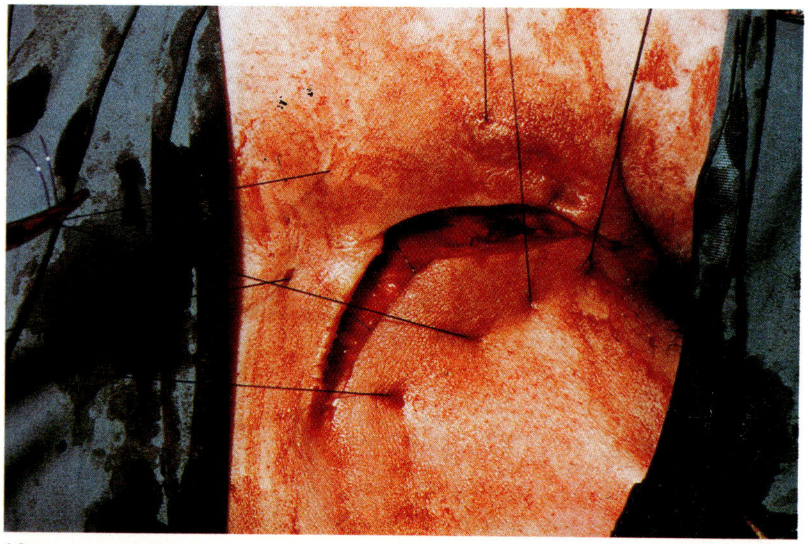

11 The problems of closure may vary depending on the loss of tissue and the need to avoid tension and dead space. In this case four sutures are shown which pass through skin, deep fascia and out through skin. These are left long.

12

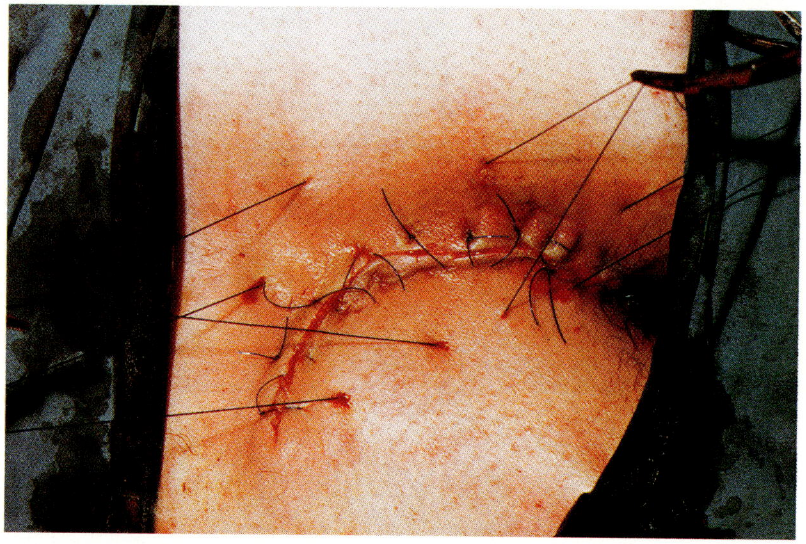

12 Interrupted mattress sutures close the skin securely.

13

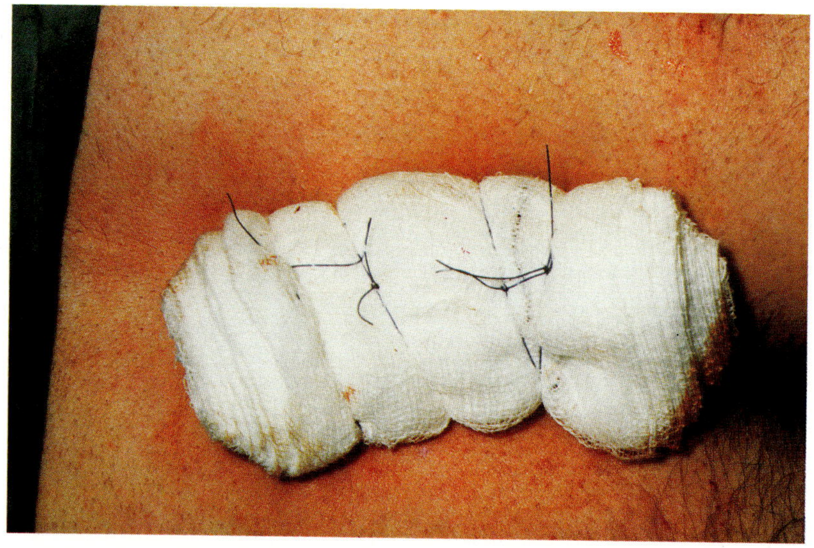

13 The long sutures are tied over a gauze pack to obliterate by pressure the dead space. This is then covered with Sleek to isolate it from the anus.

Varicose veins

The operation of Trendelenburg [sapheno-femoral ligation] with multiple ligations will be described. **Warning must be given and emphasised of the danger of damage to the femoral vein and artery leading to legal problems.** This applies also to the saphenous nerve at the medial side of the knee joint and the sural nerves in the lower limb.

1

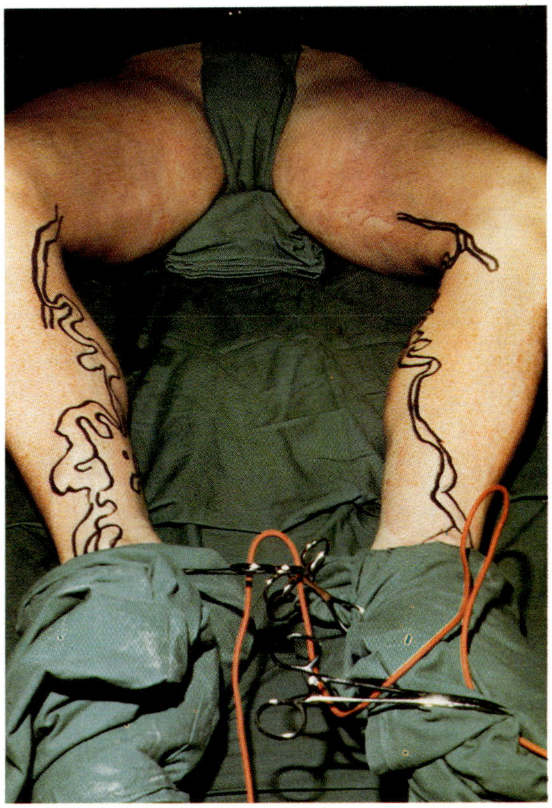

1 The prominent veins should be marked out before the appearance in theatre with the patient standing.

2 The position of the femoral artery is noted by feeling the pulsation.

3 The incision is made in the skin-crease just medial to this for about three inches.

2

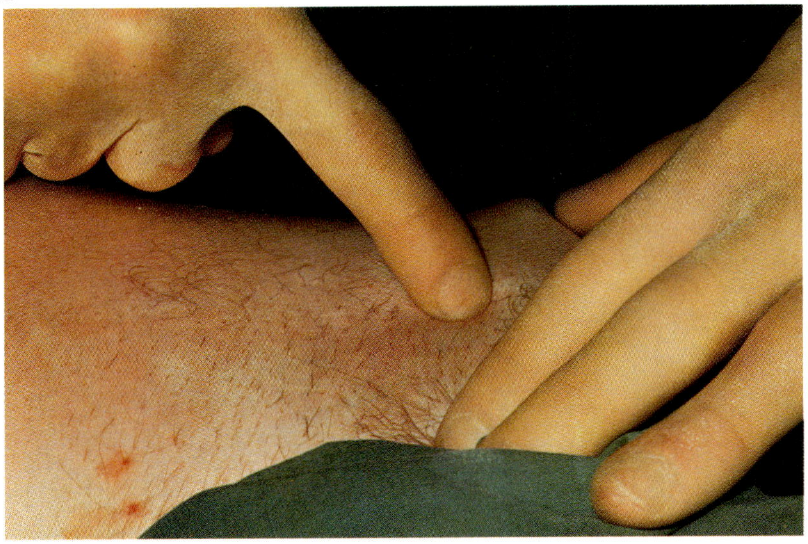

3

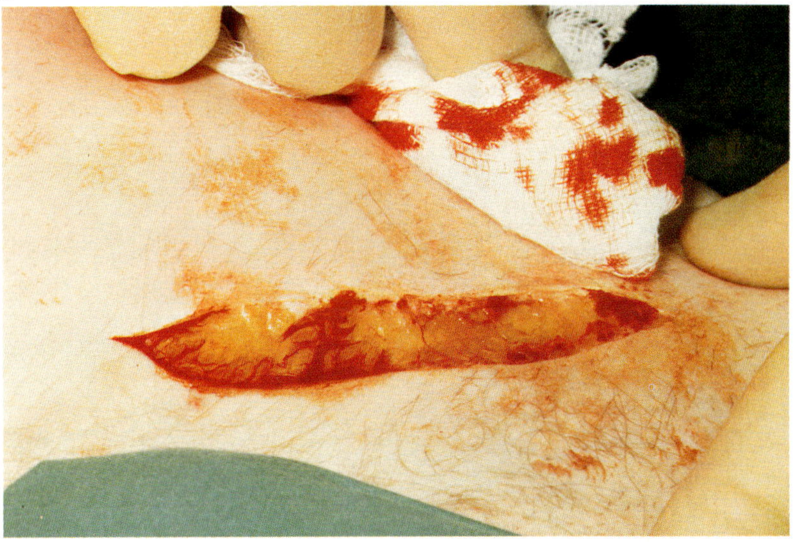

4

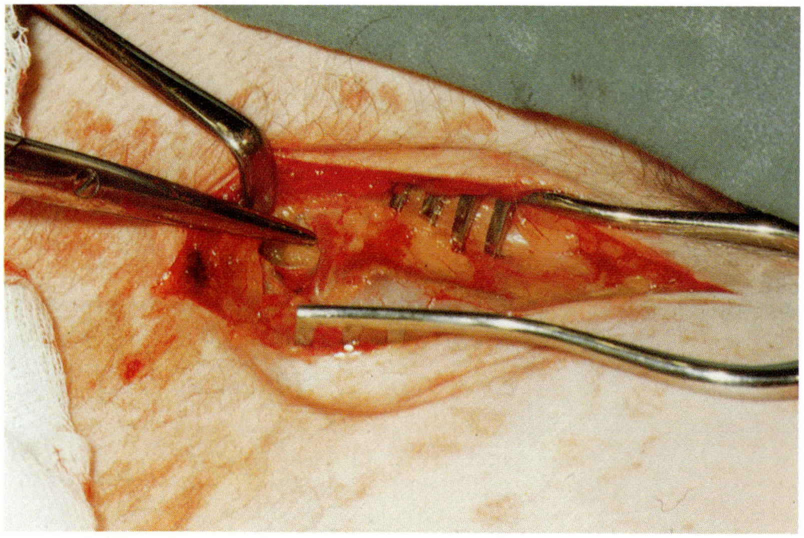

5

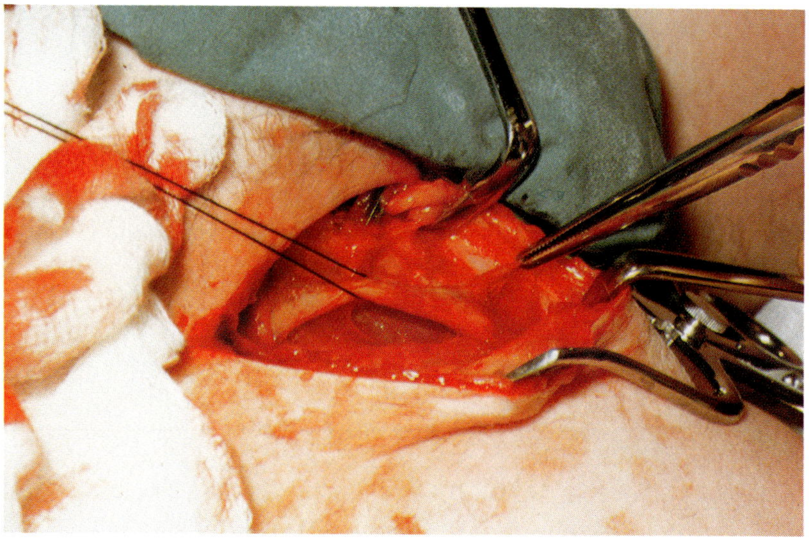

6

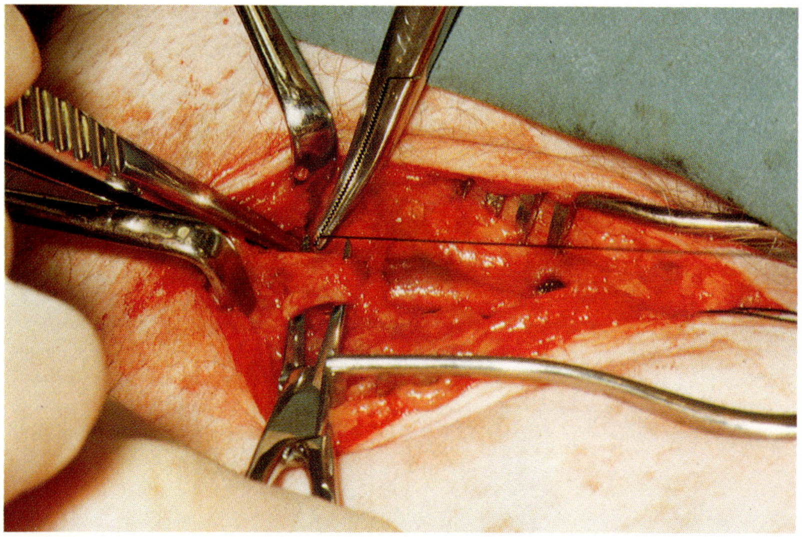

7

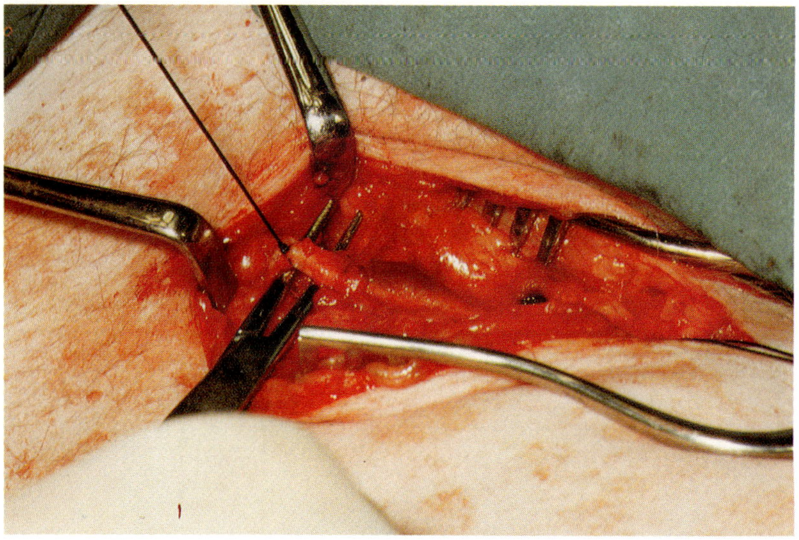

4 Dissection through the fat will reveal the long saphenous veins [L.S.V.] and a small artery may be seen crossing the vein towards the scrotum. This may be tied or carefully isolated.

5 The L.S.V. is encircled with a silk ligature and held up. Dissection is begun of the small veins, usually three of them, which are tributaries of the upper end of the L.S.V.

6 Two of these small veins are seen joining together before they enter the L.S.V. The common trunk of these two veins can then be ligated or, if desired, each ligated separately.

7 A further ligature is placed round the common trunk which is then divided.

8

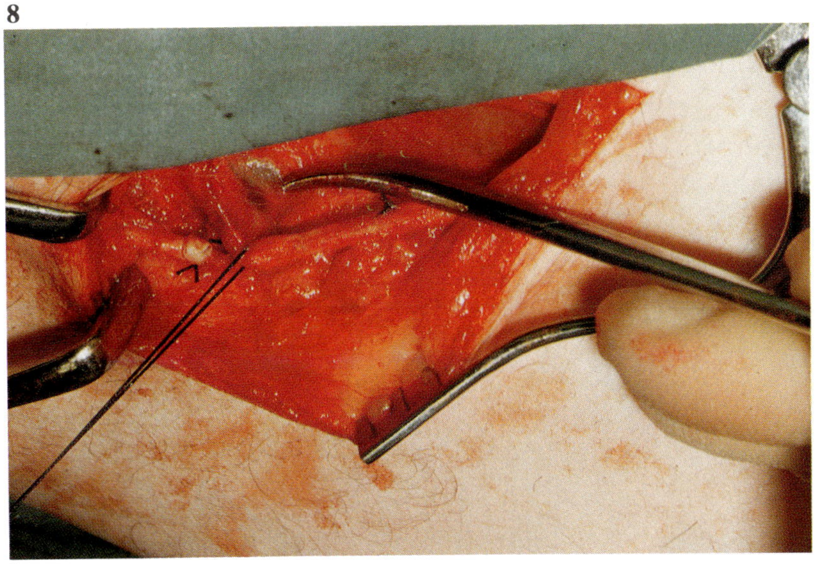

9

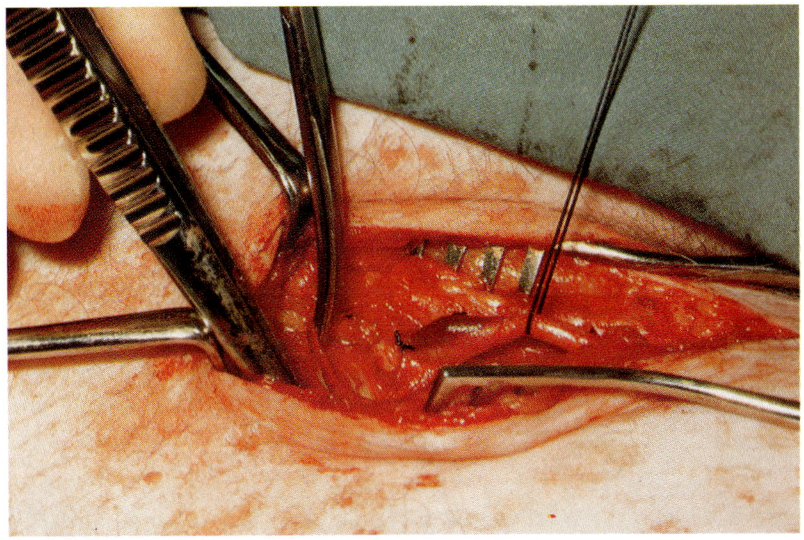

10

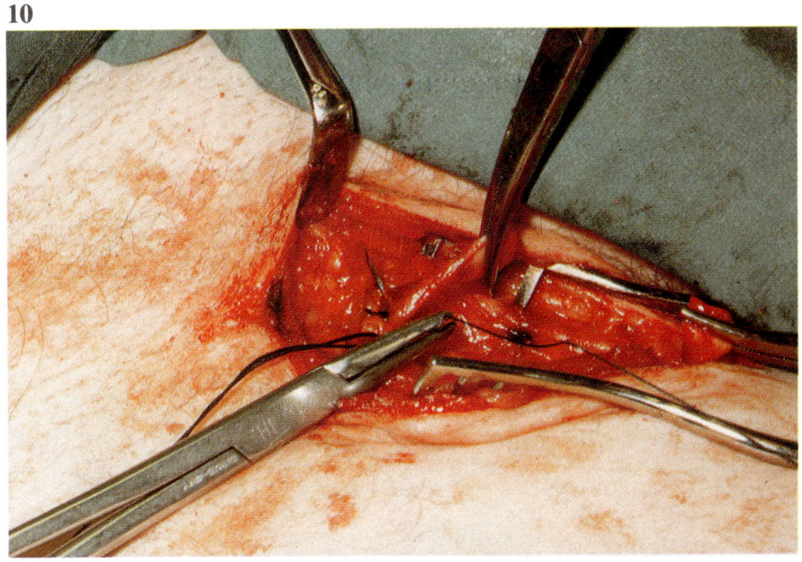

11

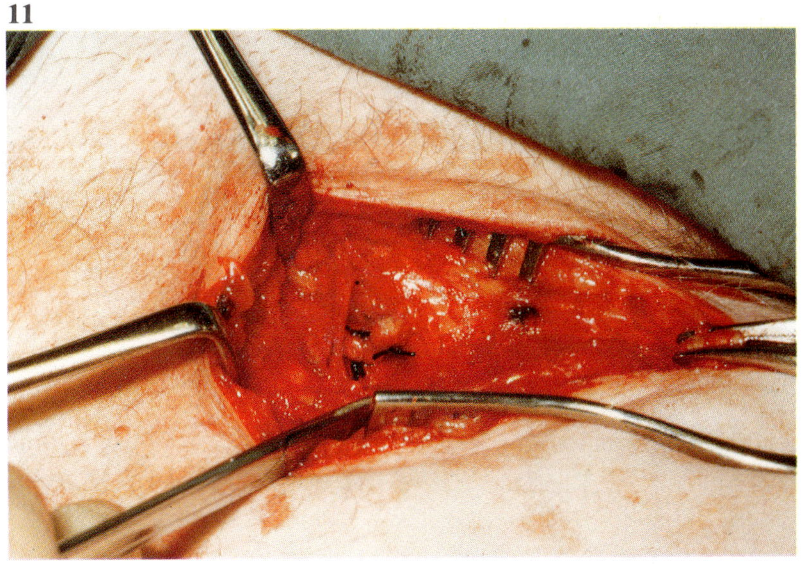

8 The third vein, superficial external pudendal, is then sought and tied.

9 The L.S.V. is now held up and the upper end is being dissected down towards its junction with the femoral vein. It is here that the danger lies and great care must be exercised in the dissection and minimal pulling of the L.S.V.

10 The L.S.V. is divided and a suture ligation made near its junction with the femoral vein. Alternatively ligation itself may be done without suture. A descending vein may be seen coming off just below the junction of the saphenous vein with the common femoral vein. The branch, if left, may lead to recurrence of varicose veins.

11 The end result is shown. The high tie ensures that no veins are left to pass down the leg and prevent further recurrence.

12

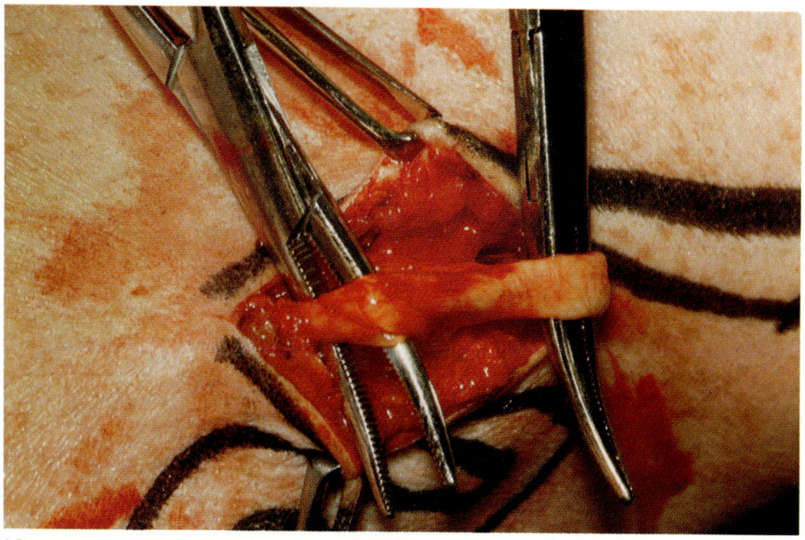

12 **Multiple incisions are made down the leg** and the veins dissected out, looking especially for veins perforating the fascia. The veins are tied.

13

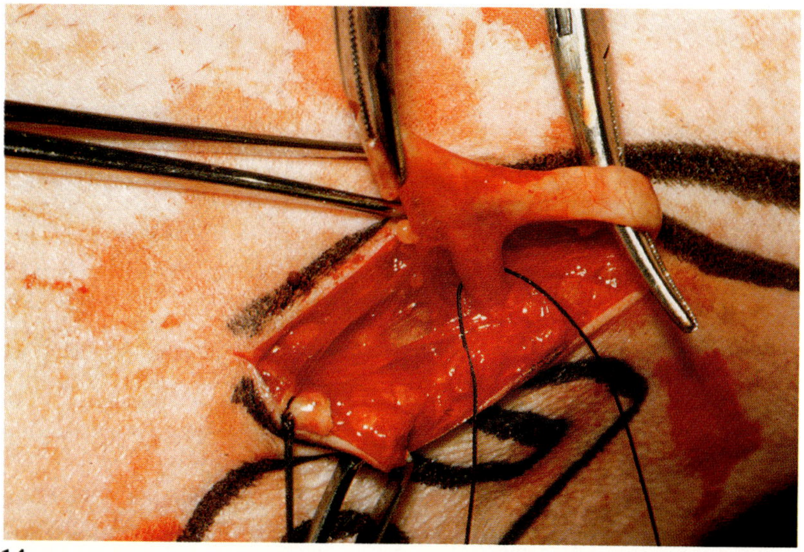

13 **A perforating vein is tied off.**

14

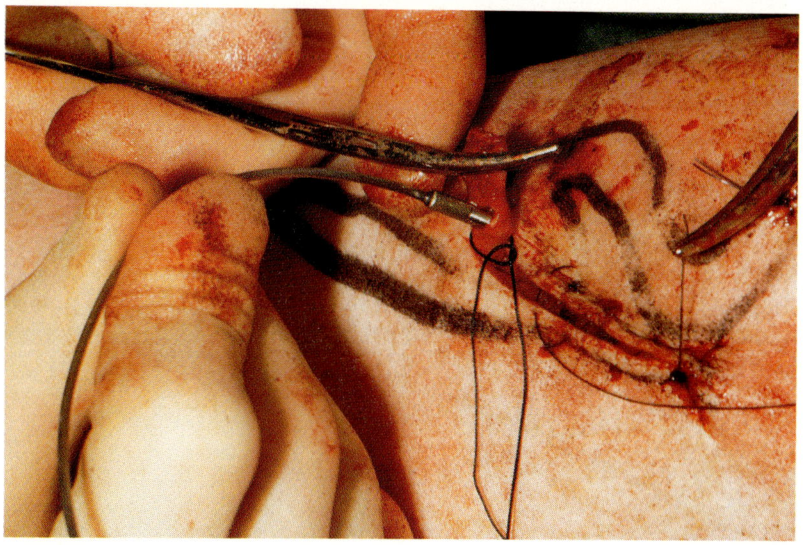

14 **The stripper is shown entering a vein.** Short lengths of veins may be stripped in this fashion. **Stripping of the whole length of the L.S.V. is not popular now as it may damage the saphenous nerve.** Stripping is probably best done above the knee.

15 **The multiple excisions are shown at the end of the operation. A pressure bandage is applied.**

15

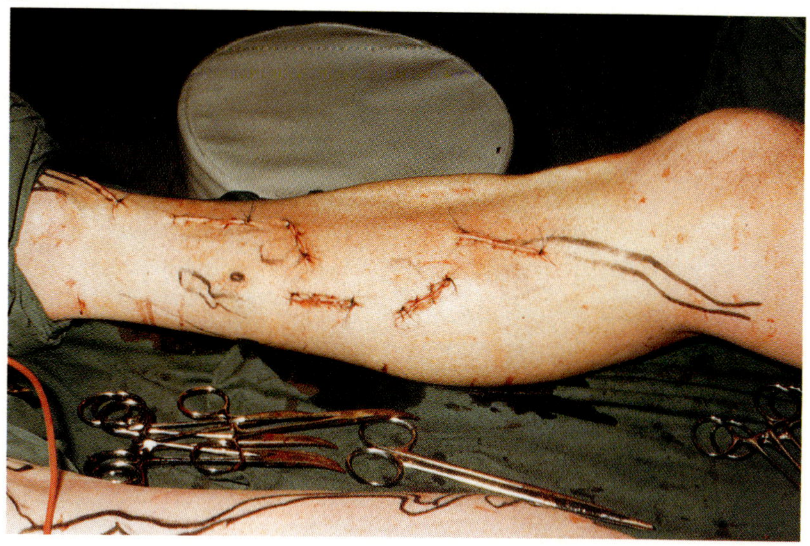

Aspiration of breast cyst

Classically, cysts of the breast occur in the last decade of reproductive life.

1

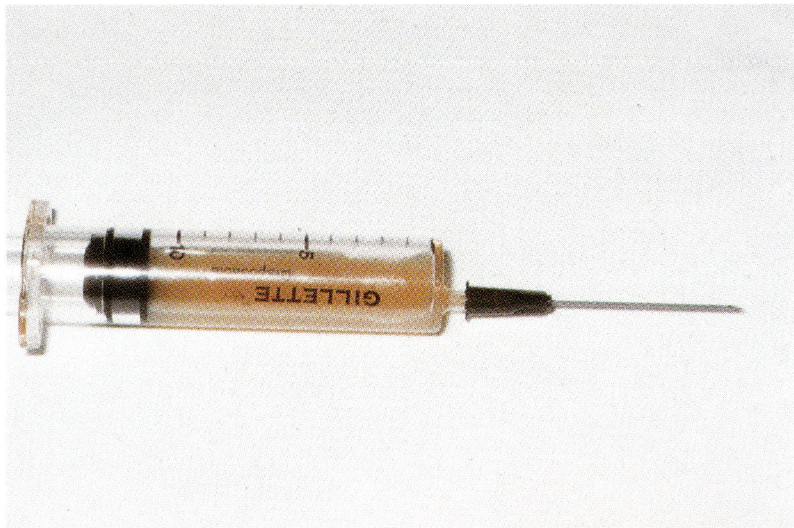

1 Aspiration using a 10 ml syringe and a 13 swg (green hub) needle immediately gives the diagnosis. As long as the aspirate is not blood-stained and there is no residual lump palpable, this is all the treatment necessary.

2

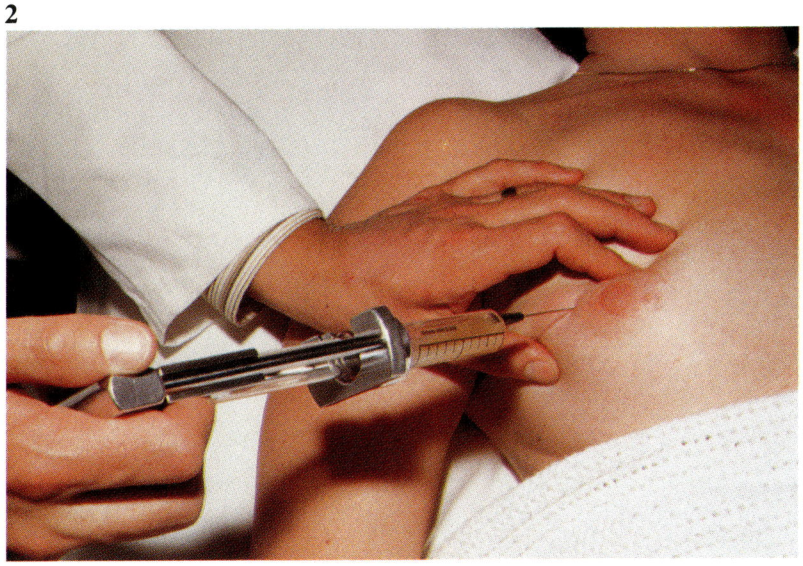

2 If the syringe is held in a holder, such as the one illustrated, one hand is released to steady the lump.

Fine needle aspiration of breast for cytology

1 Fine needle aspiration. It is not necessary to use local anaesthetic for this procedure. Such may even distort the microscopic appearances of the cells. This technique is greatly facilitated by having the 10 ml syringe in a holder. By holding the lesion with the hand so released, the surgeon can advance and withdraw the needle through the tissue, (called 'joggling') and shave off cells which are sucked into the needle by full withdrawal of the plunger of the syringe.

1

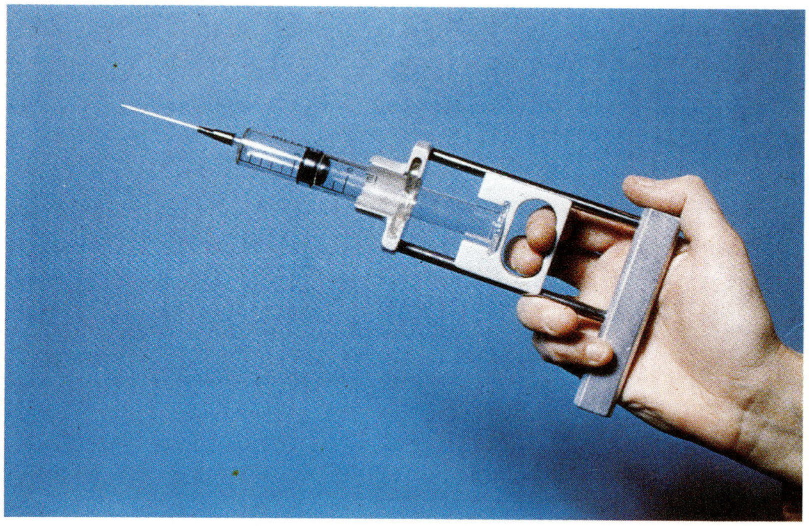

2

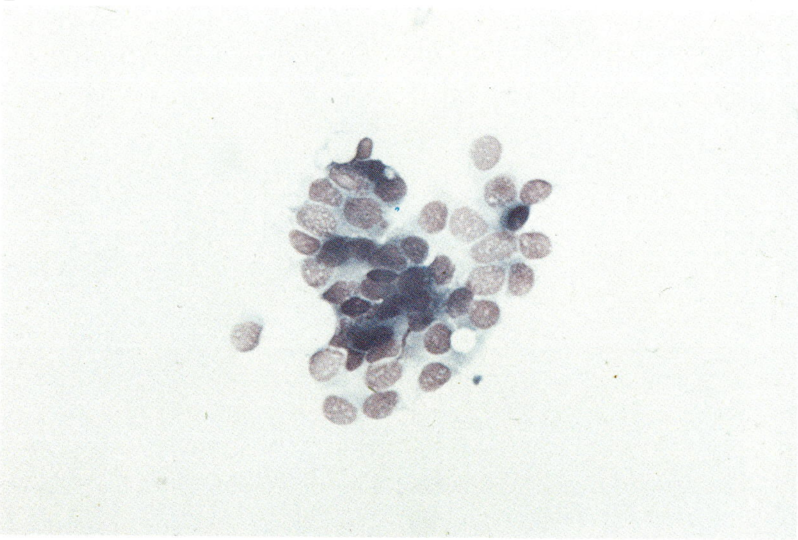

2 The quality of the smears is improved if the needle is washed through before it is used by a mixture of 0.9% saline mixed with 1000 i.u. of heparin.

Disposable needle biopsy of discrete solid tumour

1 Skin is infiltrated with plain local anaesthetic.

1

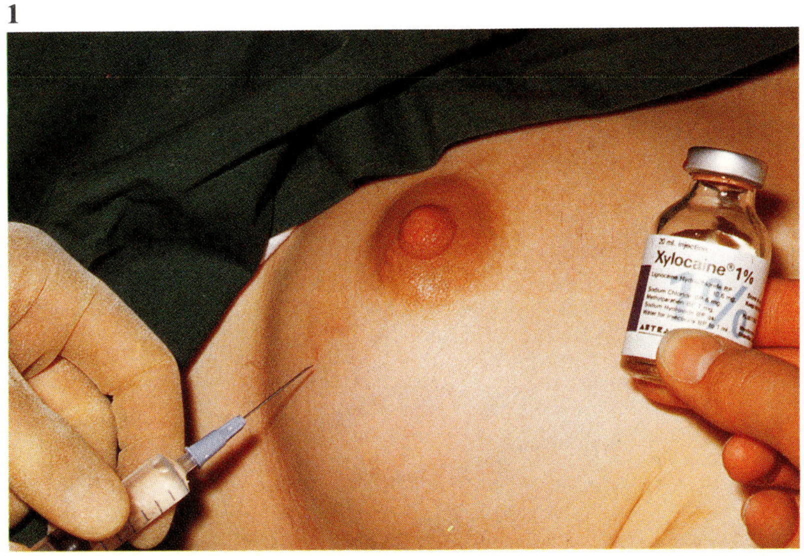

2 Small incision of skin is made over tumour with a small blade.

3 Travenol Trucut needle closed for introducing into breast.

2

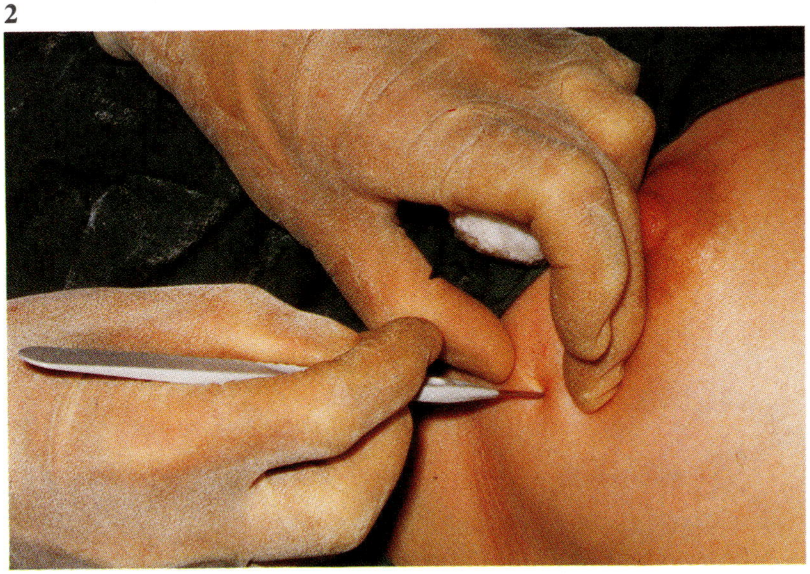

3

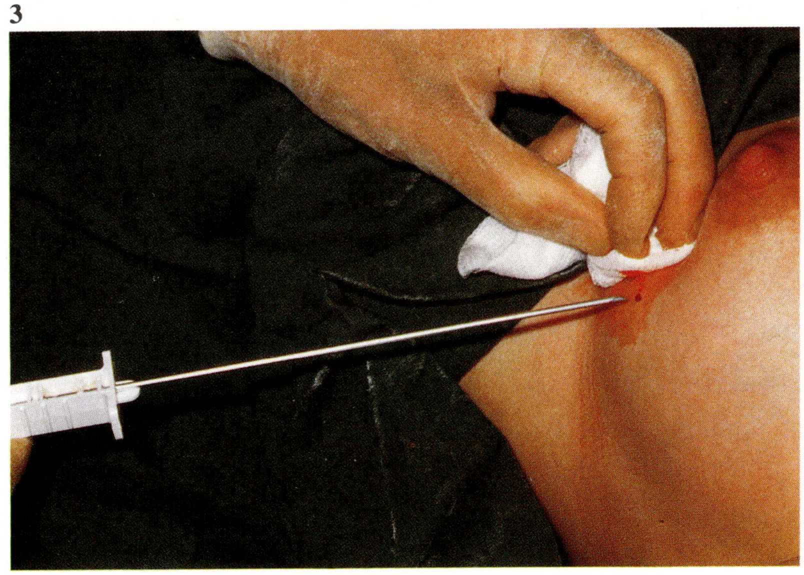

4

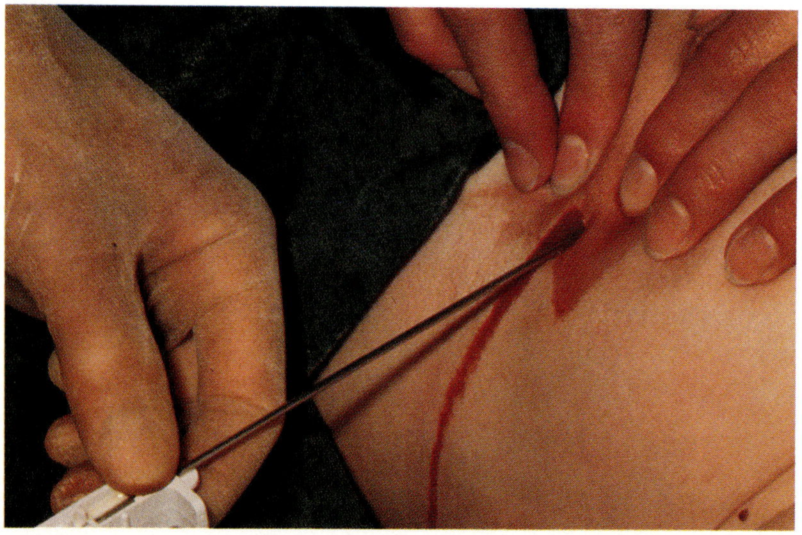

4 Central plunger of needle advanced into tumour, which is steadied by an assistant.

5

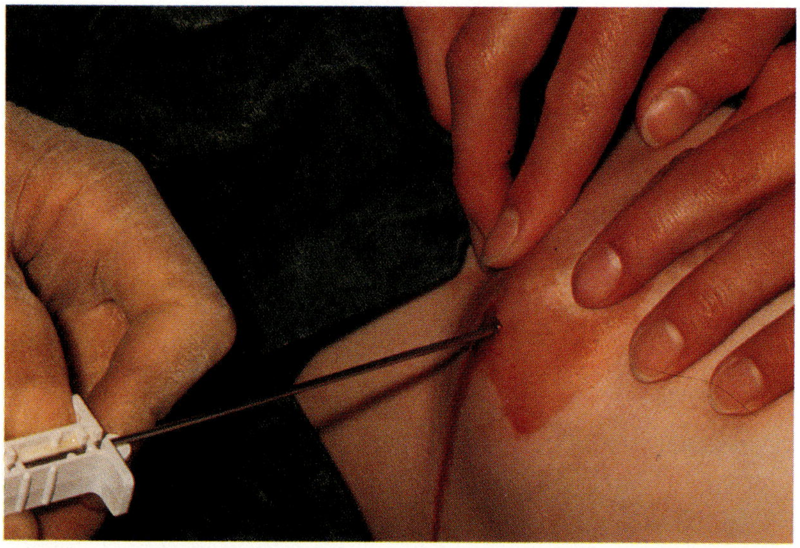

5 Outer sheath of needle advanced over plunger, cutting off small cylinder of tumour as biopsy.

6 Opened needle, after withdrawal, revealing cylindrical biopsy.

7 Specimen of tissue obtained is suitable for either frozen section or paraffin histology.

6

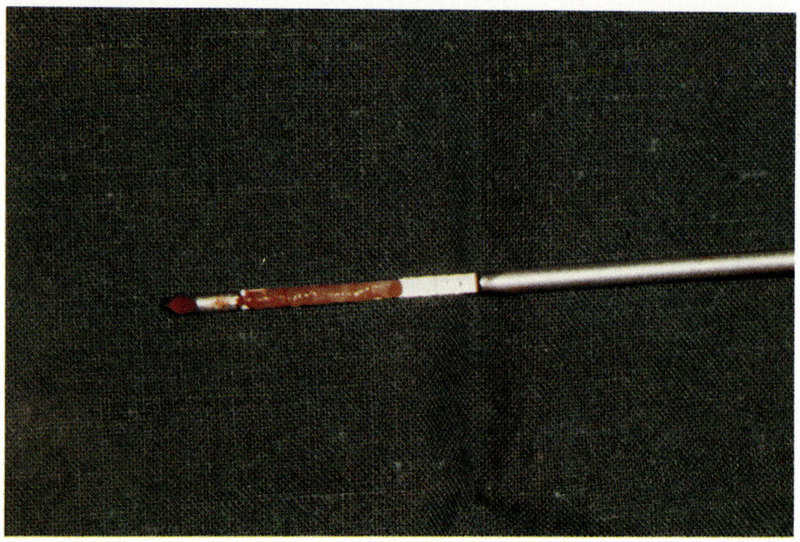

7

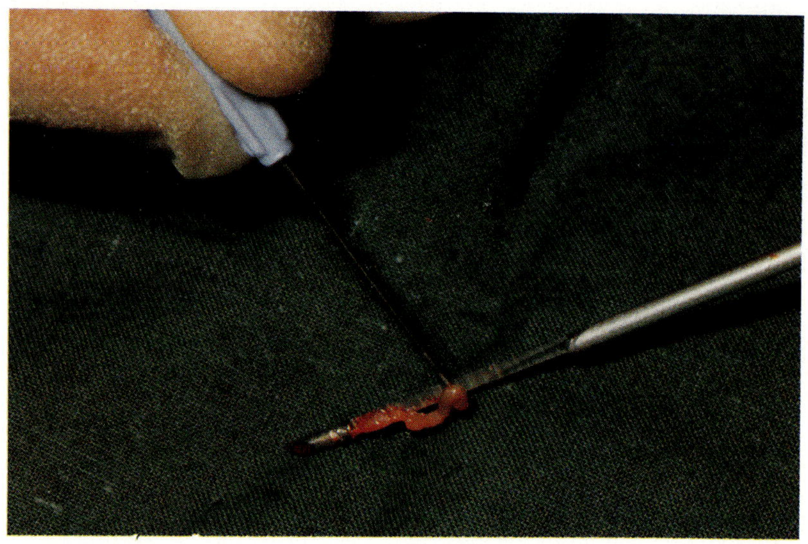

Open biopsy of breast under general anaesthetic e.g. as for fibroadenoma

1 Incision is made in skin creases, parallel with margin of areola, *not* radially.

2 After formal incision of subcutaneous fat, and haemostasis of this by diathermy, the mass to be excised is fixed either with tissue forceps or by transfixion with a catgut suture.

3 With traction on the mass, this is dissected from the remaining breast tissue. Meticulous haemostasis by diathermy is best done during this, since the bleeding points are held near the surface of the wound by the traction on the specimen.

1

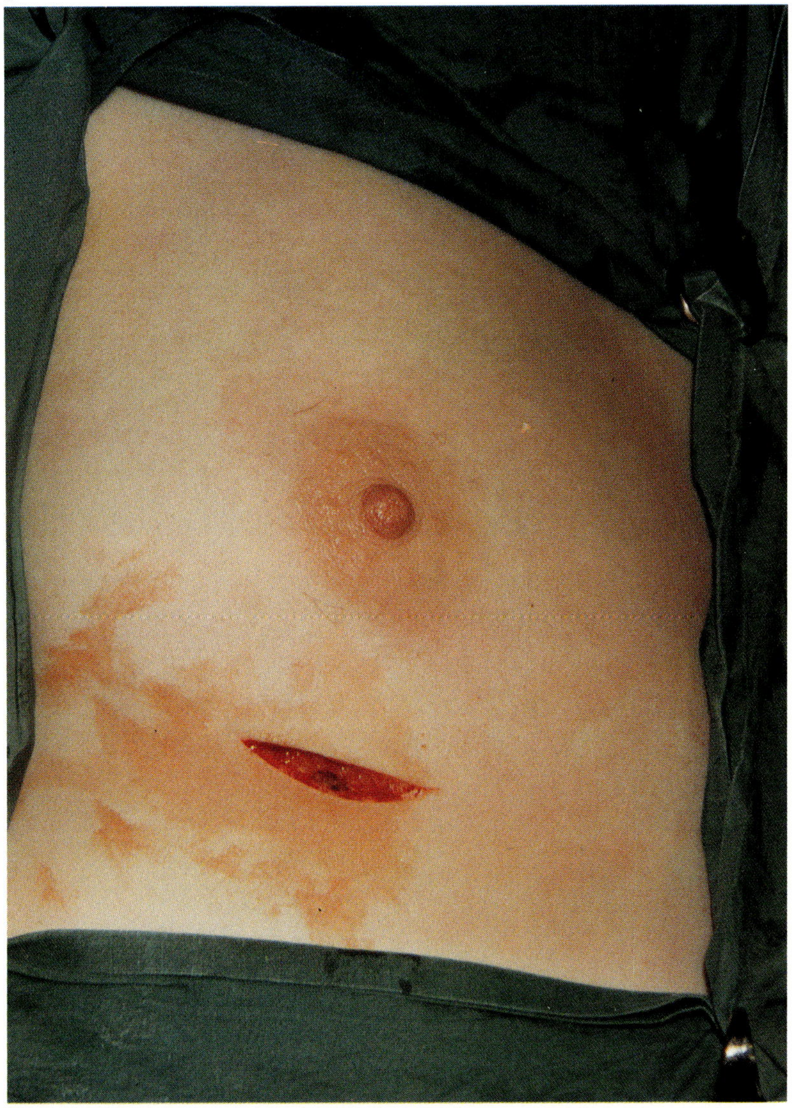

2

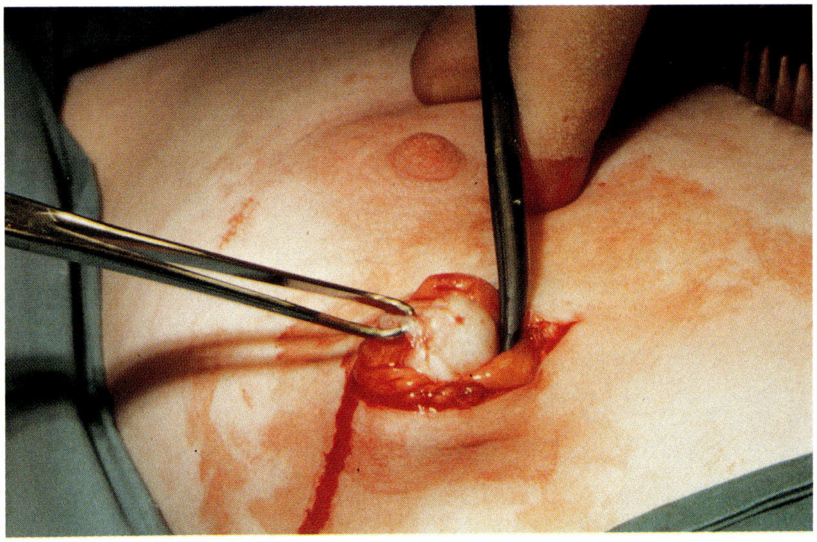

3

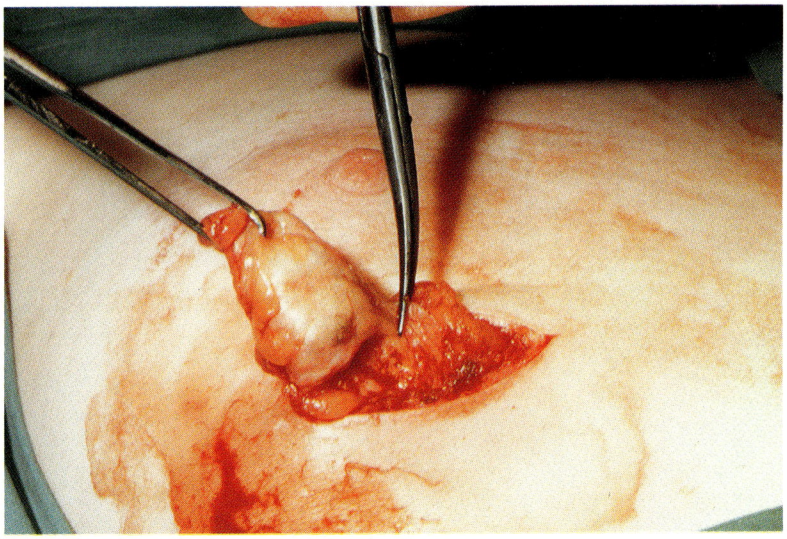

4

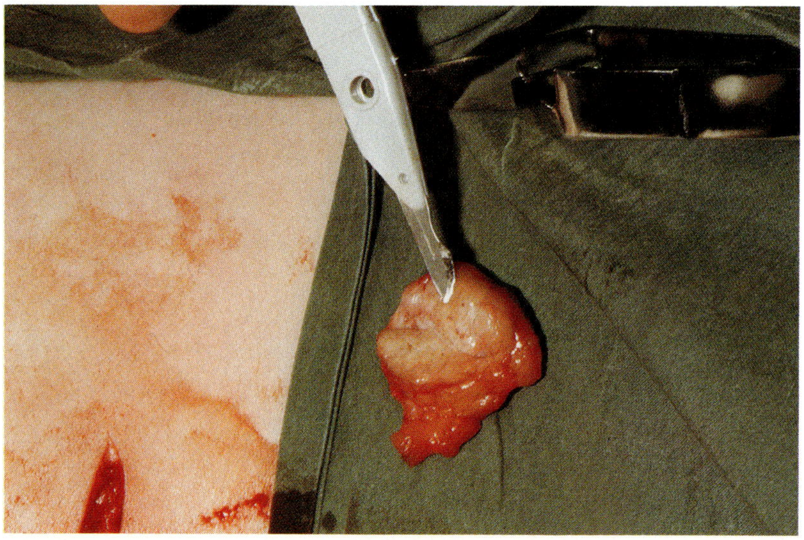

4 With the specimen removed from the breast, this may be bisected with a disposable scalpel, to assist naked eye diagnosis or to harvest part of the specimen for oestradiol receptors, should there be any possibility that the lesion is malignant.

5

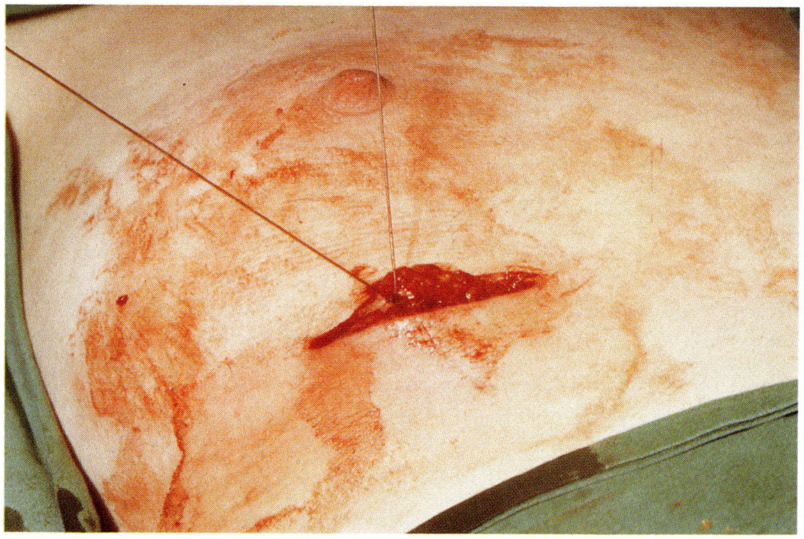

5 The resulting cavity, unless its walls fall together spontaneously, can be obliterated by interrupted chromic catgut sutures.

6 A fine monofilament Prolene sutured through the dermis gives a sound subcuticular closure, with easy painless suture removal after one week and good cosmesis in the long term.

7 A few adhesive wound closures guarantee complete and precise apposition of the incised epithelium.

6

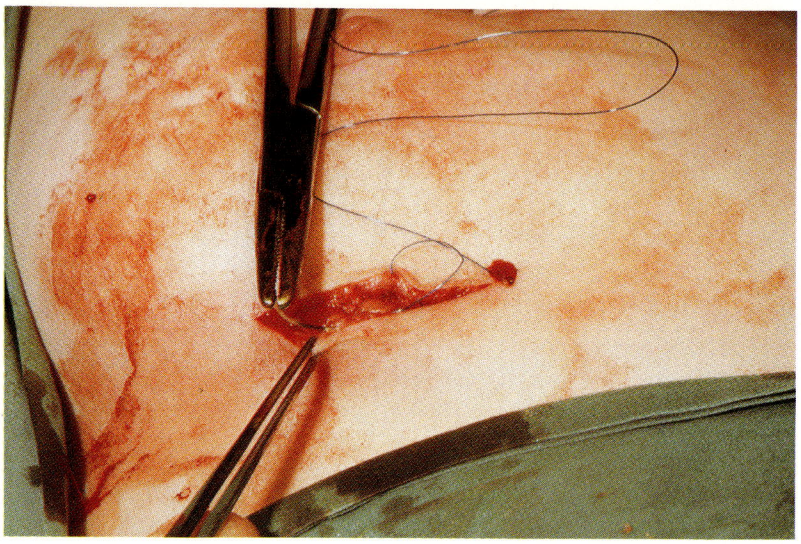

7

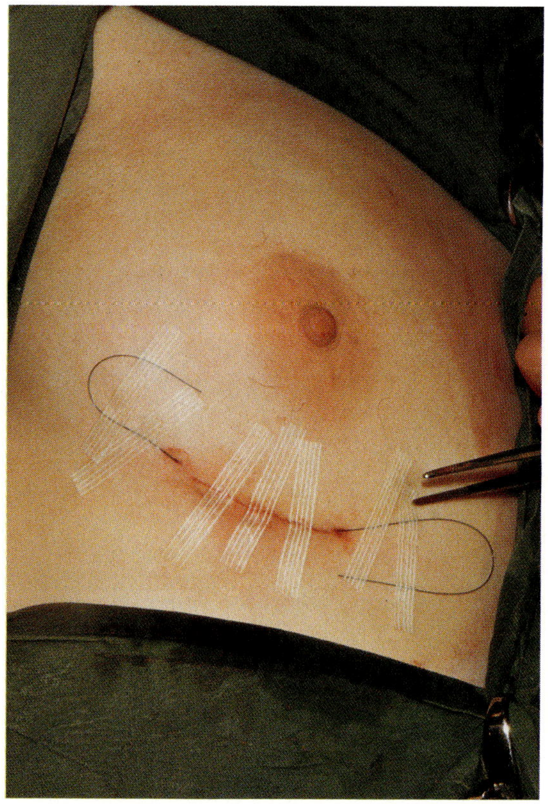

8 **An elasticated adhesive dressing over an absorbent dressing** provides some firm postoperative pressure and minimises tendency to ecchymosis and haematoma in this vascular organ.

8

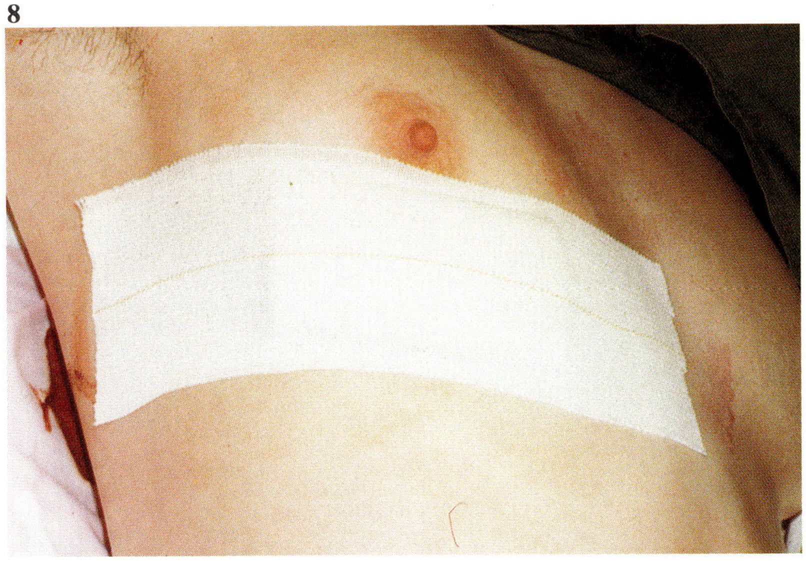

Drainage of breast abscess

1 **When the signs of an abscess are present in the breast, it is useless persisting with antibiotics.** Incision is essential.

1

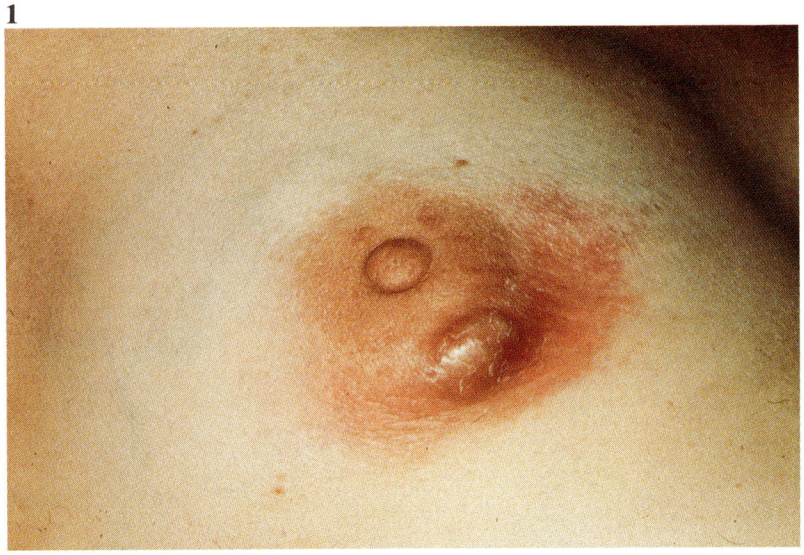

2 **This is best done under general anaesthetic.** The incision is made in the skin crease, to improve the ultimate cosmetic end result. After evacuation of pus, the wound should be packed and left open. A swab is taken for bacteriology.

2

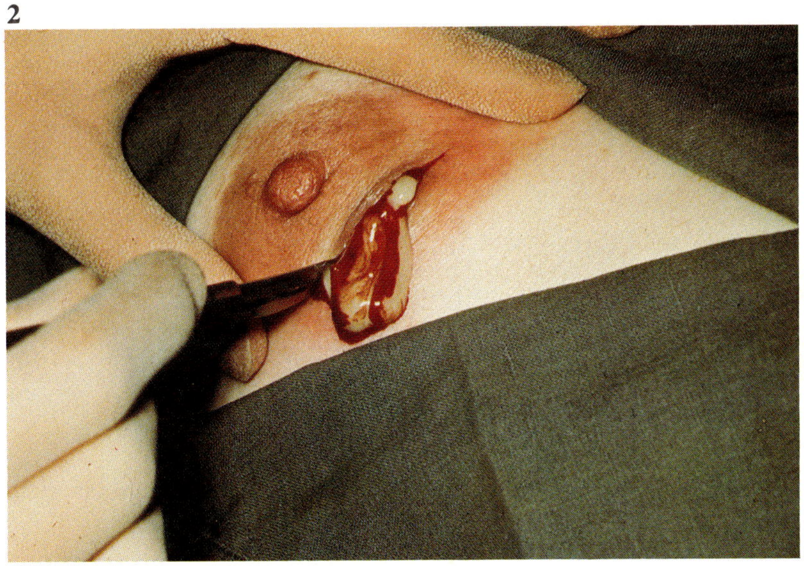

Subareolar mammary duct excision for duct ectasia

1

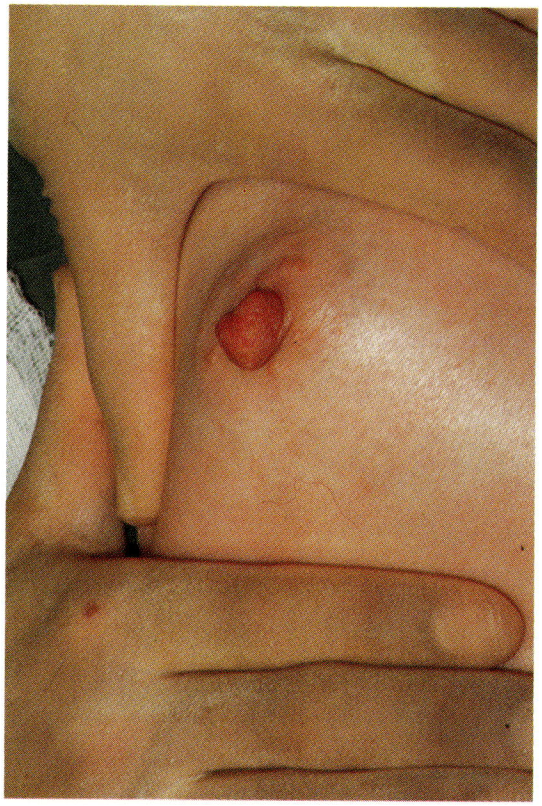

2

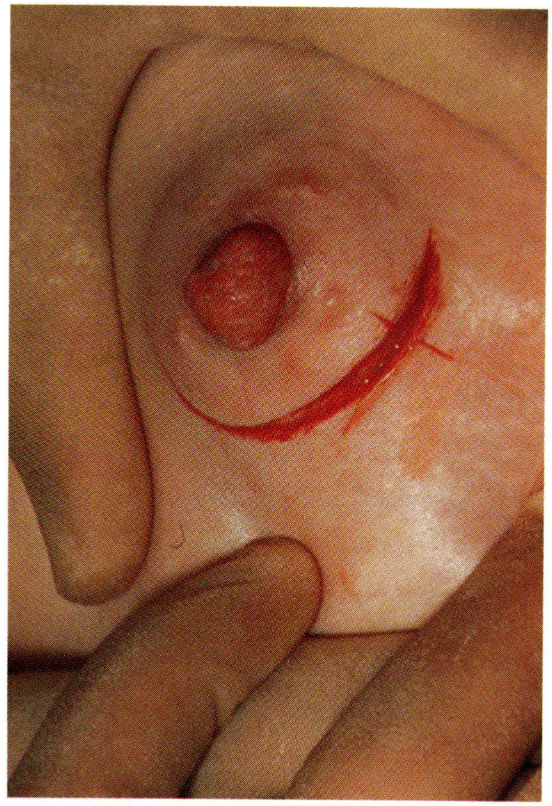

1 Using two hands the assistant tenses the skin of the breast so that the margin of the areola is fixed.

2 The inferior 180° of the margin is incised cleanly and continuously, after three or four short linear excoriations have been made across the lower half of the areolar margin (to facilitate the closure).

3 The areola is elevated as a full thickness flap.

3

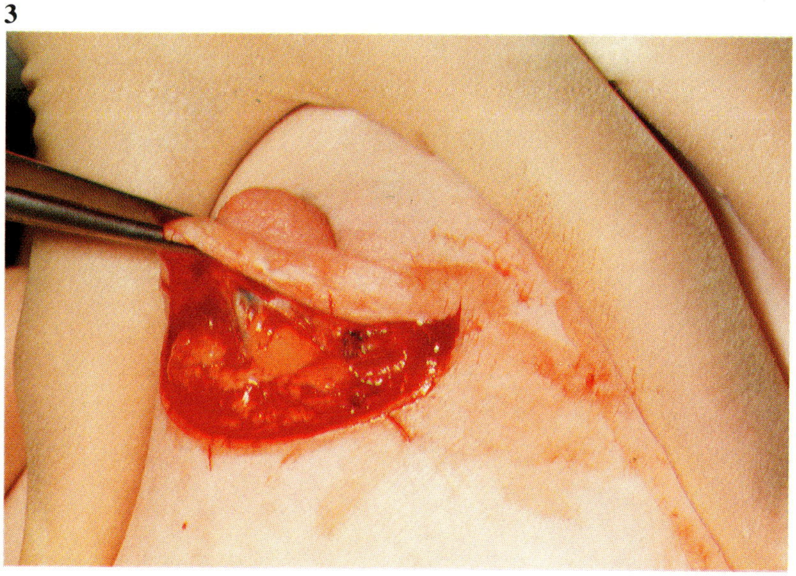

4

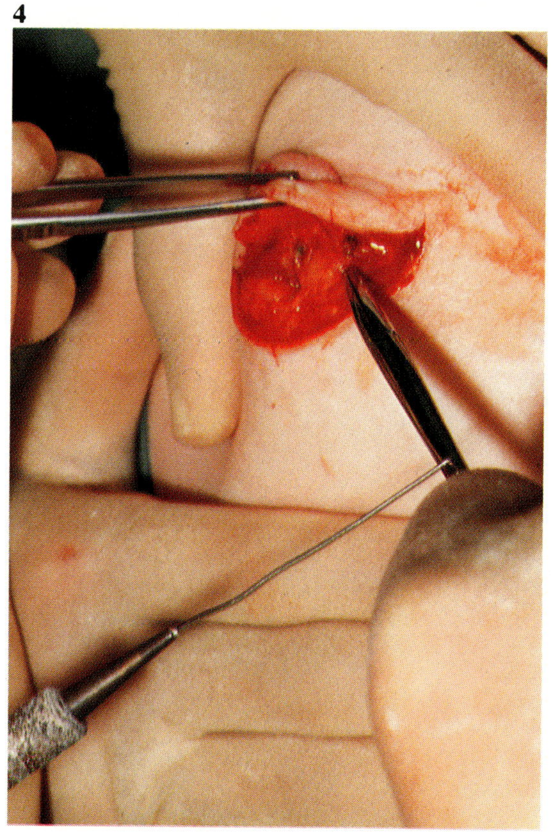

4 Haemostasis by diathermy is restricted to the breast side of the dissection to minimise risk of ischaemia to the areola and nipple.

5

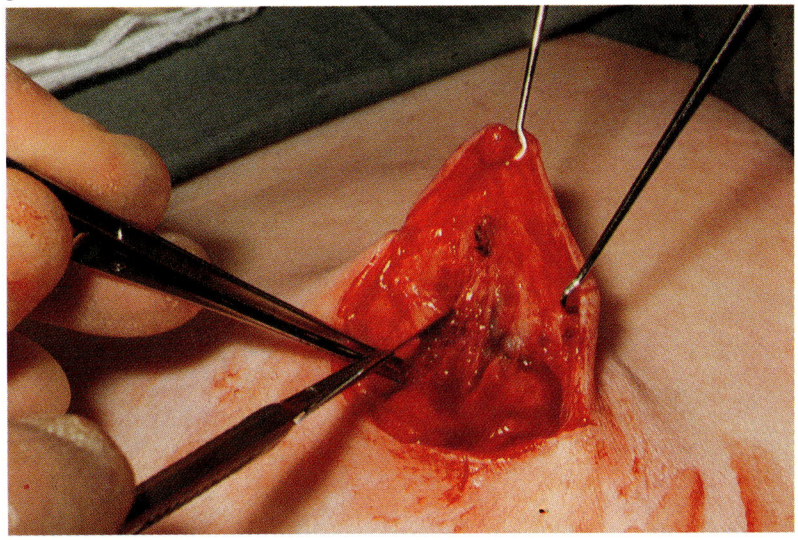

5 It is vital that the plane of the flap reaches the summit of the collecting ducts of the nipple, without button-holing. Recurrence of symptoms after this operation can frequently be traced to duct remnants left under the skin of the summit of the nipple.

6

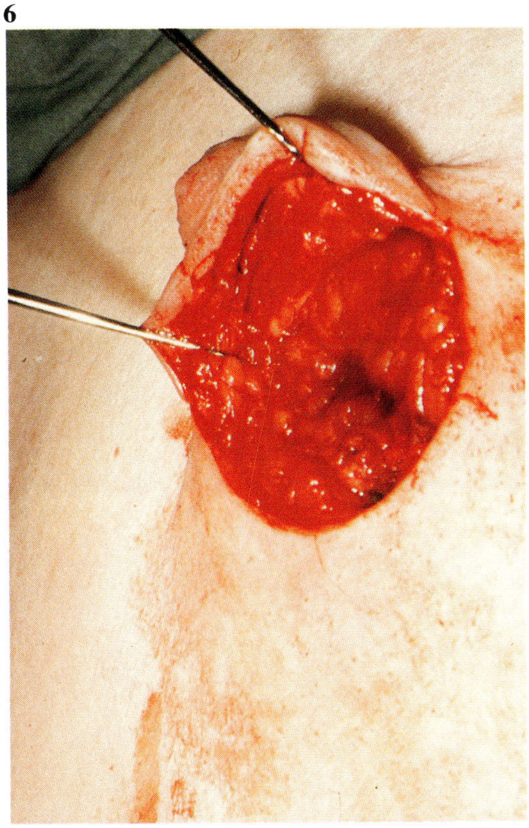

6 The dissection is complete when full retraction of the areola exposes a circle of underlying breast tissue.

7

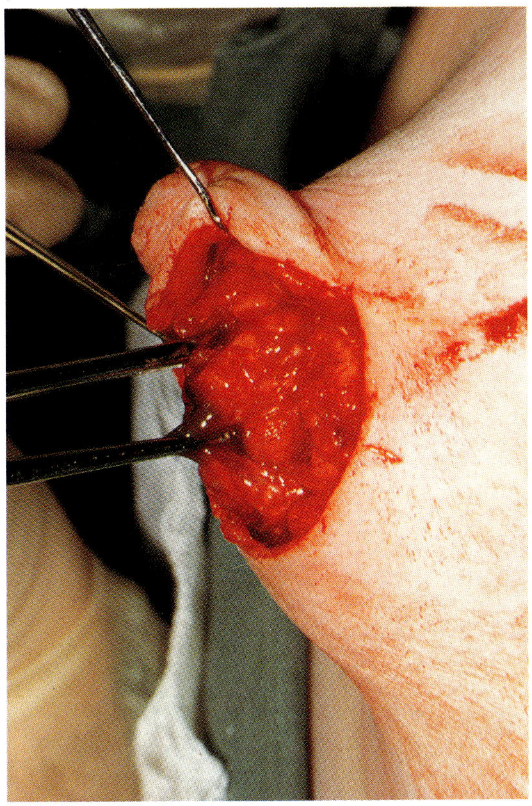

7 Using two Allis tissue-holding forceps placed symmetrically near to, but on opposite sides of, the nipple, the subareolar ductal system is stabilised for excision.

8

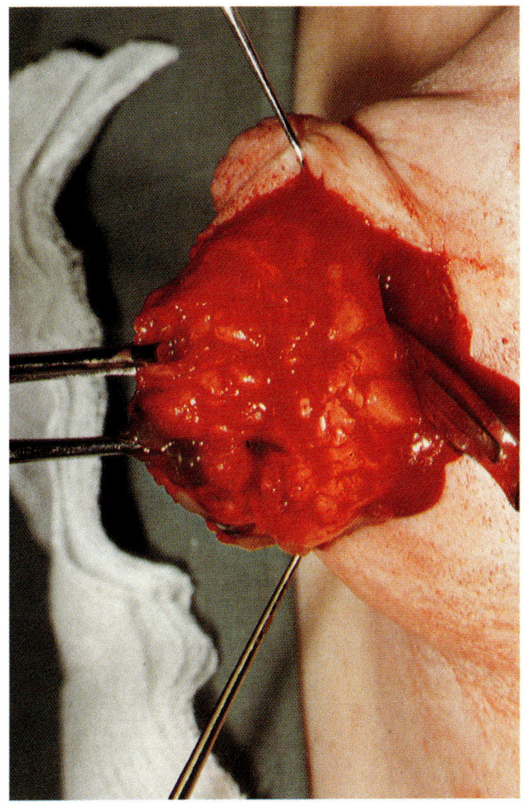

8 The disc of tissue which consists of the major ducts is demarcated by the margin of the areola. A scalpel is used to incise the circular margin of the disc of tissue being removed, the tissue being retracted continuously by means of the Allis forceps held by the assistant.

9

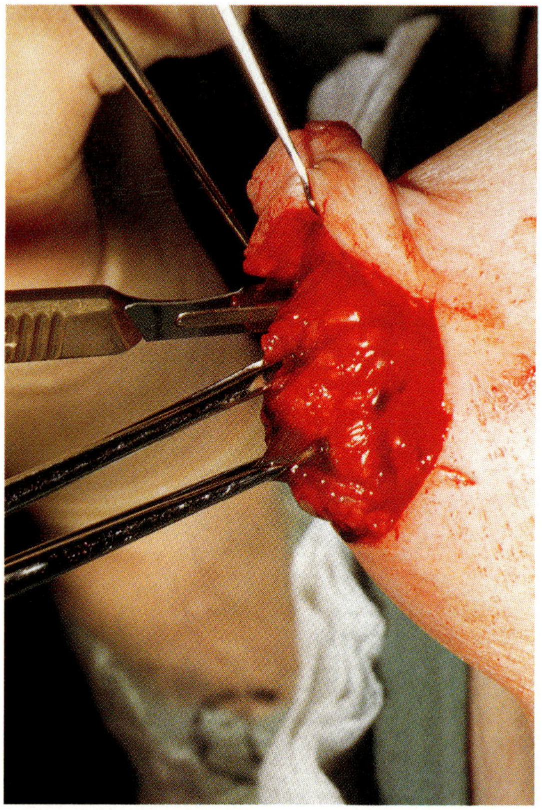

10

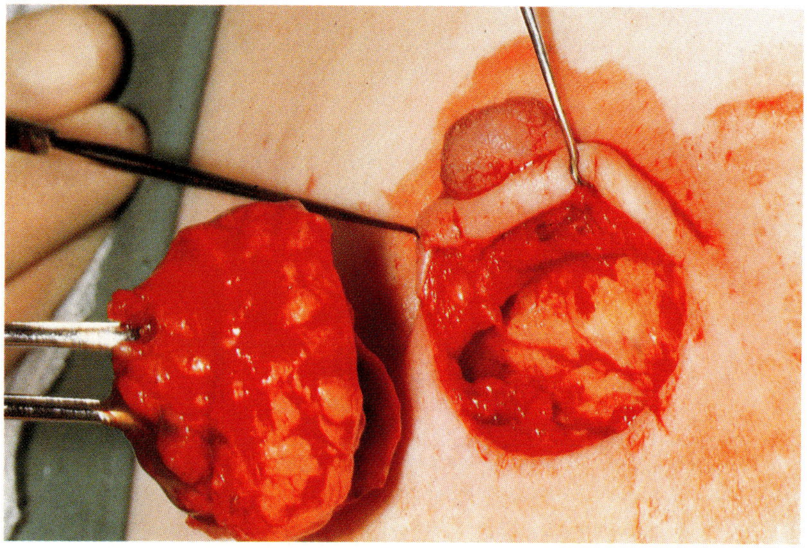

9 The duct excision is completed by cutting across the base of the disc of tissue, a place which is 2-3 cm deep to the front surface of the breast.

10 Excision of the ductal system leaves a crater-like defect.

11 Haemostasis is best effected with diathermy.

12 Using chromic catgut mounted on a trochar pointed needle, the size of the crater can be diminished considerably and easily by approximating its edges. Usually no more than three interrupted sutures are required.

13 The scratch marks across the areolar margin are approximated to achieve perfect alignment.

14 The closure is done with least risk of damaging the areola by using interrupted sutures of 3/0 monofilament Prolene, placed as mattress sutures, with the knots outwards, and on the areolar side through dermis only, not penetrating the epidermis.
(See also Michrodochectomy, **15**).

15 Care must be taken at this time that the skin of the nipple is *everted*.

16 Healing of the nipples in an everted way can be encouraged by dressing the wound with a non-adherent gauze with a nipple-sized window cut in it.

17 Usually the long-term end result leaves little concavity of the breast.

11

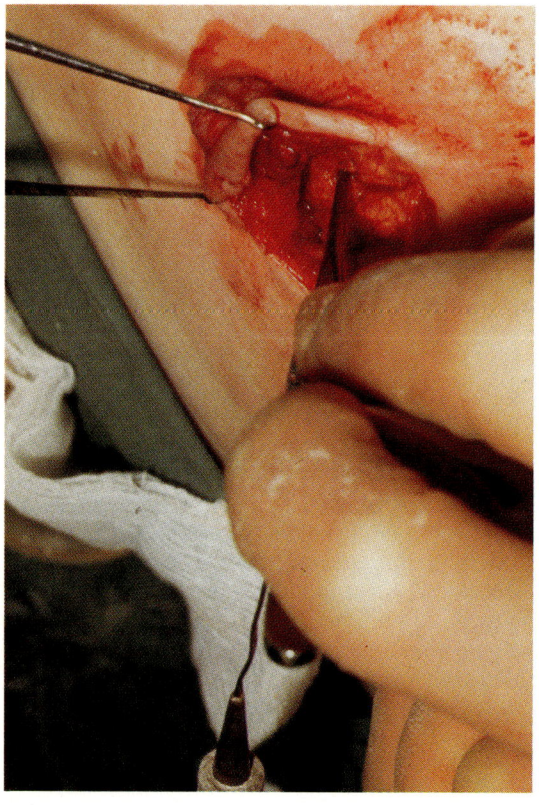

12

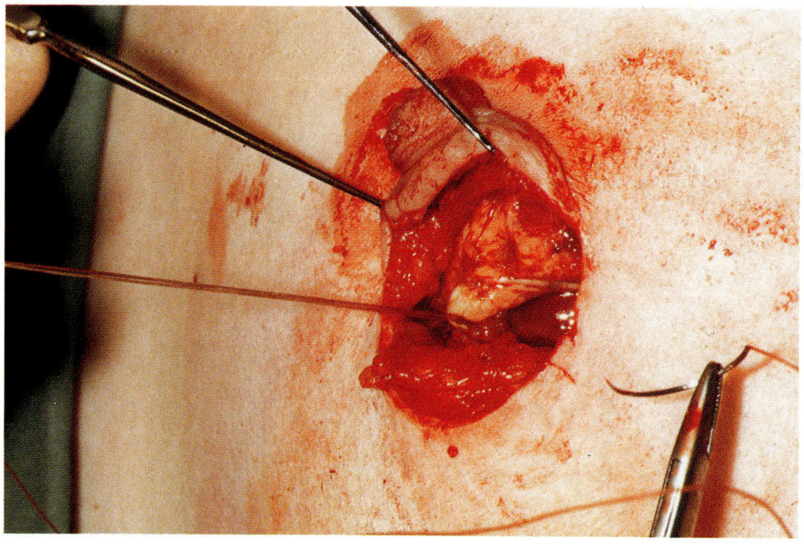

13

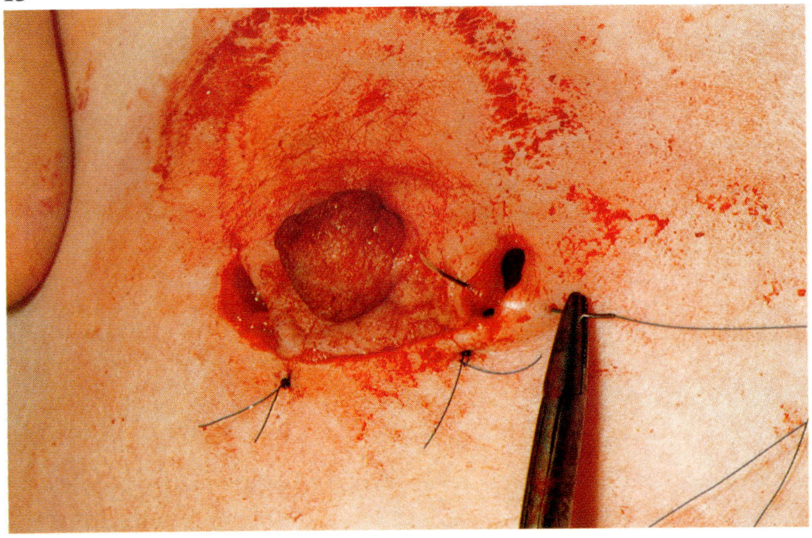

14

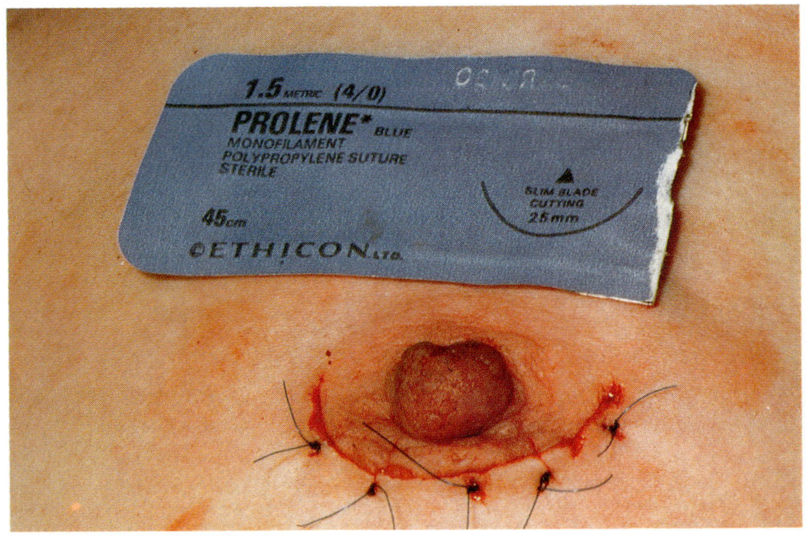
1.5 METRIC (4/0)
PROLENE* BLUE
MONOFILAMENT
POLYPROPYLENE SUTURE
STERILE
SLIM BLADE CUTTING 25mm
45cm
©ETHICON LTD.

15

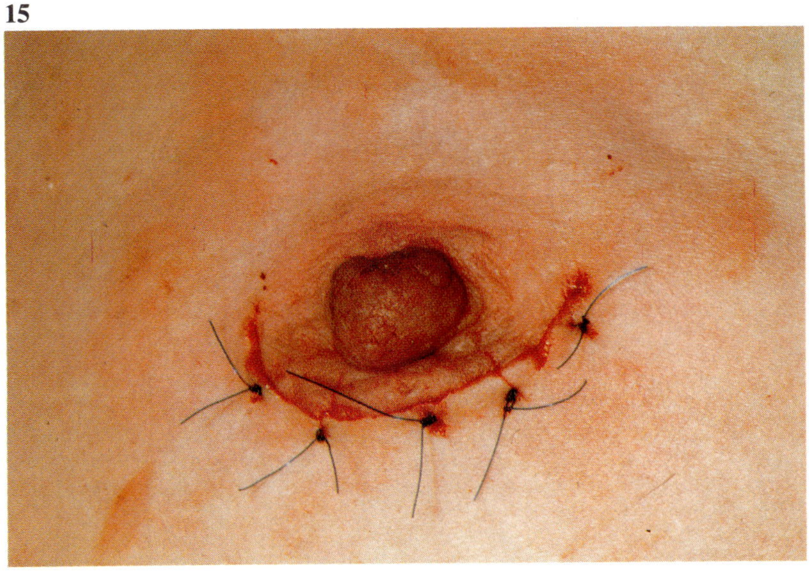

16

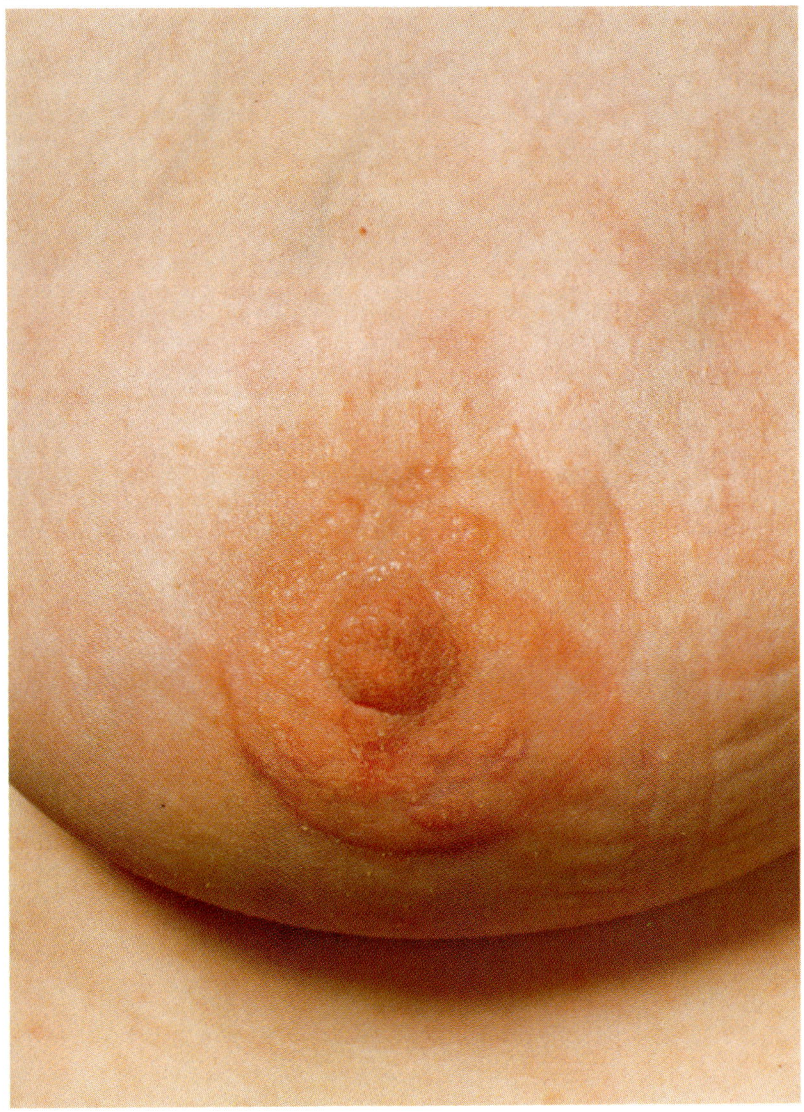

17

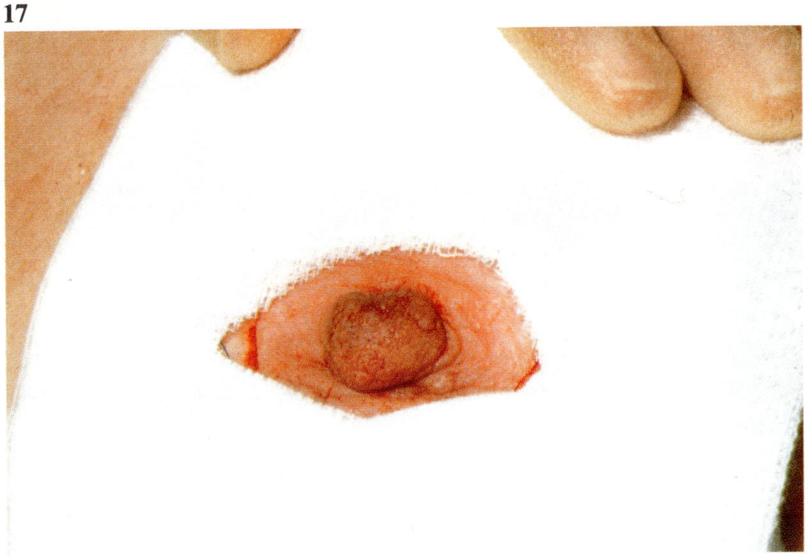

Michrodochectomy: To establish cause of blood-stained nipple discharge coming from a solitary duct

1 The major ducts deep to the areola are firmly compressed with two hands. This must not be done before surgery, or discharge may be lost.

2 The blood-stained nipple discharge is expressed.

3 The opening of the leaking duct is explored gently with an appropriate sized lachrymal probe.

1

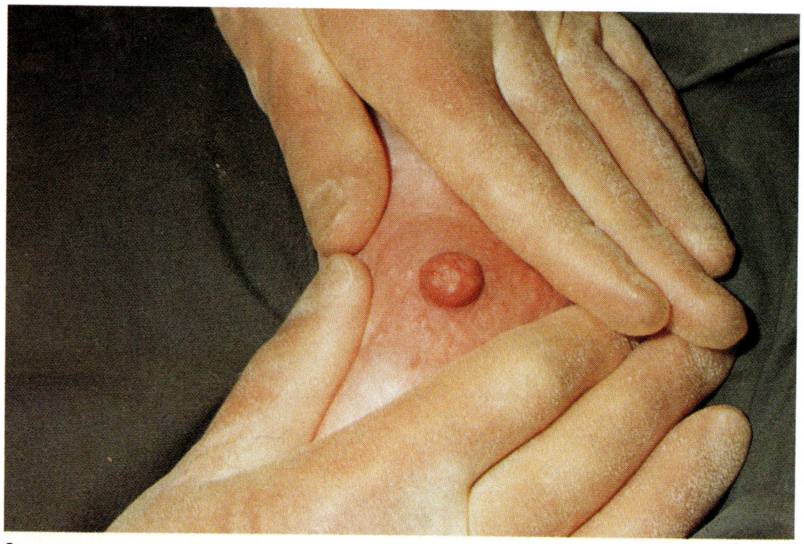

2

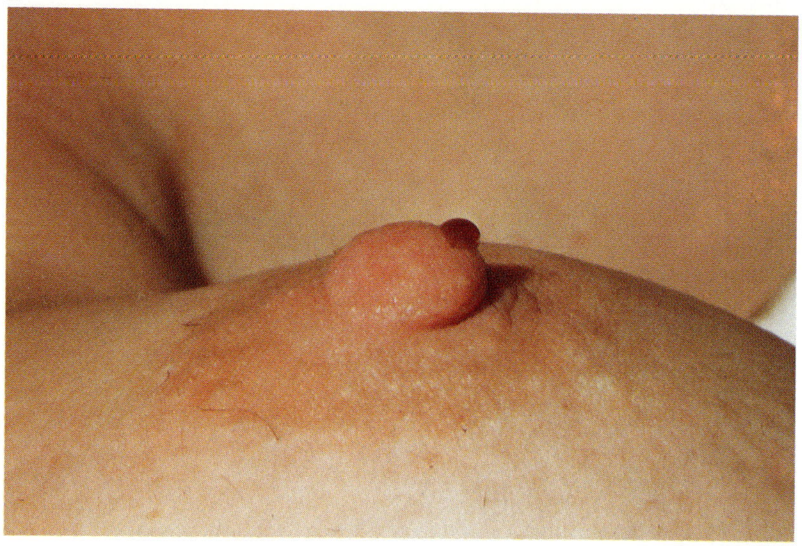

3

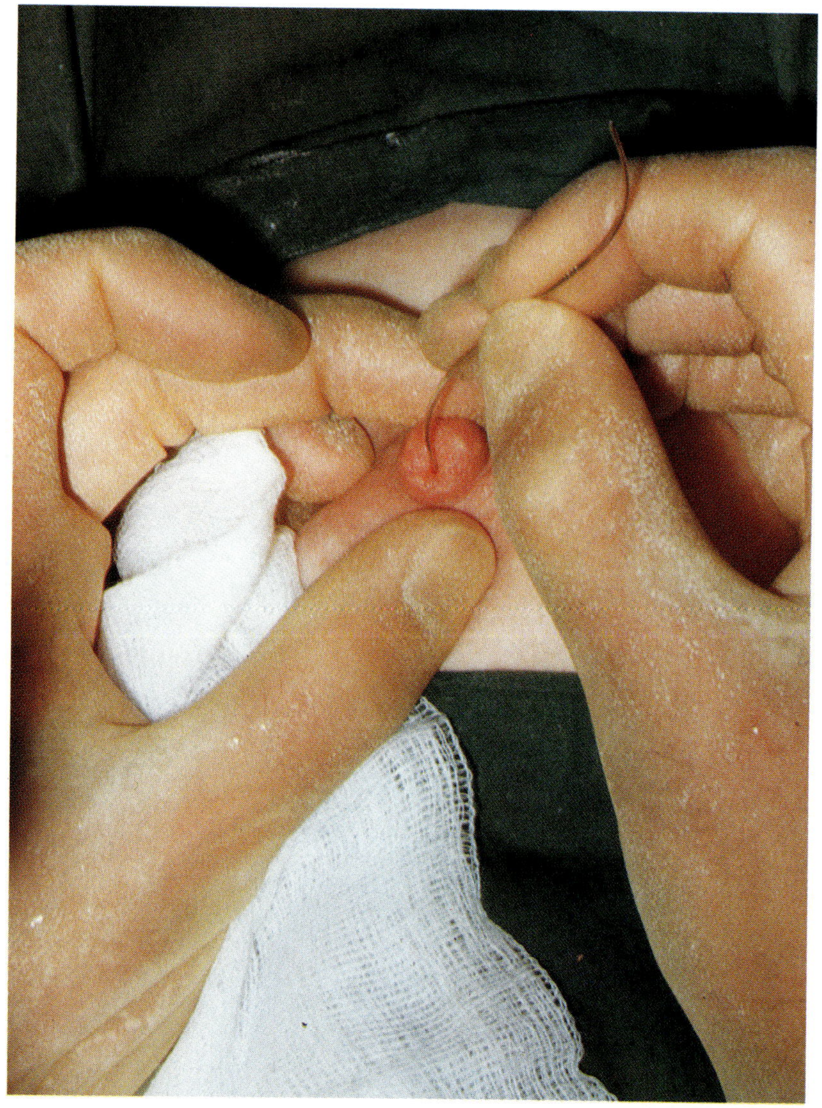

4

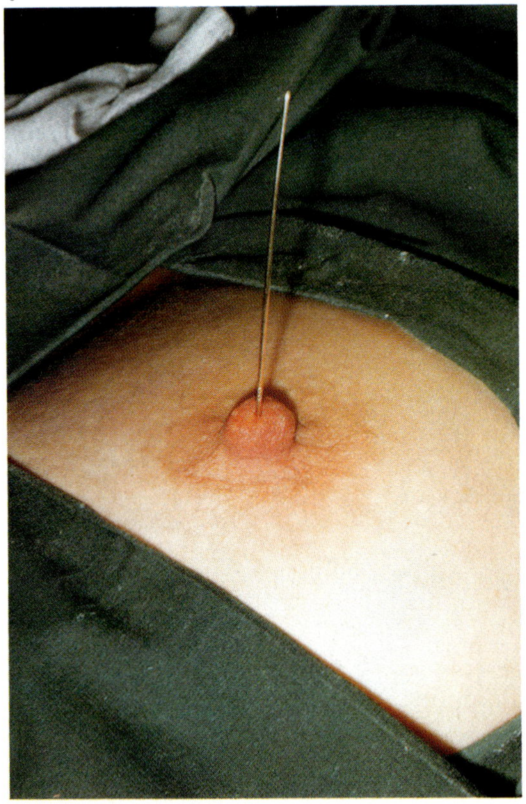

4 The site of the bleeding duct is identified by the direction the probe passes, having been introduced into the lumen of the duct without force.

5

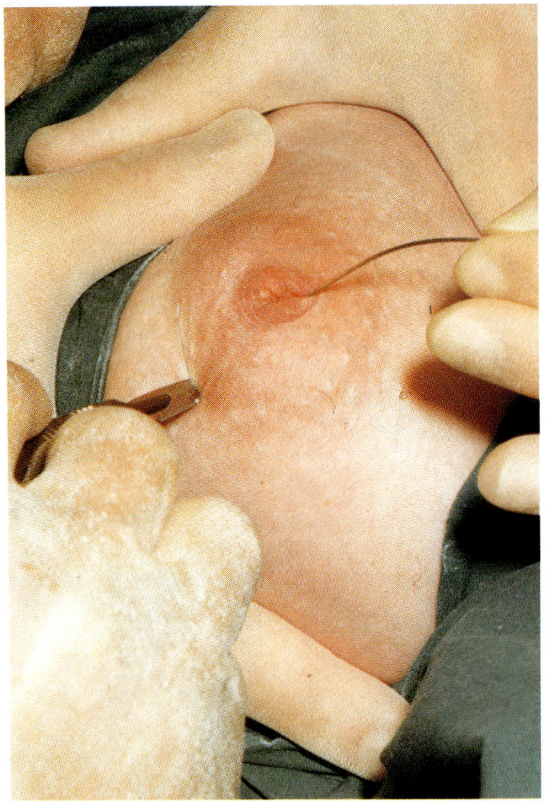

5 The incision is made in the radius of the margin of the areola under which the probe has passed, with the probe held in position within the duct by the scrub nurse, and the assistant tensing the skin of the centre of the breast using both hands.

6

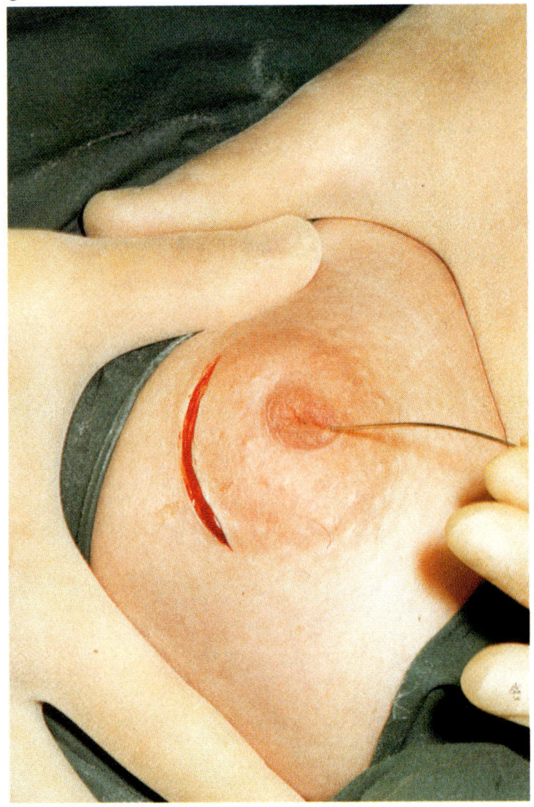

6 The incision needs to be about 5 cm long, i.e. about one third of the whole circumference of the areola.

7

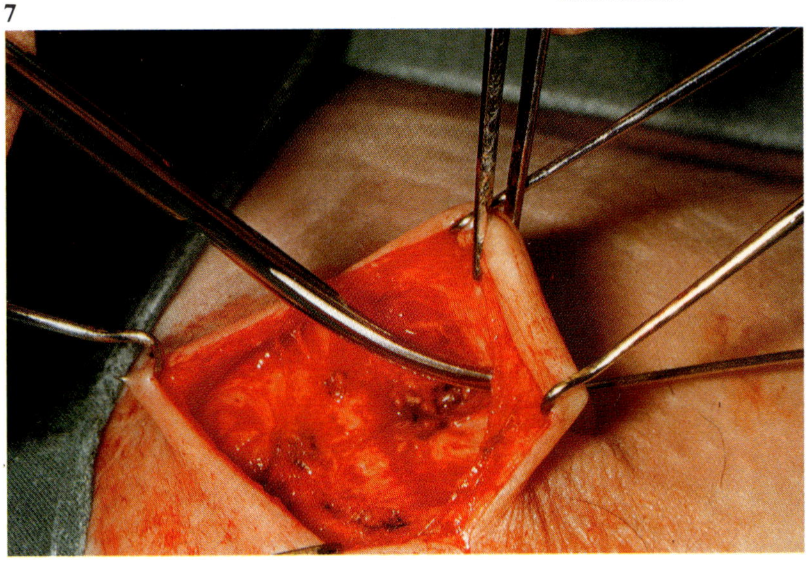

7 The skin on the outside, and the areola on the inside, of the incision are carefully dissected off the breast so that by progressive undercutting two flaps are raised, retracted on fine skin hooks.

8

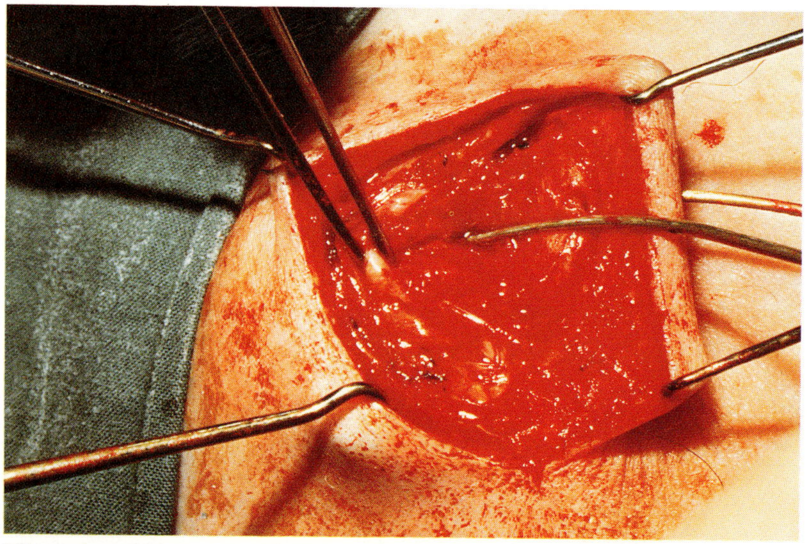

9

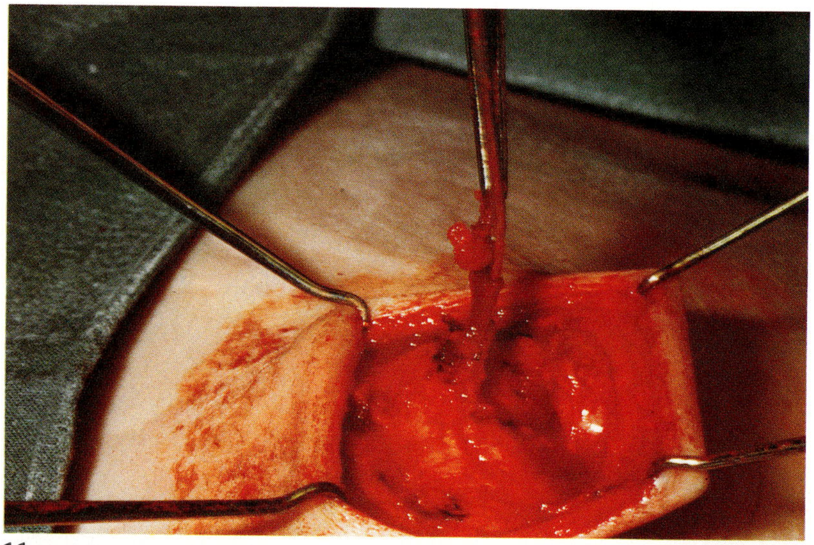

10

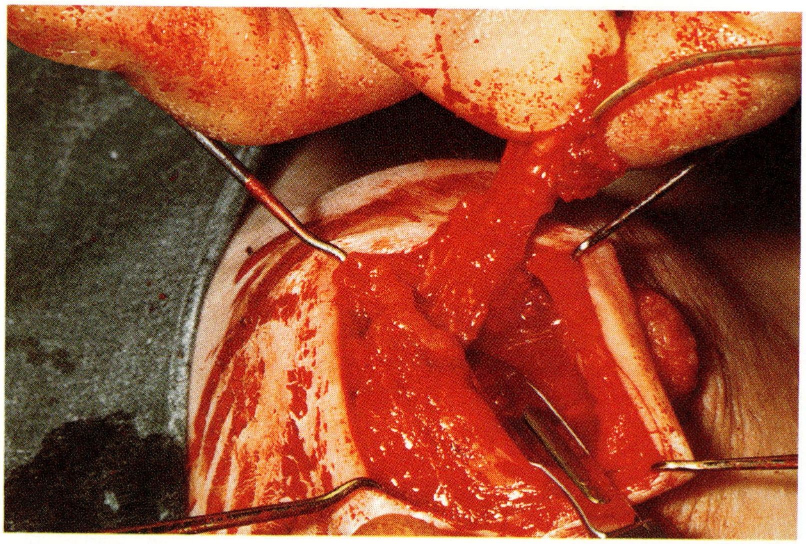

11

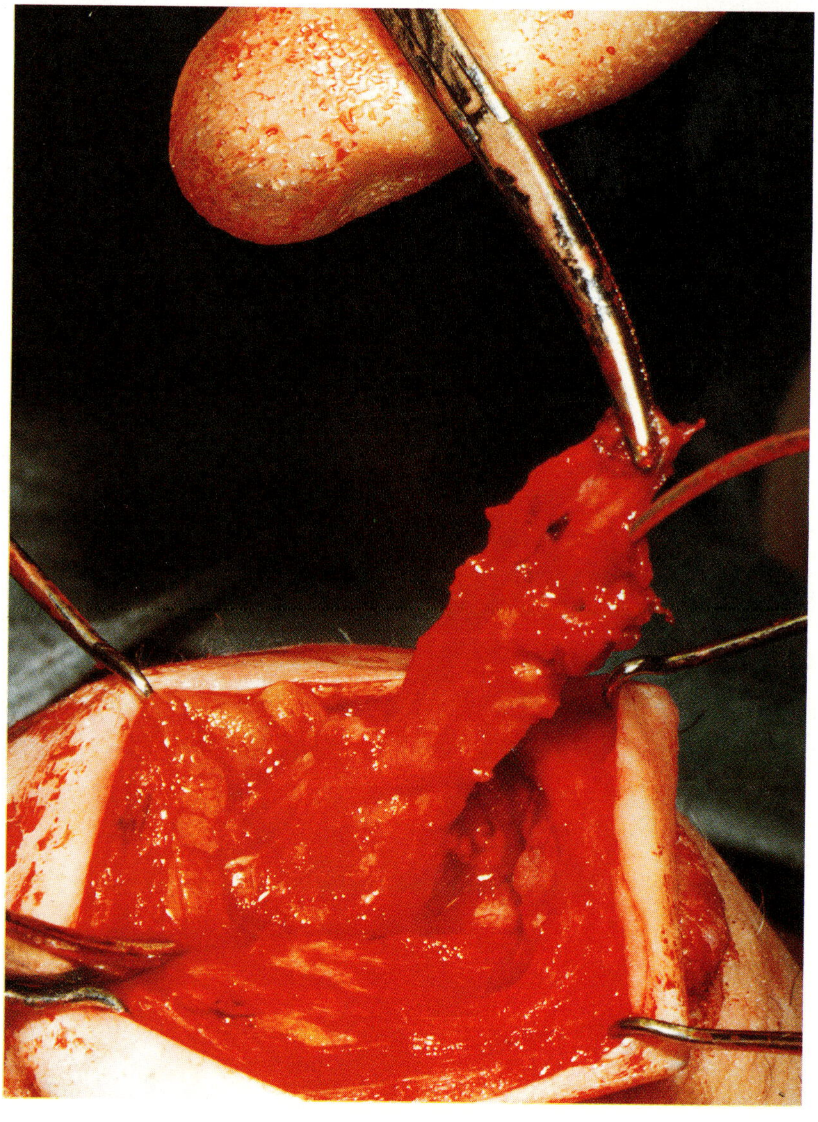

8 A point is reached where elevation of the flap of areola reveals the metal shaft of the probe, i.e. the leaking duct is opened just deep to the skin of the summit of the nipple. The original probe is slowly withdrawn from the nipple, and at the point where its tip is at the skin a second similar probe is passed into the duct from the wound.

9 With the probe in the duct, the single duct is dissected from the bundle of major ducts which make up the nipple.

10 As the dissection is continued towards the periphery of the areola, it is taken increasingly wide of the stented duct. This enables any tributaries of the main duct to be harvested with the specimen for microscopic examination.

11 Beyond the margin of the areola, i.e. under the flap of the skin, the dissection is widened so that the specimen assumes a club-like shape.

12

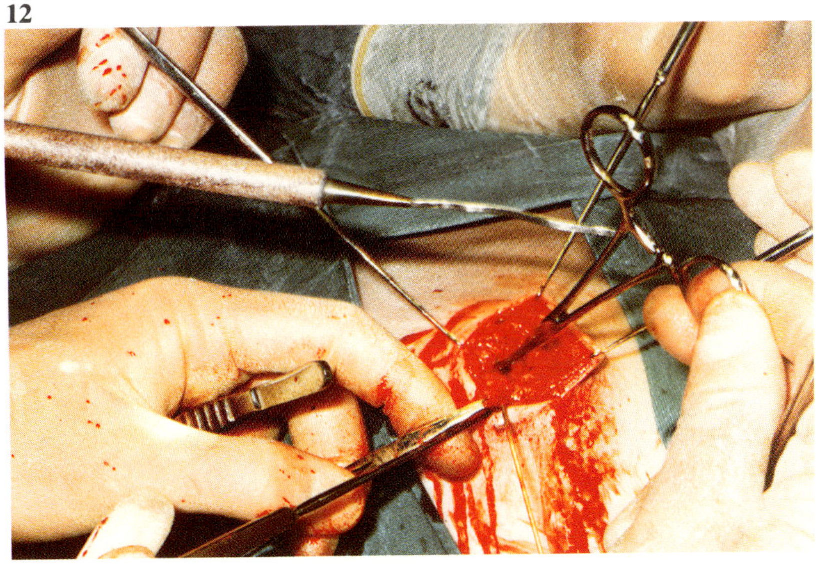

13

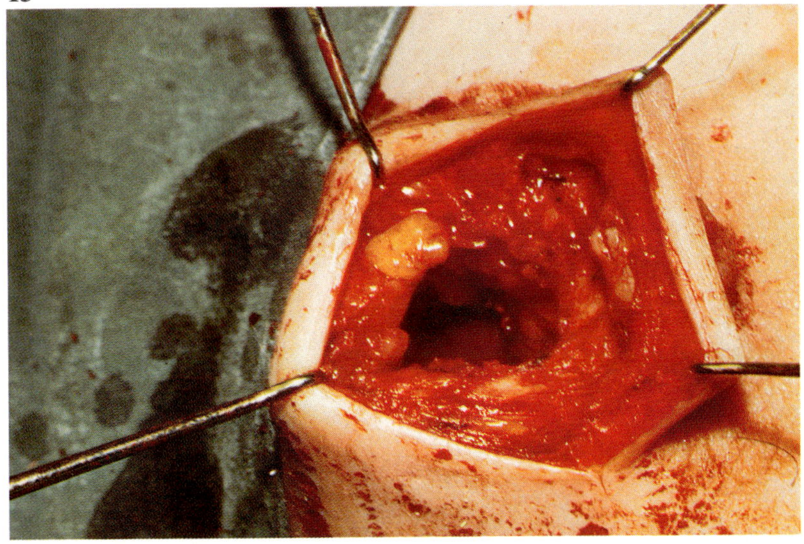

14

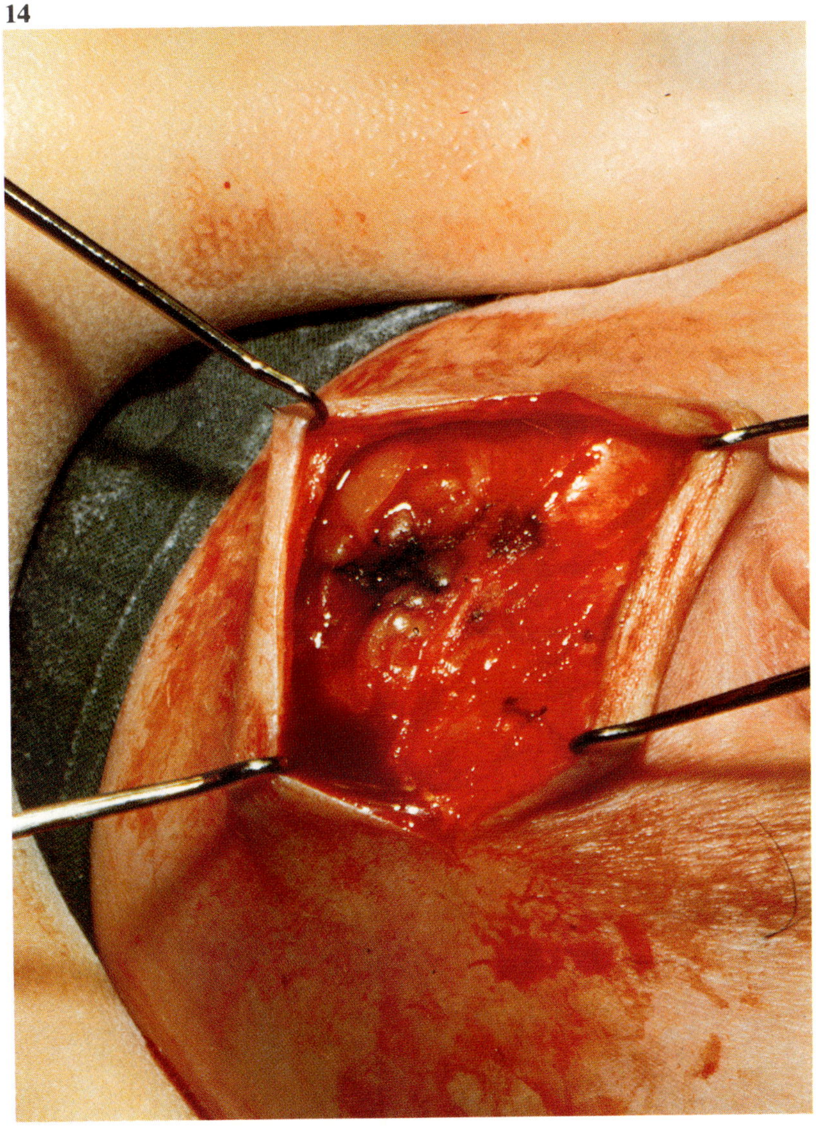

12 Meticulous haemostasis is performed with diathermy *before* the specimen is finally removed.

13 A cavity results after the duct is excised.

14 The cavity may close simply by its sides falling in, or this can be effected by using one or two fine chromic catgut sutures. Using these, special care needs to be taken not to dimple the overlying skin.

15 The skin is closed with interrupted 3/0 monofilament Prolene sutures, placed as mattress sutures, but with their areolar components passing only through the dermis.
(See previous operation, **14**).

15

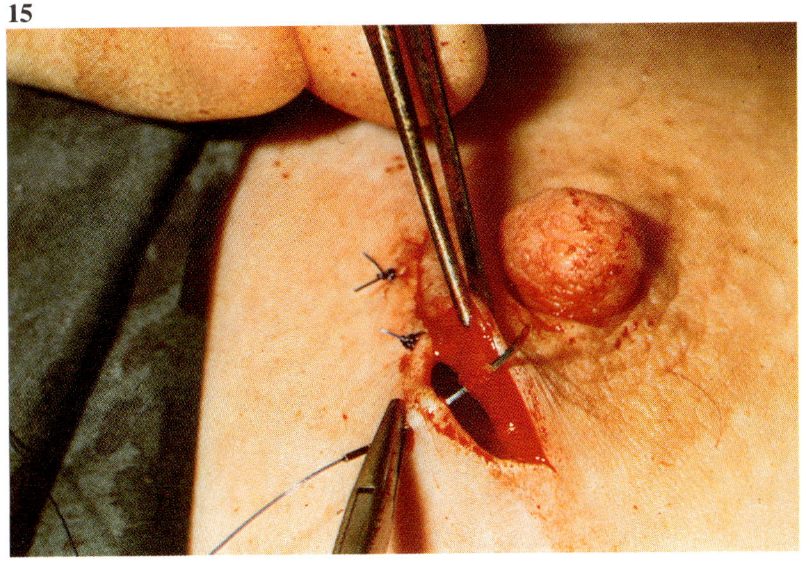

16

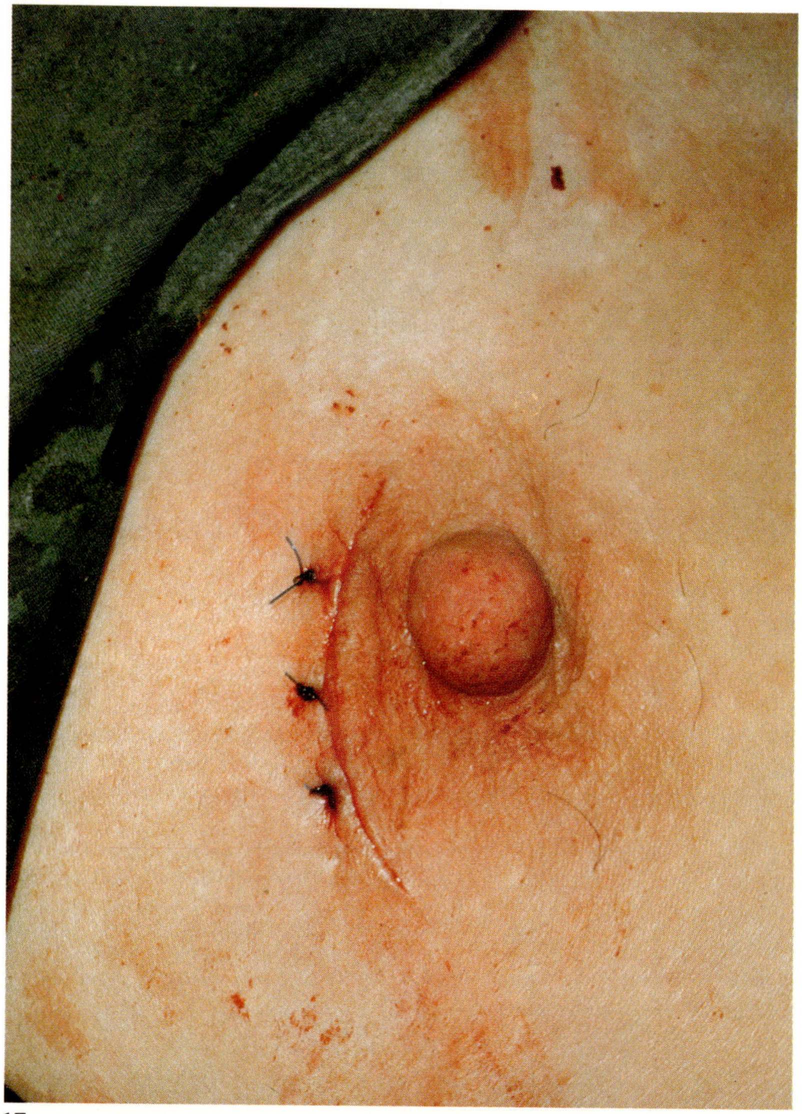

16 The circumareolar incision comes together and heals better than a radial incision. The resulting scar is cosmetically superior. It affords peri-operative access which is at least as good, if not better, than the apparently more obvious radial incision. A pressure dressing is applied.

17

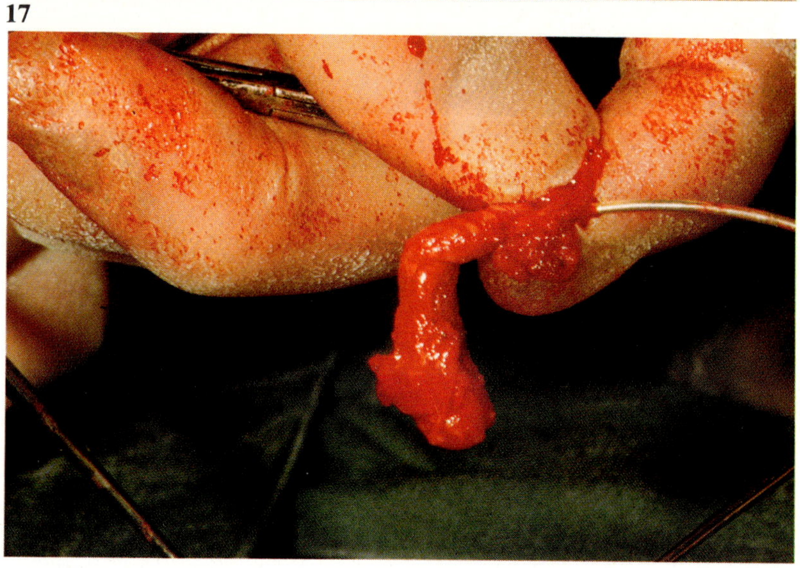

17 The lumen of the duct can still be identified after the specimen has been excised.

18 The size and shape of the excised duct are seen, just before it is fixed with formalin.

18

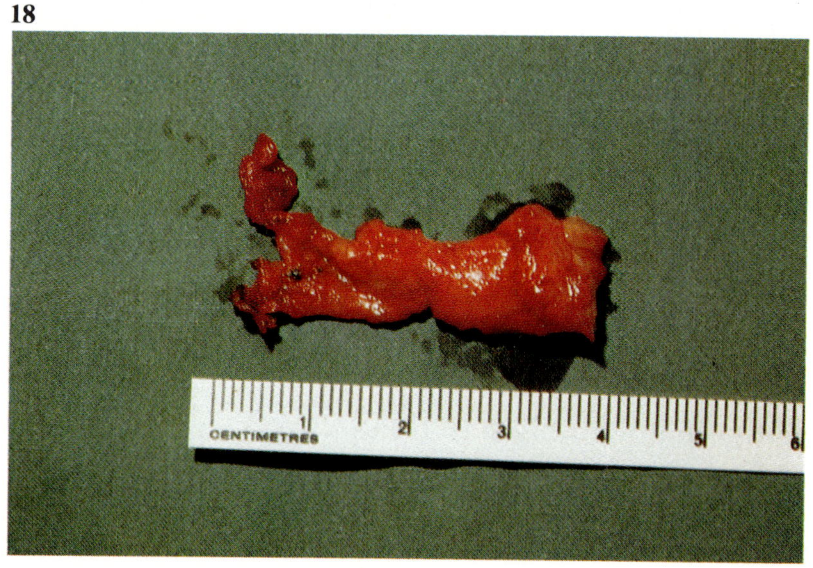

Localising technique for impalpable breast lesions

1

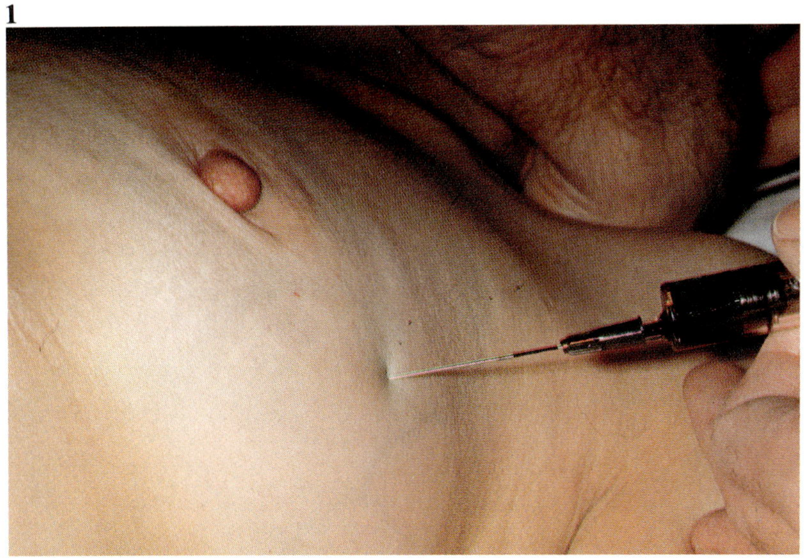

1 One ml of mixture of 45 per cent Hypaque with two drops of Patent Blue Violet Vital Dye is injected into the breast – a half to one hour before surgery.

2

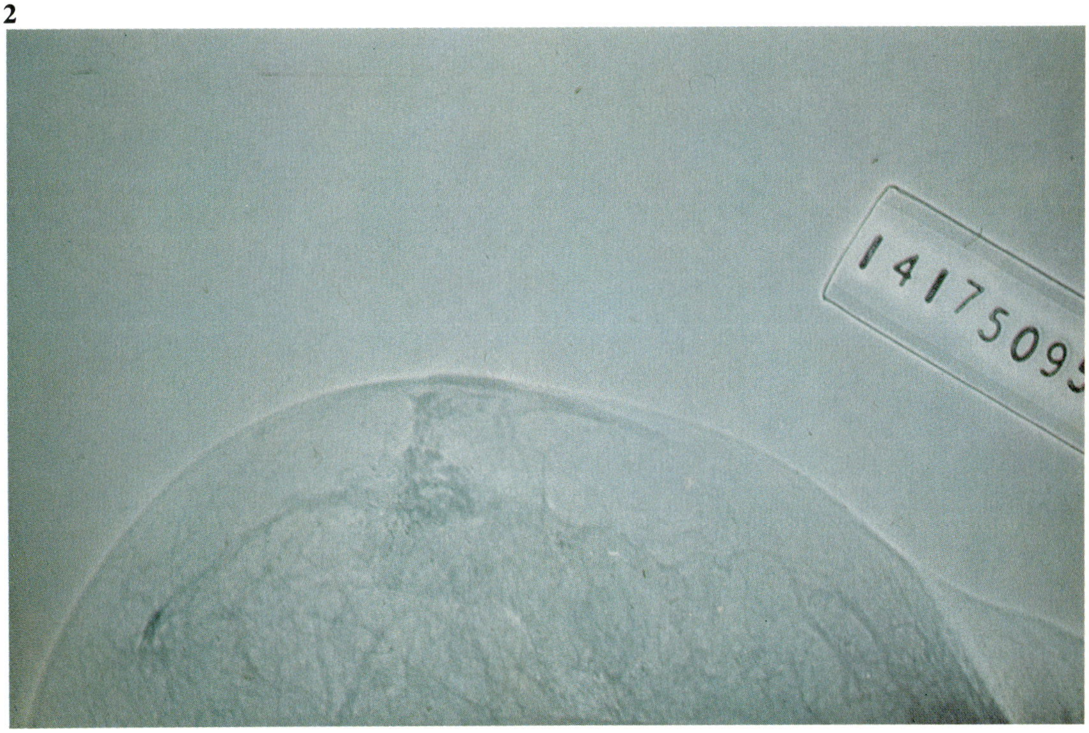

2 Mammogram showing the suspicious focus and the relationship of the contrast dye to it.

3

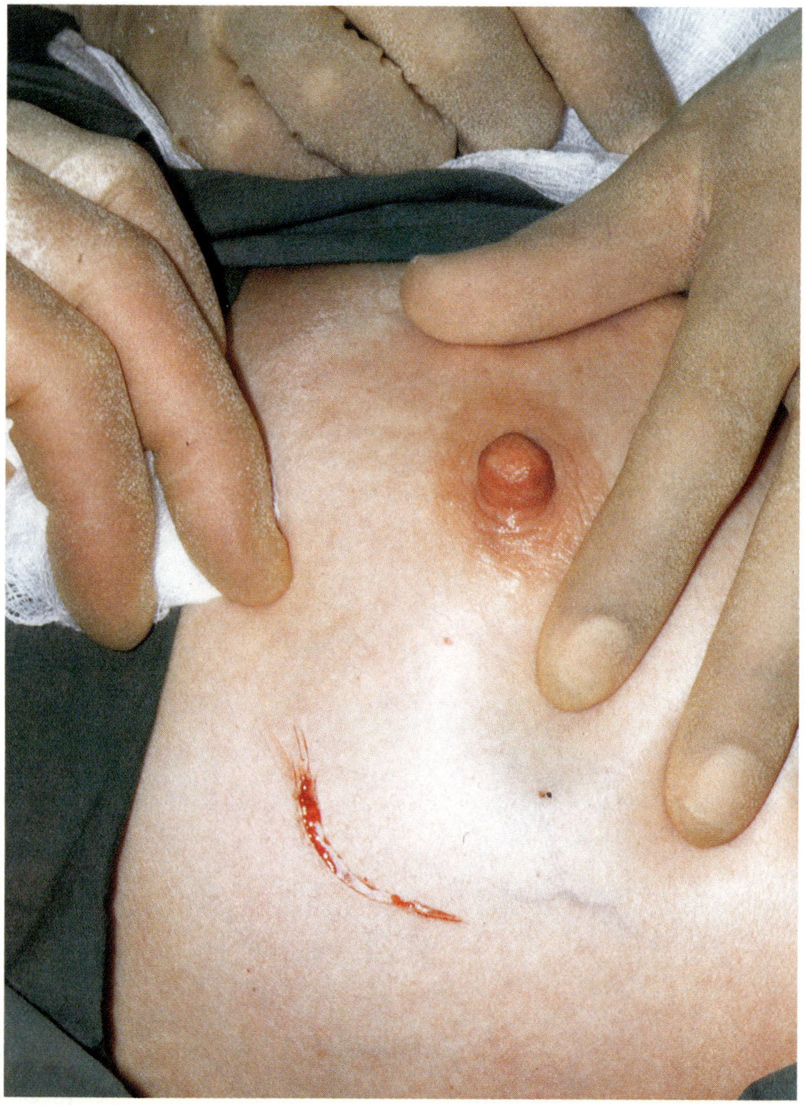

4

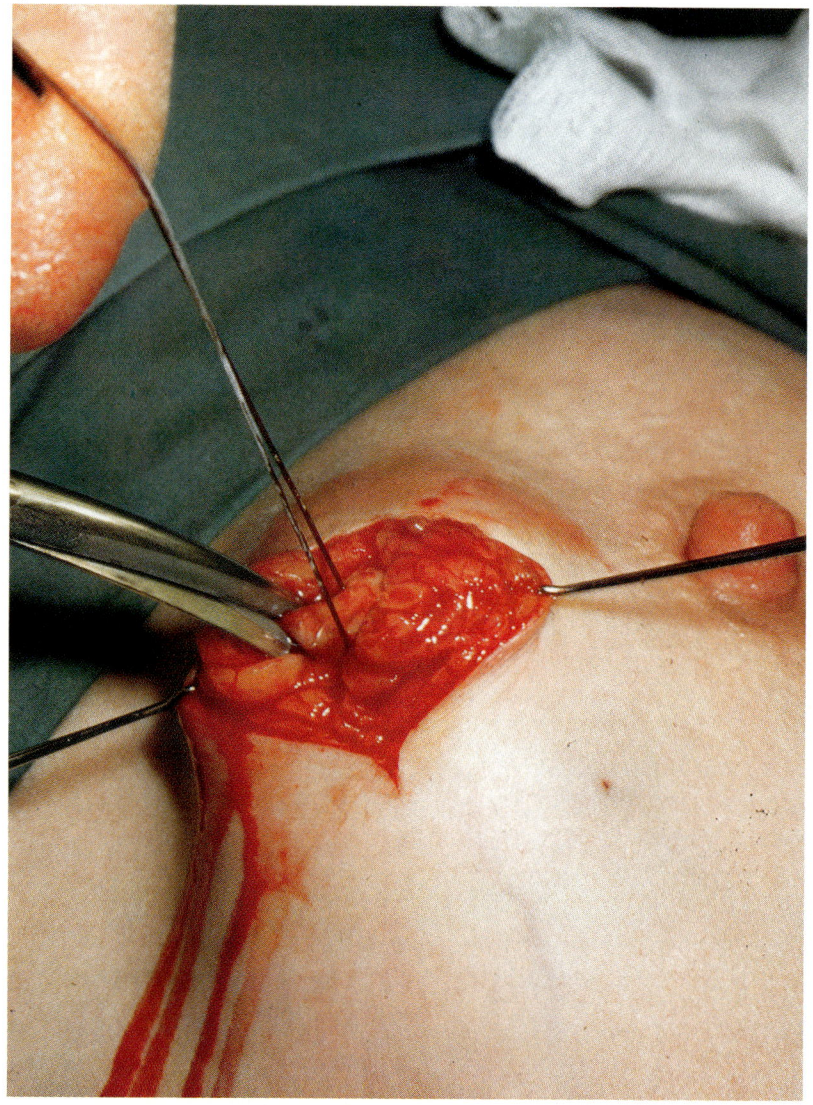

5

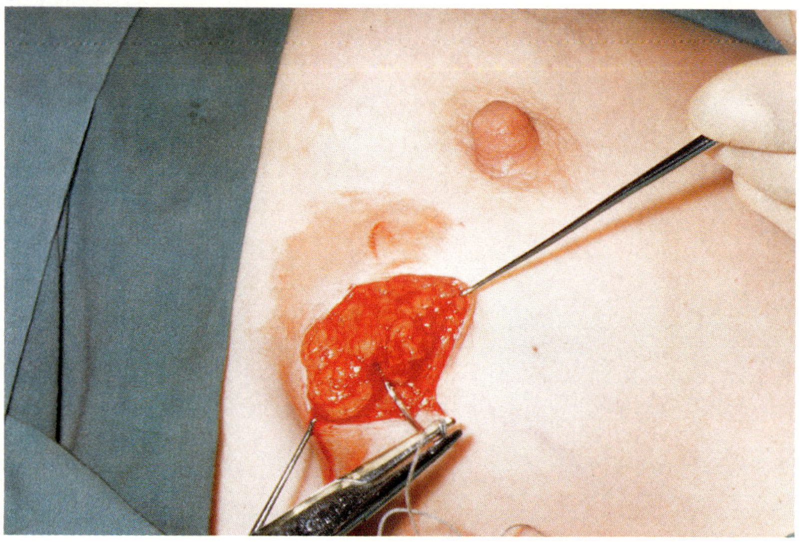

3 A skin crease incision is made with reference to needle puncture site, in a position giving best access to suspicious lesion.

4 After incision of the subcutaneous fat, the site of suspicion is transfixed with strong catgut on a large cutting needle.

5 By traction on the catgut the biopsy is dissected out with scissors.

6

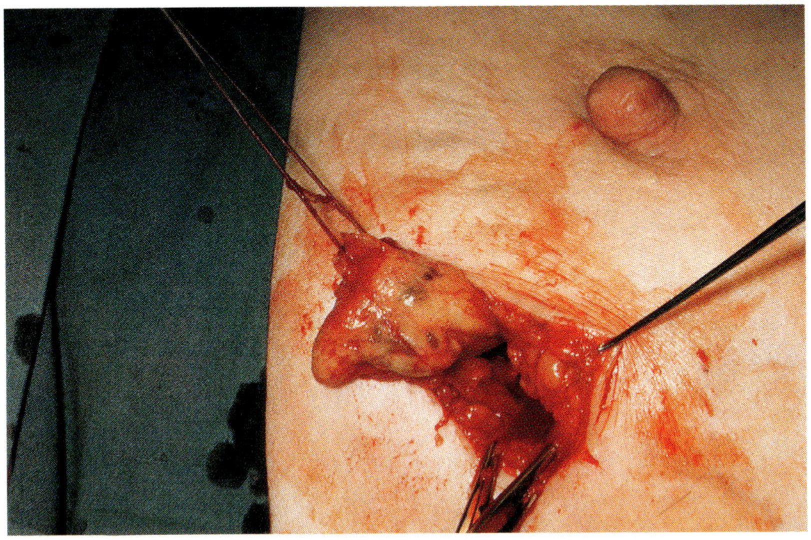

7

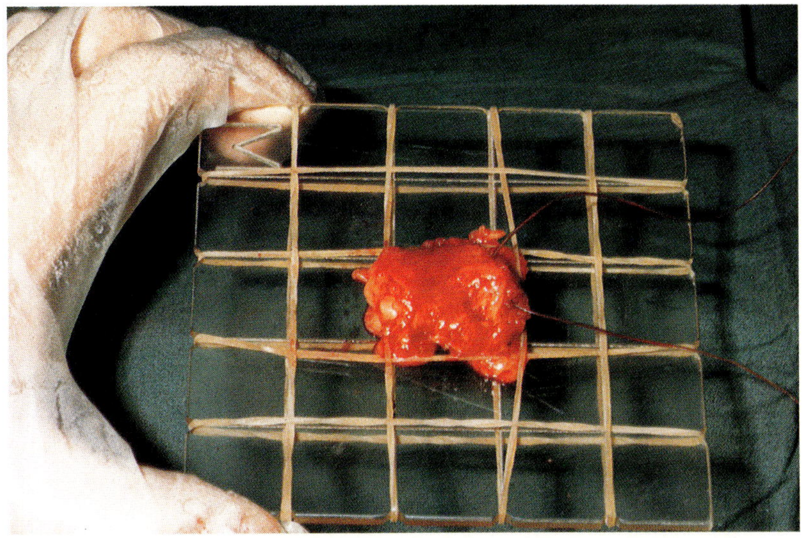

8

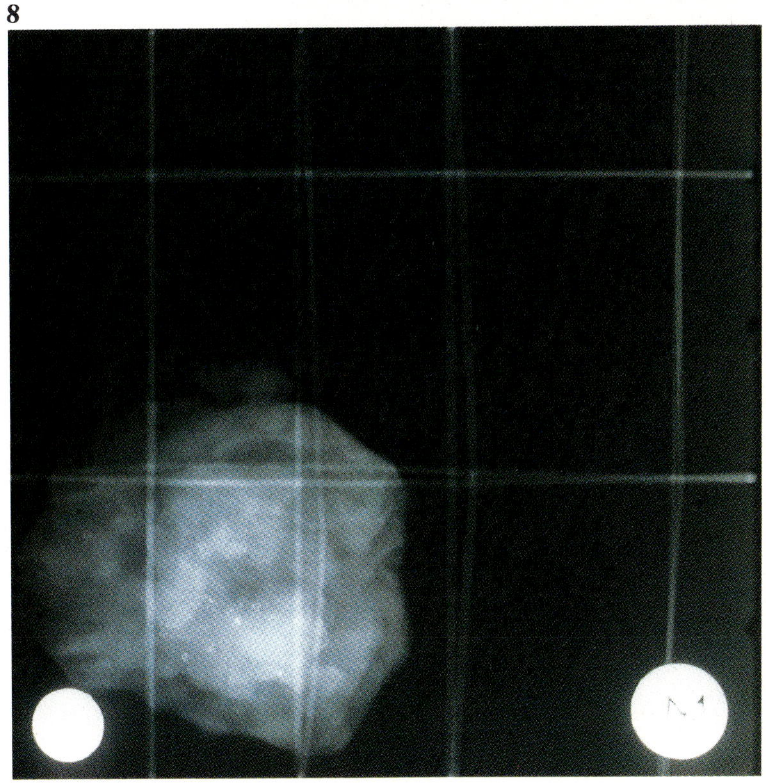

6 Haemostasis is performed before the biopsy is completely removed from the breast.

7 The excised specimen is mounted on a perspex grid for radiological examination to confirm that the suspicious focus has been removed.

8 Radiograph of the specimen, confirming to surgeon that biopsy was of correct tissue, and guiding pathologist as to where to make blocks.

Lower axillary clearance *without* mastectomy

1

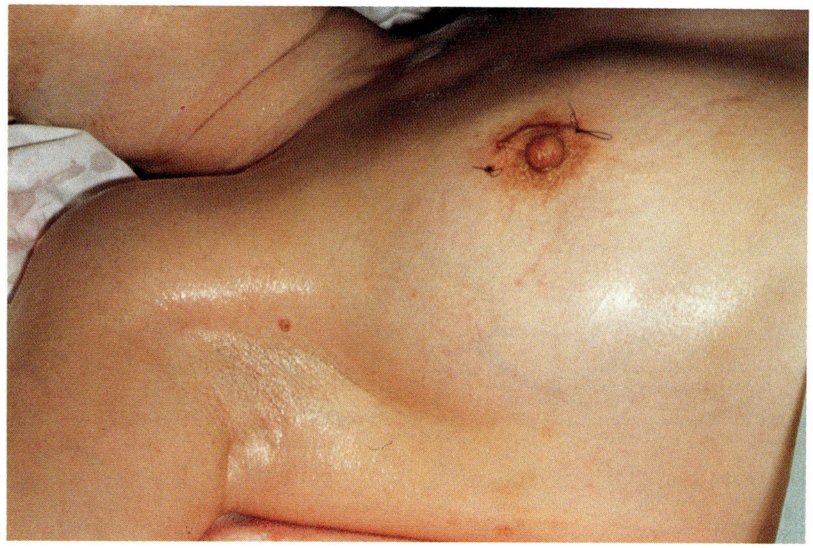

1 The patient lies supine on the operating table with the arm abducted.

2

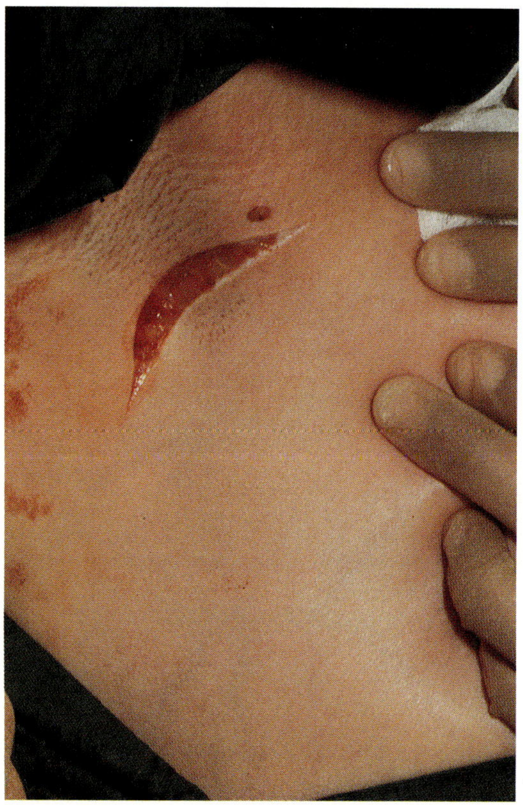

2 The incision is made in a skin crease across the 'floor' of the axilla.

3

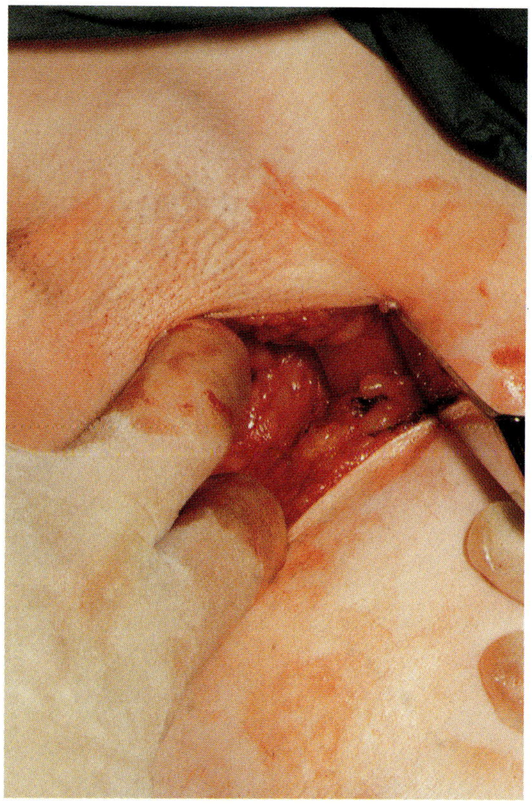

3 The lateral border of pectoralis major is identified and retracted medially with a large Langenbeck or small Morris retractor.

4

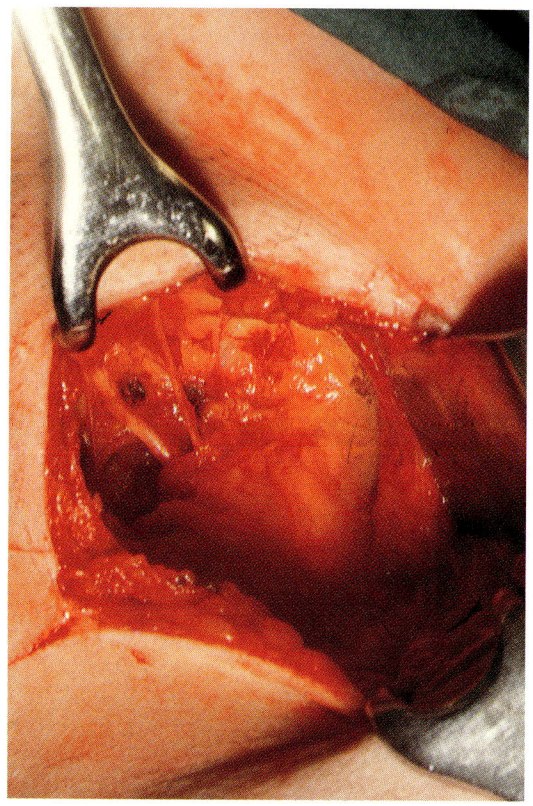

4 After division of the clavipectoral fascia, the axillary vein can usually be seen through the axillary fat.

5

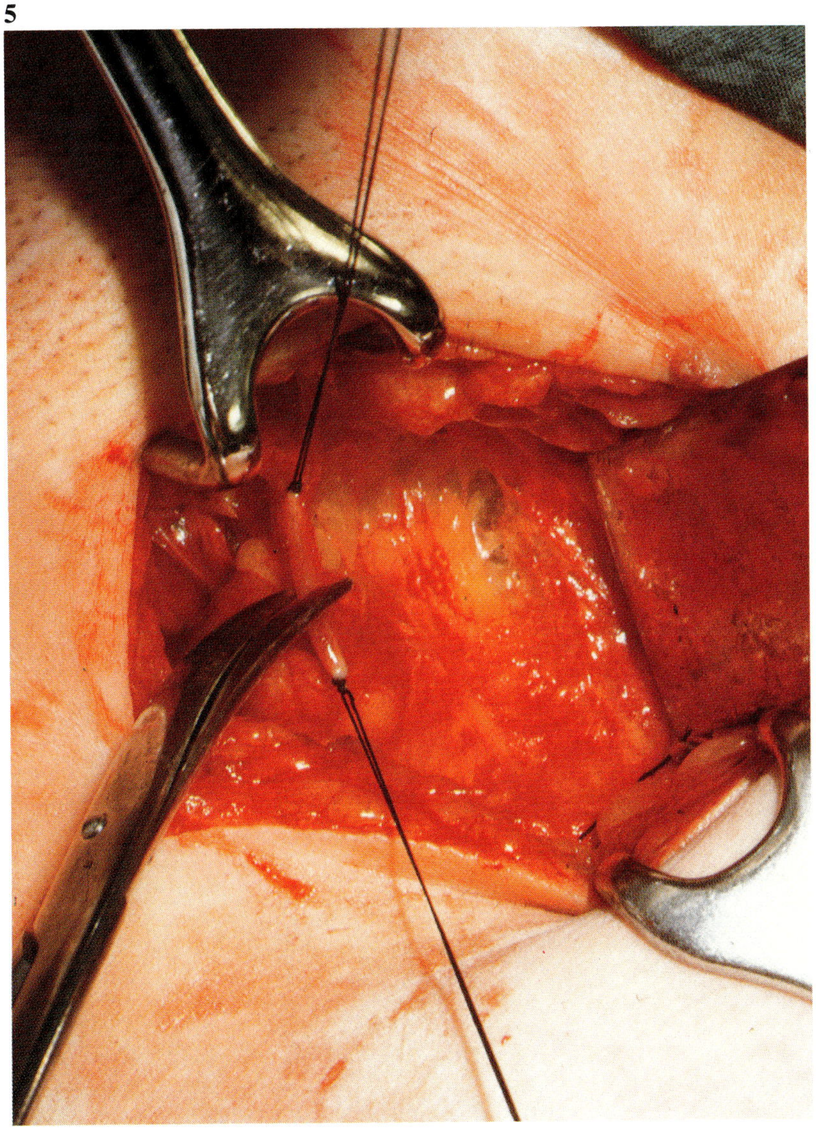

6

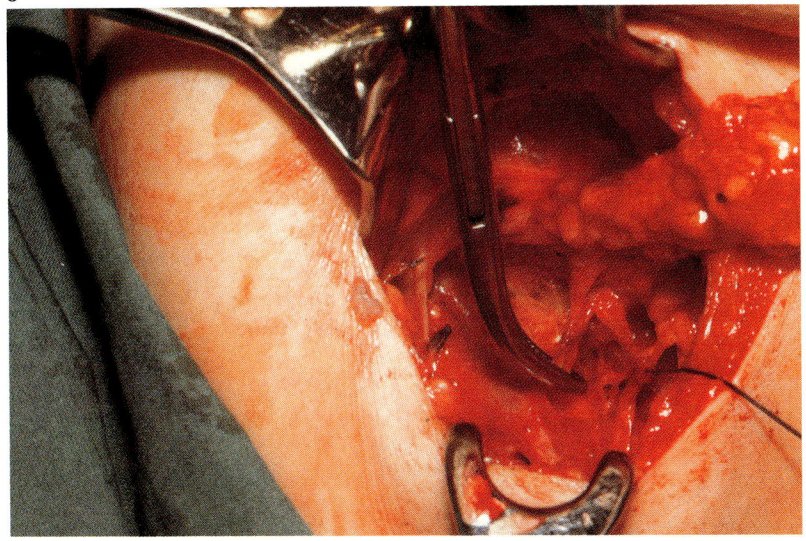

7

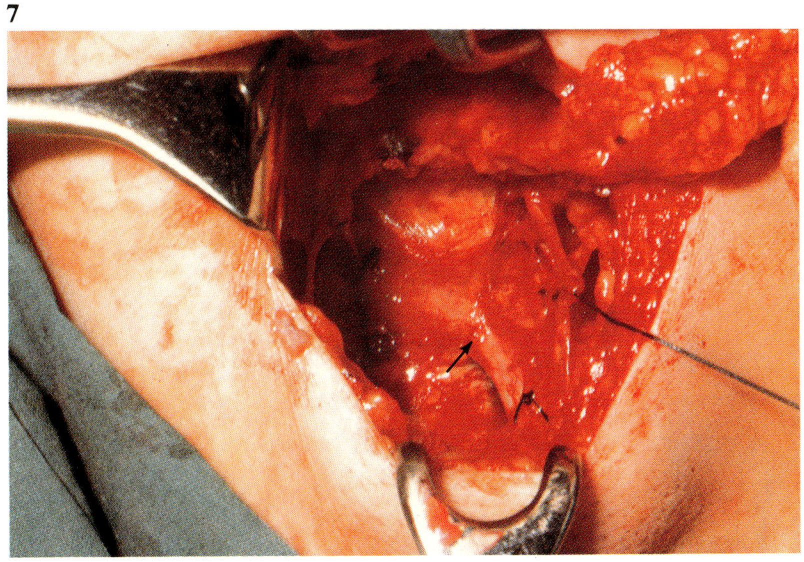

5 The tributaries of the axillary vein entering its inferior aspect are sequentially defined, ligated with fine braided non-absorbable ligatures and divided, with the exception of the *subscapular* which is preserved, with its nerve.

6 As the block of tissue is dissected out, the haemostasis of vessels away from the axillary vein can safely be done with diathermy.

7 As the axillary contents are cleared from the angle between the axillary vein and the lateral border of pectoralis minor, down the medial wall of the axilla, the *nerve (arrowed) to serratus anterior* will usually be seen and should be preserved to prevent winging of the scapula.

8

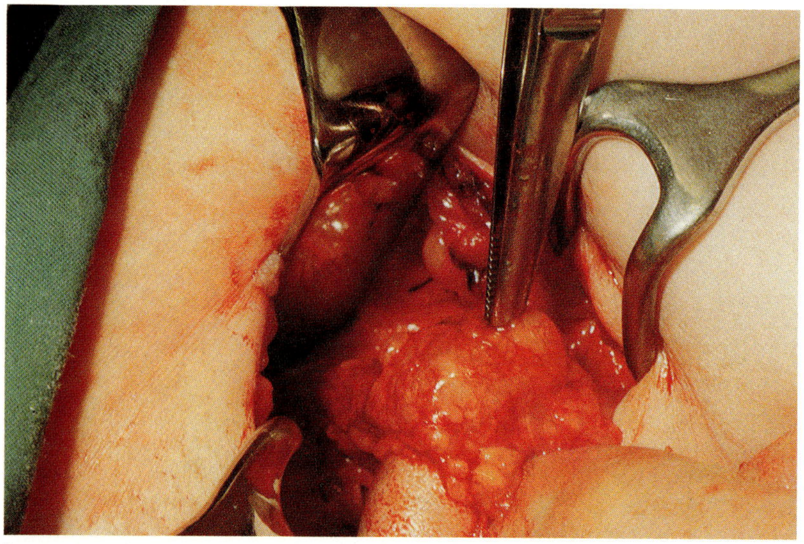

9

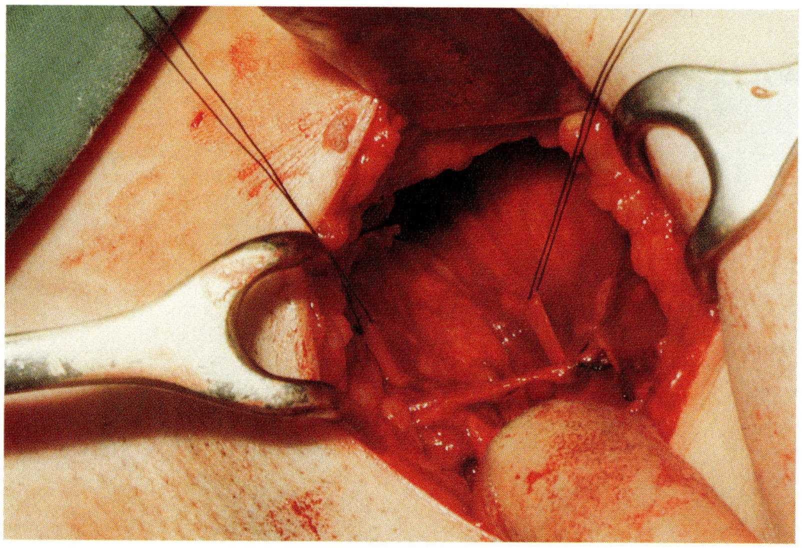

10

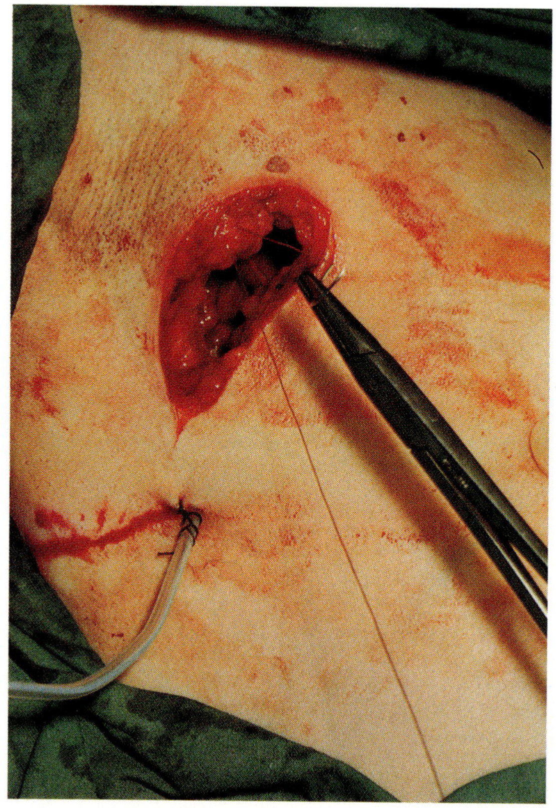

11

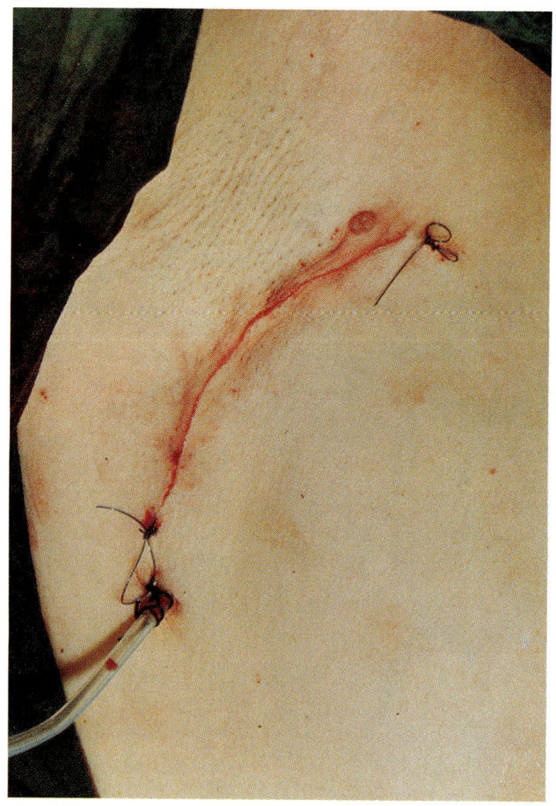

8 The lateral part of the dissection separates the axillary contents from the deep surface of the narrow, thin part of *latissimus dorsi* whose nerve reaches it on this surface and should be preserved. The muscle is often difficult to identify, although the fact that the dissection is medial to it is often confirmed by finding a plexus of veins which lie just medial to it.

9 The intercostobrachial nerve which supplies sensation to the medial side of the upper arm and skin of the upper lateral chest wall is always seen here running across the axilla. If the axillary contents can be removed without dividing this the patient is spared anaesthesia and hyperaesthesia of the territories it supplies, but its sacrifice, if essential, is not disabling.

10 A small suction drain reduces the formation of haematoma and seroma in the postoperative period. Interrupted catgut sutures to the subcutaneous fat refashion the floor of the axilla.

11 Subcuticular monofilament Prolene gives a neat and comfortable closure of the skin.

Palmar fasciectomy

The nodules of palmar fascia thickened by Dupuytren's disease in the elderly need removal if they are a nuisance to the patient. The exact indications vary widely with the individual.

The cause of contraction is unknown but there is a strong familial tendency especially in the male line. Usually, the ring and little fingers are affected first and the condition may spread to affect other parts of the palm and the other digits. There is great variation in the degree of affliction and in the scope of the surgery required for relief.

A limited fasciectomy is illustrated in the following pictures.

1

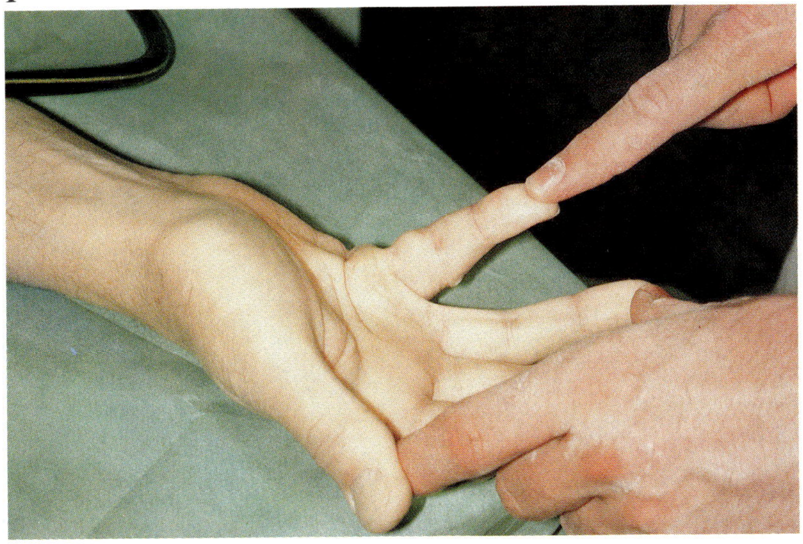

1 This patient's little and ring finger will not extend because of the contractions and thickening of the palmar fascia.

2 Any operation on Dupuytren tissue should be performed under a tourniquet so that the exact anatomy of the palm can be defined and no important structure damaged.

3 A lead hand is an essential tool for the operation to provide the necessary stability of the many joints in the operative field.

2

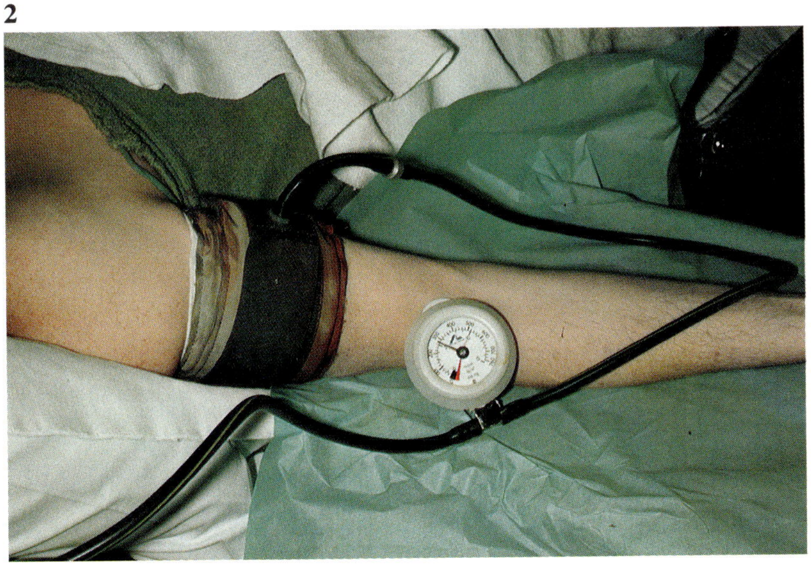

3

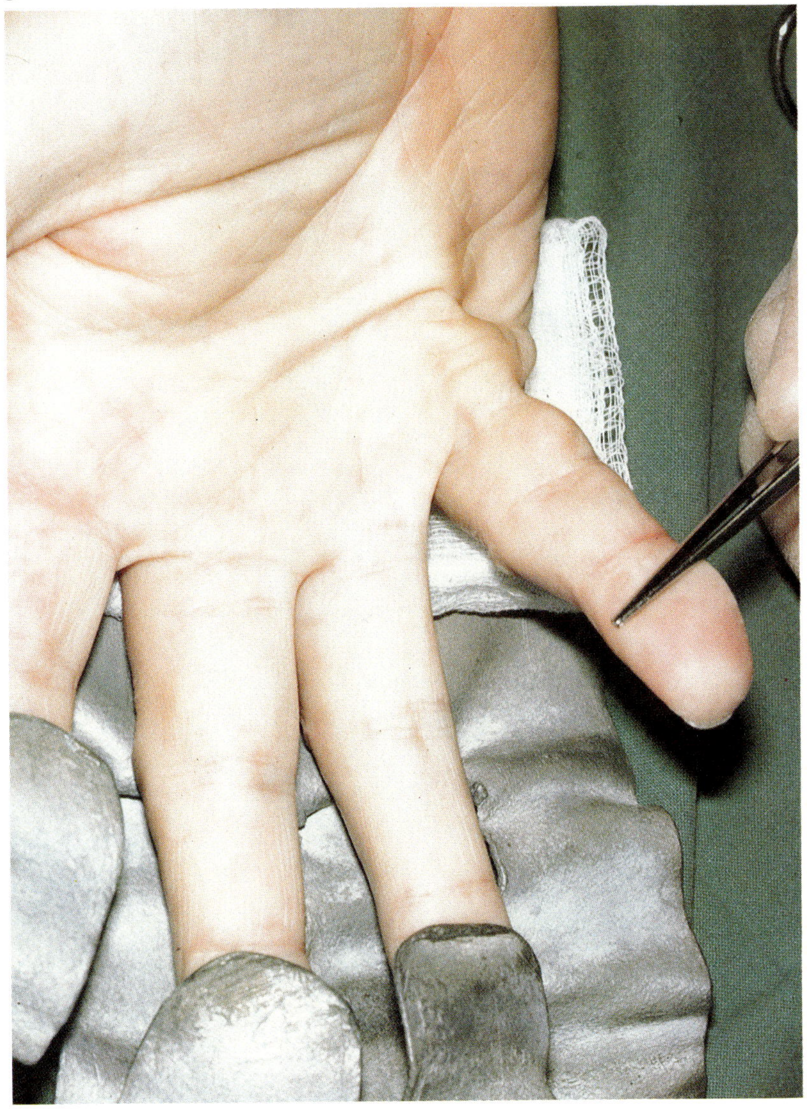

4

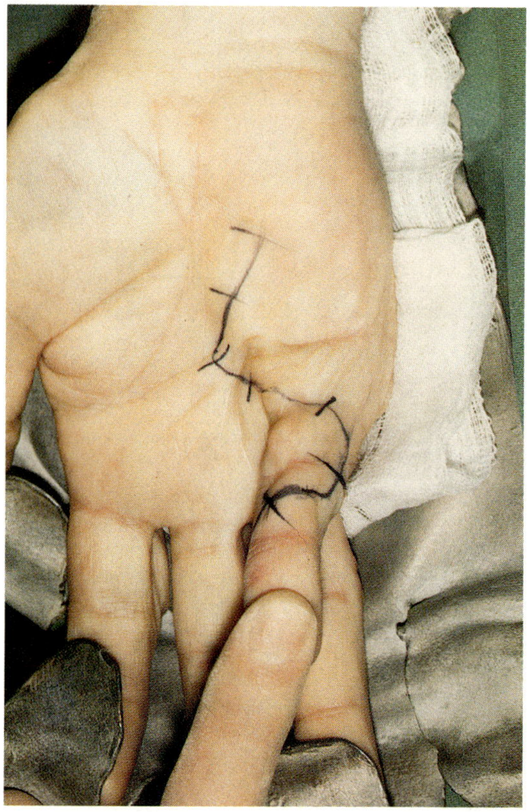

5

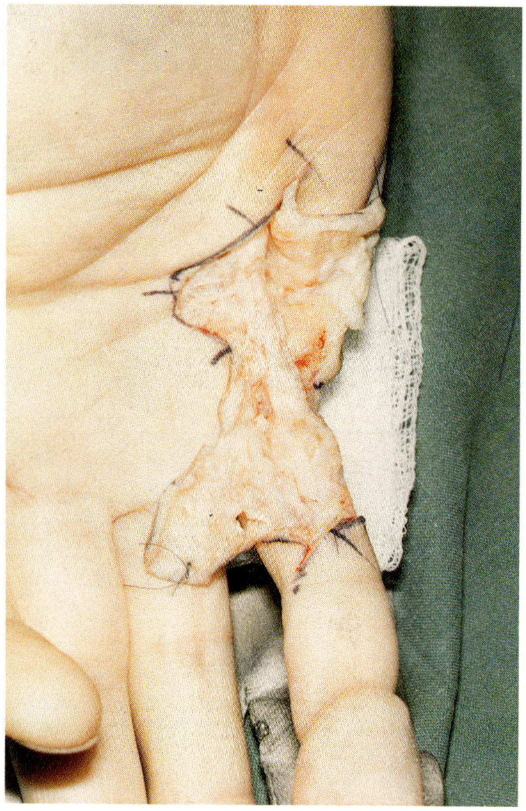

6

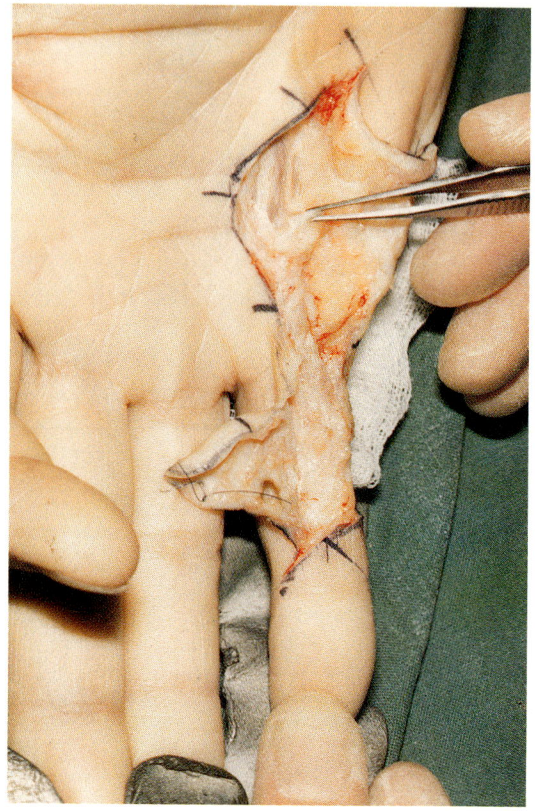

7

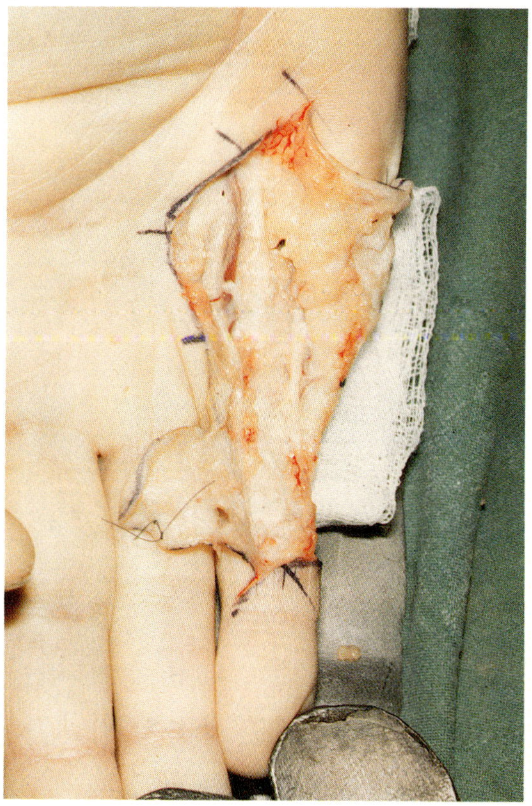

4 The skin incision is planned and then marked on the skin. The angles at the points of the flaps should not be less than 60° and longitudinal incisions in the line of the tendons should be avoided.

5 The skin flaps are raised carefully, the plane of dissection being just deep to the dermis. The contracted palmar fascia should be fully exposed.

6 The proximal limit of the Dupuytren disease is defined and the junction between normal and abnormal palmar fascia is divided transversely.

7 The abnormal palmar fascia is removed from the underlying neurovascular and tendinous structures by very careful dissection extending distally. The extensions of the thickened fascia which pass into the fingers are also removed. Particular care with the digital nerves and vessels is required alongside the phalanges.

8

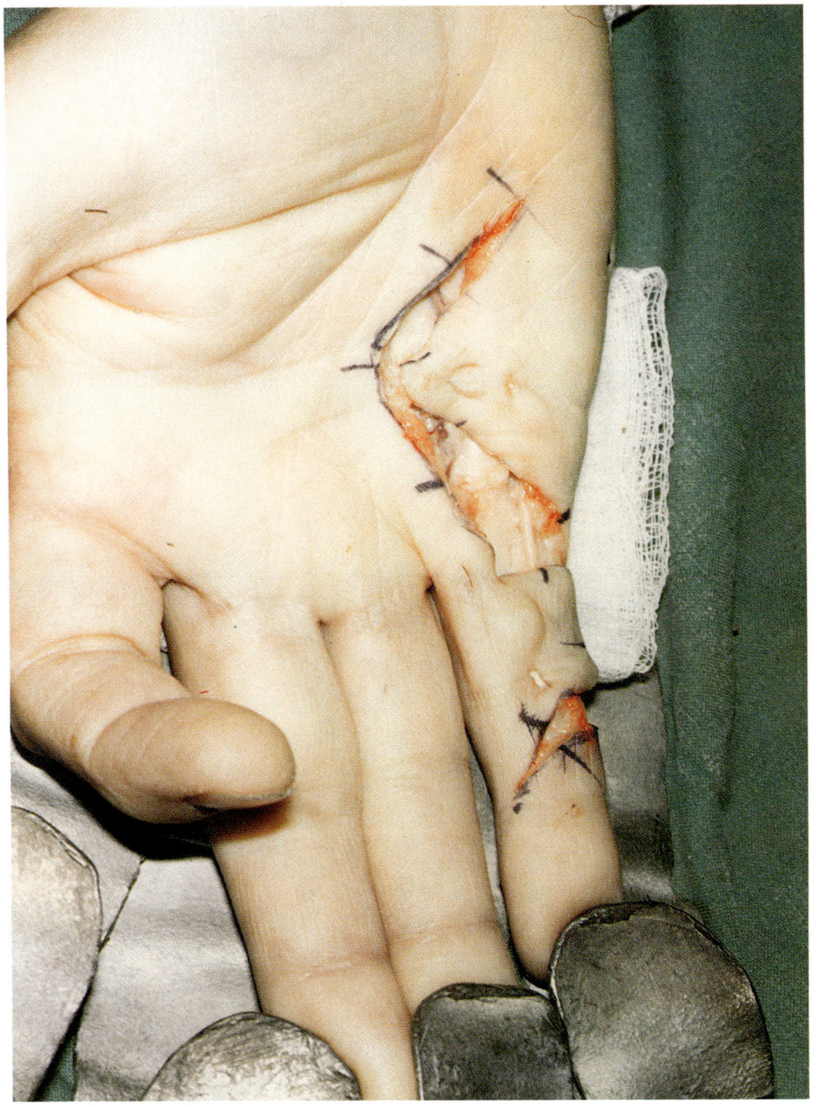

9

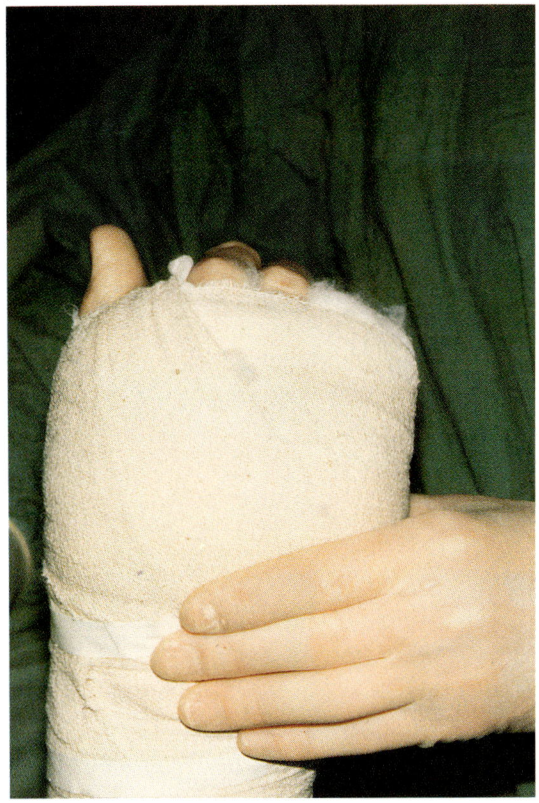

10

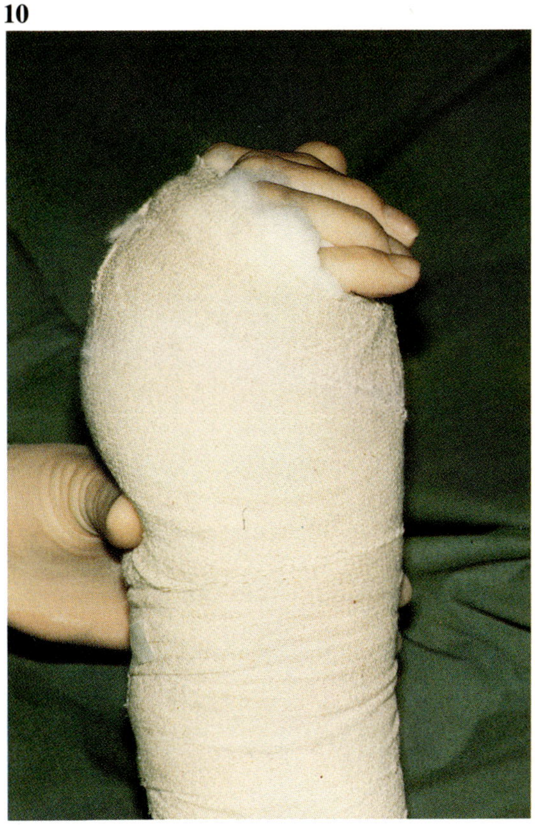

8 The skin flaps are sutured with wide loose stitches to avoid tension and possible necrosis at the points of the flaps.

9 Gauze or non-adherent dressings are laid over the wound and are held in place by a very bulky layered dressing of wool and crepe bandages. This gives light pressure on the wound and diminishes haematoma formation.

10 The bulky dressing should be carefully applied to hold the hand in the position of function. That is: the wrist is slightly dorsiflexed; the thumb is in opposition; the metacarpophalangeal joints are flexed to a right angle; the interphalangeal joints are extended.

The arm should be elevated for 24-48 hours to diminish swelling. The dressings can be reduced to a minimum at 10 days to allow vigorous active and passive movements of the digits.

De Quervain's stenosing tenovaginitis

This condition may be caused by non-suppurative tenosynovitis of the tendons of extensor pollicis brevis and abductor pollicis longus. There is thickening of the extensor retinaculum and there may be inflammatory changes in the tendon sheaths. Free fluid may also be present.

These changes lead to a tender swelling at the tip of the radial styloid with painful movements of the thumb [both passive and active]. The condition is most often seen in middle-aged women.

1 The operation is best performed under a tourniquet with regional or general anaesthesia. A 3 cm longitudinal incision over the tip of the radial styloid gives good exposure but a transverse incision heals with a less conspicuous scar. The local subcutaneous vein should be retracted as well as small branches of the radial nerve.

2 The extensor retinaculum is recognised deep to the subcutaneous fat. The tip of the radial styloid process is identified.

3 A longitudinal incision is made into the extensor retinaculum over the radial styloid and the underlying tendons visualised. The retinaculum can be 1-5 mm in thickness.

1

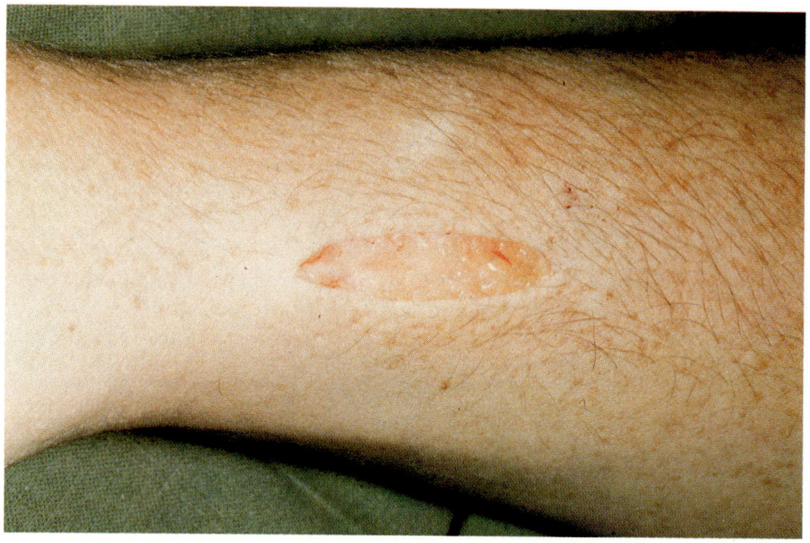

3

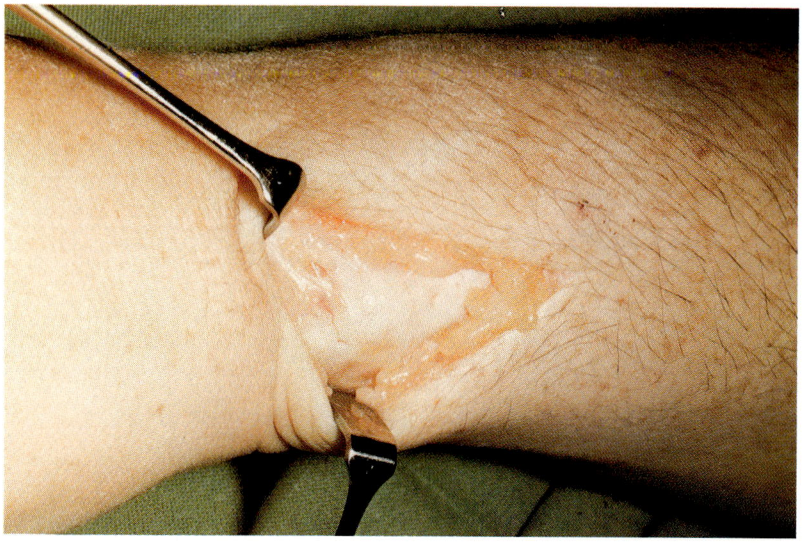

2

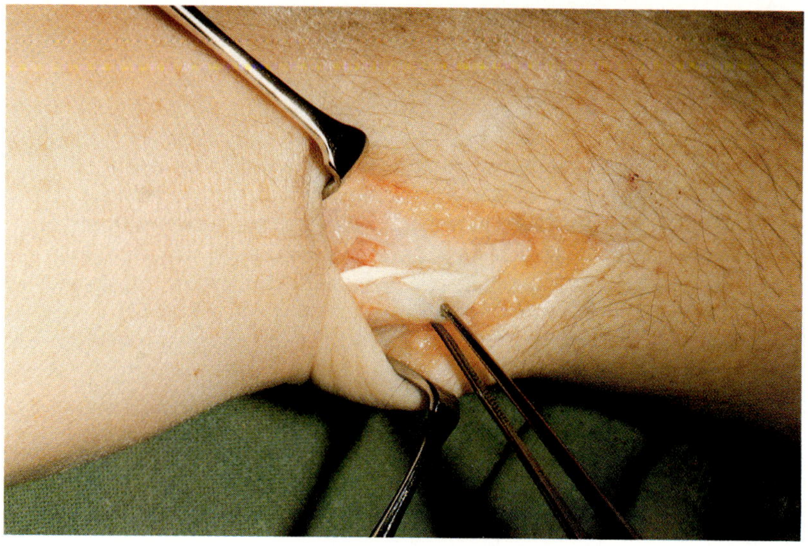

4 The tendons of extensor pollicis longus and abductor pollicis longus are identified. A third or fourth tendon may be found in this compartment of the extensor retinaculum as an anatomical variant.

If any fluid or inflamed synovium is found this can be cultured and biopsied. The retinaculum is not repaired but the fat and skin are closed in separate layers. A small padded dressing is applied. Full function is to be expected as soon as the wound has healed at 10-14 days.

4

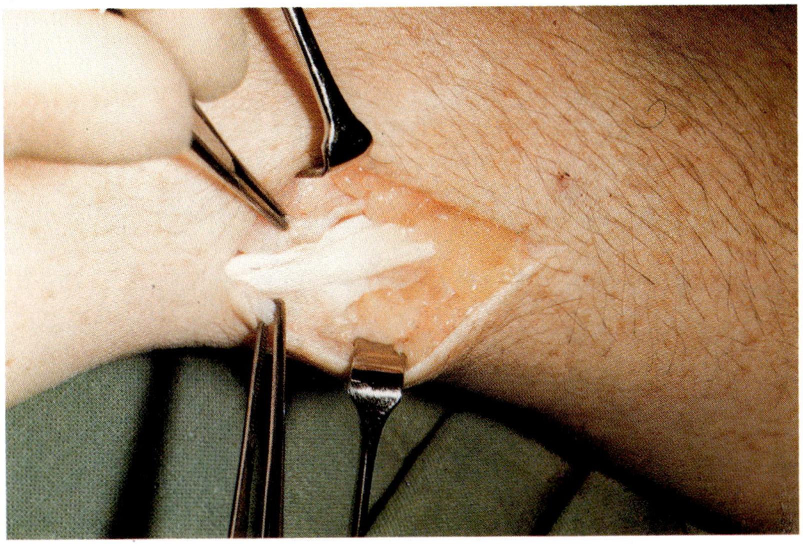

Removal of head of radius

This operation is indicated when a fracture of the radial head is likely to impede elbow movement or forearm rotation. It is commonly performed within a day or two of injury or else several weeks later after an unsuccessful trial of early active movements.

1

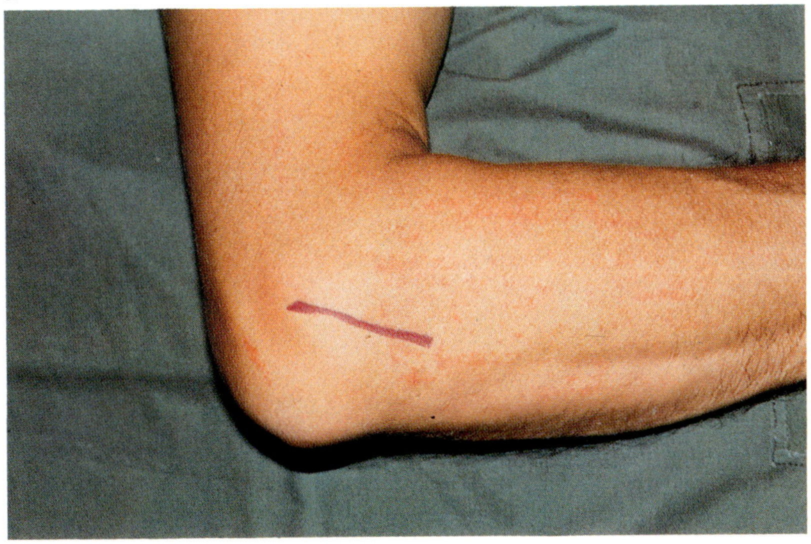

1 A tourniquet is used and a 10 cm incision is made on the outer side of the elbow extending distally from the lateral epicondyle and angled slightly posteriorly. The most convenient posture of the arm for the surgical approach is with the elbow flexed to a right angle and the arm lying across the chest.

2

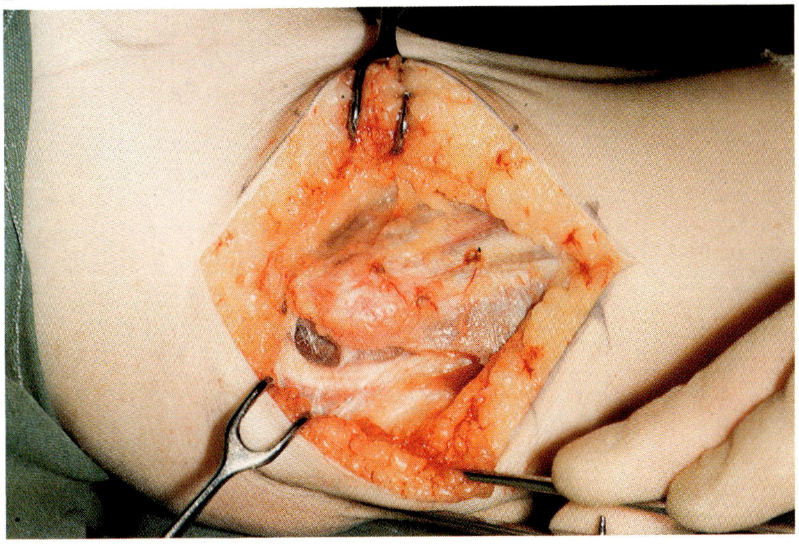

2 The incision is deepened through the subcutaneous fat to expose the deep fascia. At this level in the arm the radial nerve runs anterior to the elbow before passing posteriorly through the supinator muscle 2-3 cm distal to the neck of the radius.

3 An incision is made mid-laterally in the fibro-muscular tissue overlying the radial head. This should not extend more distally than the neck of the radius in order to preserve the radial nerve.

The head of the radius is then exposed. The fracture is usually obvious but the whole circumferential margin of the radial head can be examined by retracting the margins of the wound and fully pronating and supinating the forearm.

3

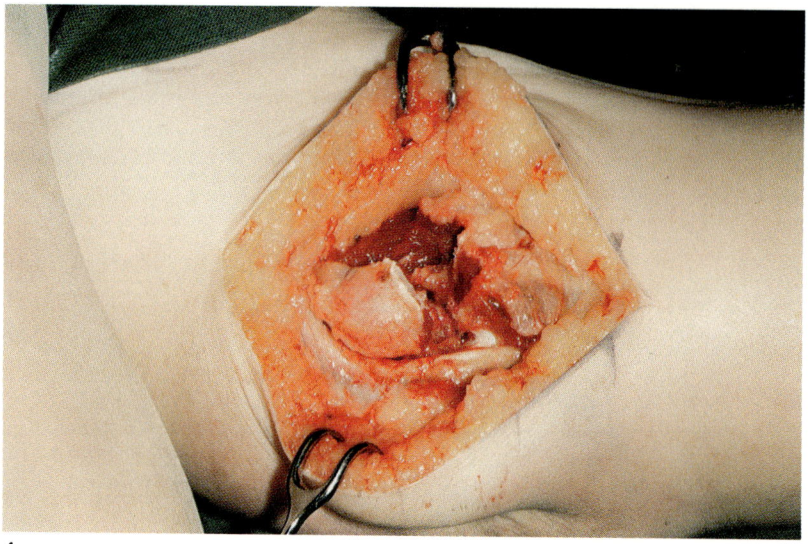

4 The fragments of the radial head can be picked out of the wound. If the neck of the radius requires division this can be performed by a power saw, or by the careful use of a small thin osteotome. The line of division is perpendicular to the axis of the radial shaft.

If a saw or oestotome is not required due to the fracture line in the radial neck being in a suitable plane, the raw surface can be made smooth.

The interior of the elbow joint is inspected to make sure that no fragments of the radial head are left behind. If in doubt the available fragments are assembled on a swab to check for missing segments.

4

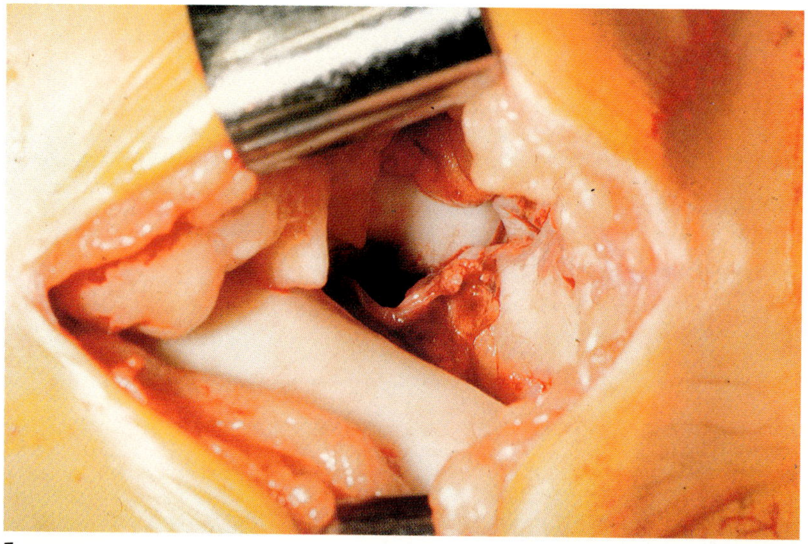

5 The wound is closed by absorbable sutures to the deep tissues. The skin is closed by interrupted sutures with or without sterile adhesive tapes. A wool and crepe compression bandage is applied with the elbow flexed to 90°. The torniquet is released and a triangular sling applied.

The skin stitches are removed at 10 days and the compression bandage reduced. Thereafter the patient is encouraged to perform regular active exercise to regain movements. Rotation exercises for the forearm are particularly important.

5

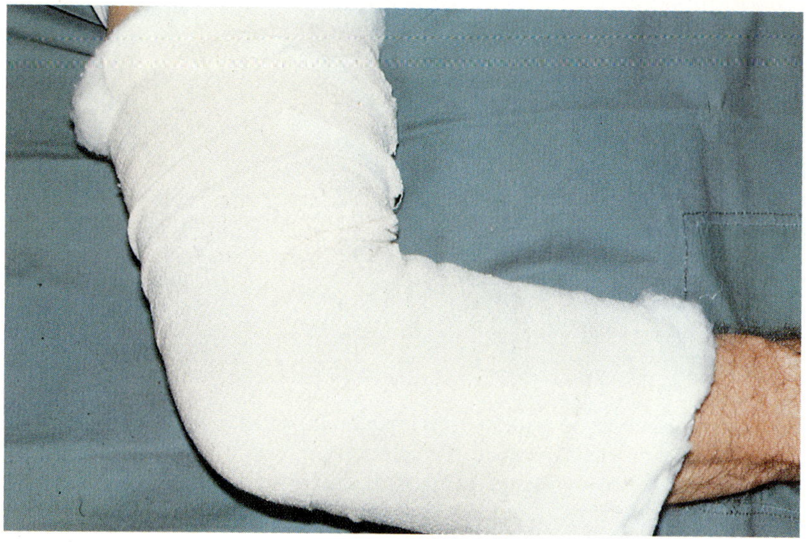

Bunionectomy

This operation can be performed with or without a tourniquet, but as most bunions are removed from older people there are advantages in avoiding tourniquets for fear of provoking vascular damage in the thigh or calf. Local or general anaesthesia can be used, preferably the latter.

The bunion may reform after 10 or 20 years from continued irritation of the patient's shoes.

If the foot is ischaemic the need for surgery should be reassessed. Specially made shoes may be a better option.

1

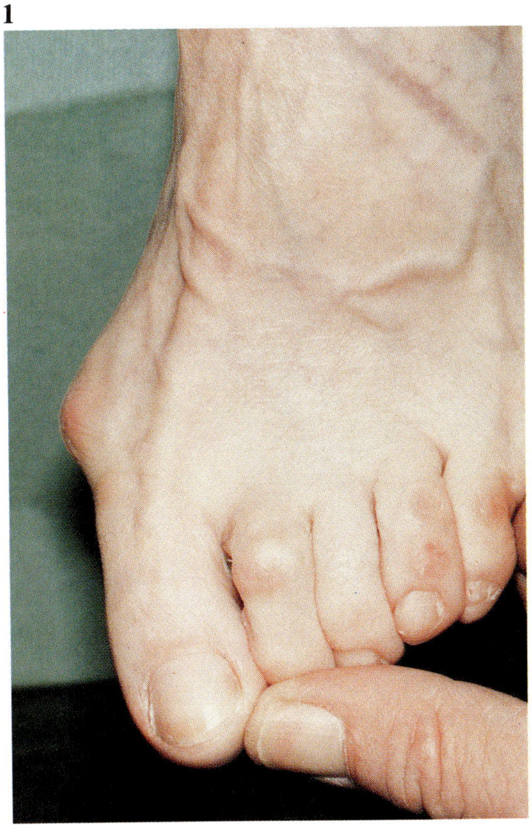

1 This bunion is not particularly large but the patient had difficulty in finding suitable shoes. Exclude ischaemic disease before operating.

2

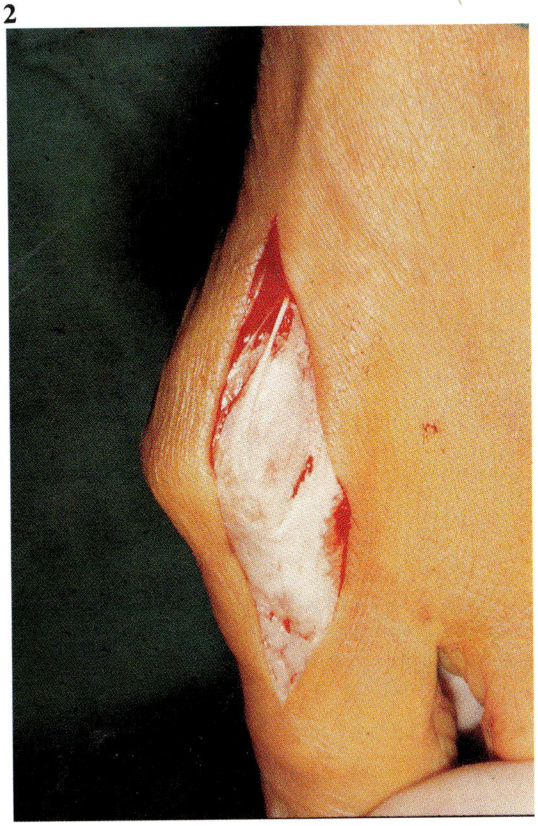

2 The longitudinal incision lies dorsomedially over the 1st metatarsophalangeal joint. This position of the scar minimises pressure from the shoes in the postoperative period.

Bleeding is diminished by the patient being tipped slightly head down to empty the leg veins, and by the assistant forcibly flexing the big toe. The dorsomedial cutaneous nerve should be avoided.

3

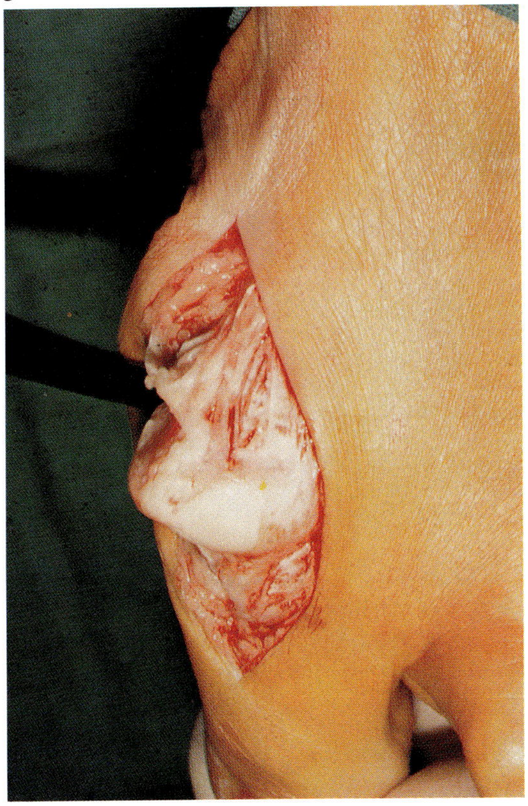

3 Further dissection close to the medial side of the 1st metatarsal head will fully expose the exostosis by detaching the medial ligament of the 1st metatarsophalangeal joint. The tendon of extensor hallucis longus must be protected on the lateral side of the wound. The demarcation between normal articular cartilage and the exostosis is usually obvious as this is a groove.

4

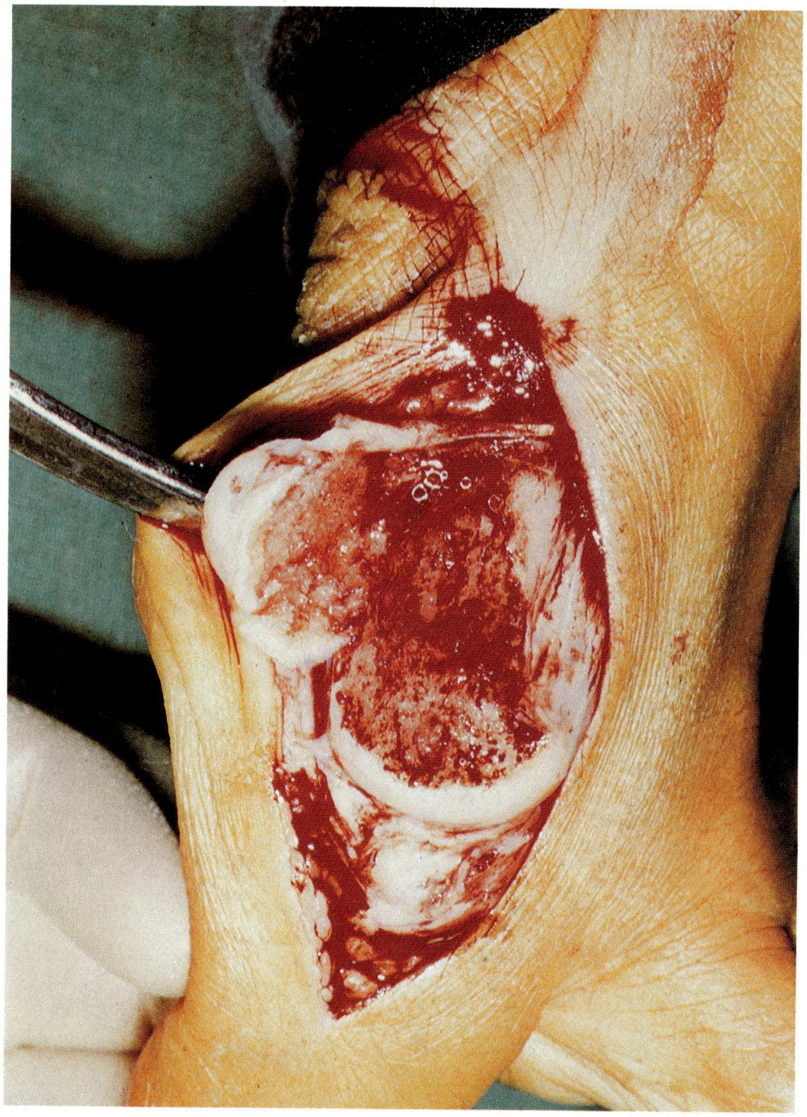

5

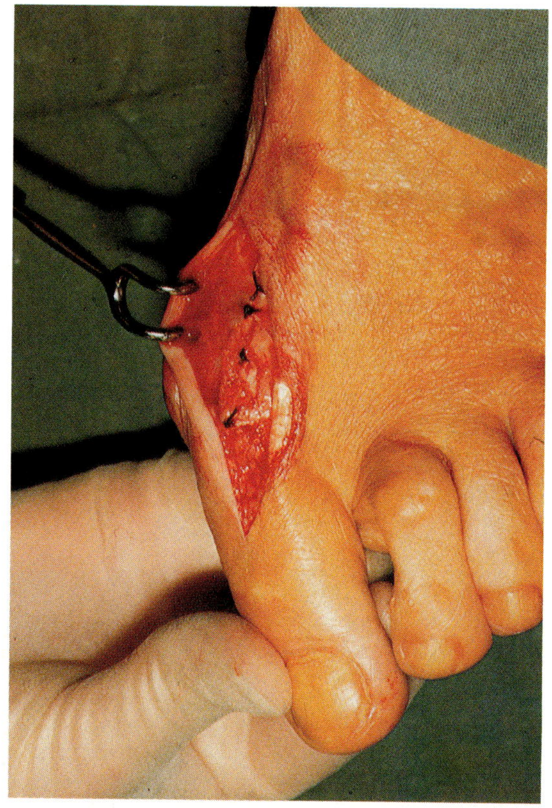

6

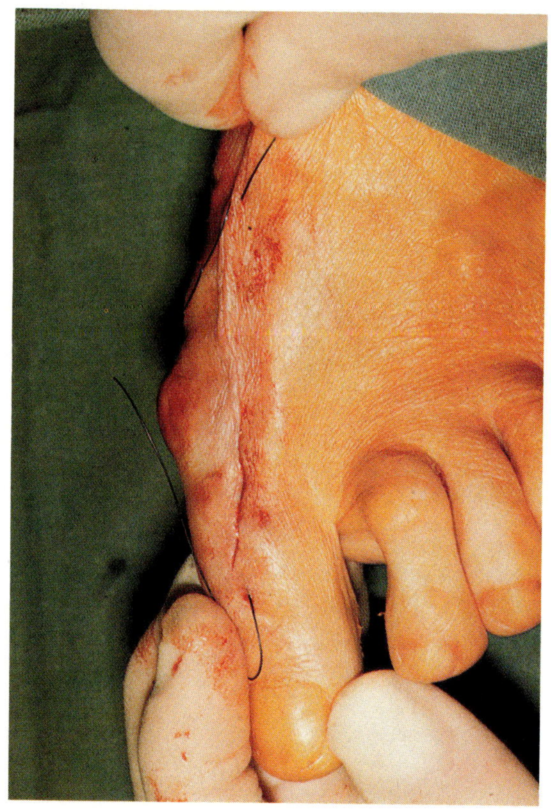

4 A bone lever can be inserted between the soft tissues and the flexor surface of the first metatarsal head. This acts as an efficient retractor.

An osteotome has been used to remove the greater part of the exostosis but the sharp edges must be removed separately as they can be very irritating to the patient if left behind.

5 The soft tissues are closed by catgut. A wide variety of methods are advocated for repairing the medial capsule of the 1st metatarsophalangeal joint but these are of doubtful value.

6 A subcuticular nylon suture has been used to close the skin. The suture line can be reinforced by sterile adhesive tapes.

7

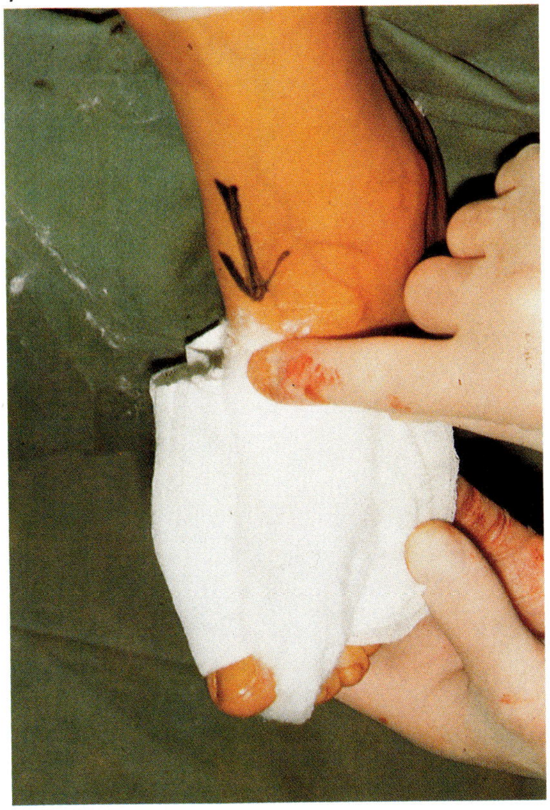

7 Gauze dressings have been applied to the wound and a strip of wool has been placed between the first and second toes to correct any valgus inclination of the big toe during the healing phase.

8

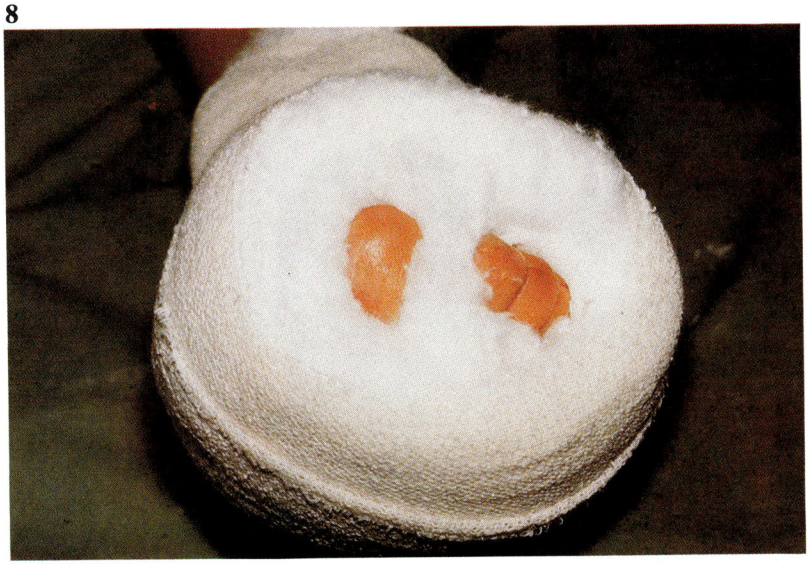

8 Plenty of wool is wrapped around the forefoot and is held by a firm crepe bandage. This diminishes the formation of a wound haematoma and provides protection for the forefoot.

The patient can stand on her heel after 24 hours but should keep the foot elevated in bed or on a chair for long periods while healing takes place over the next 10 days. Postoperative swelling persists for a few weeks so that capacious shoes or slippers are needed until the foot is slim enough to fit into normal shoes.

Keller's arthroplasty

This operation is used to relieve the combined effects of a bunion and valgus deviation of the big toe. It can also be used for hallux rigidus. It shortens the big toe as well as straightening it.

An immediate secondary effect is to cause the patient to lose flexion and extension of the big toe for a few weeks until the tendons have shortened.

Many surgeons have their own individual variation in the performance of the operation but whatever is done deformities of the big toe are likely to recur after 10 years or so.

1

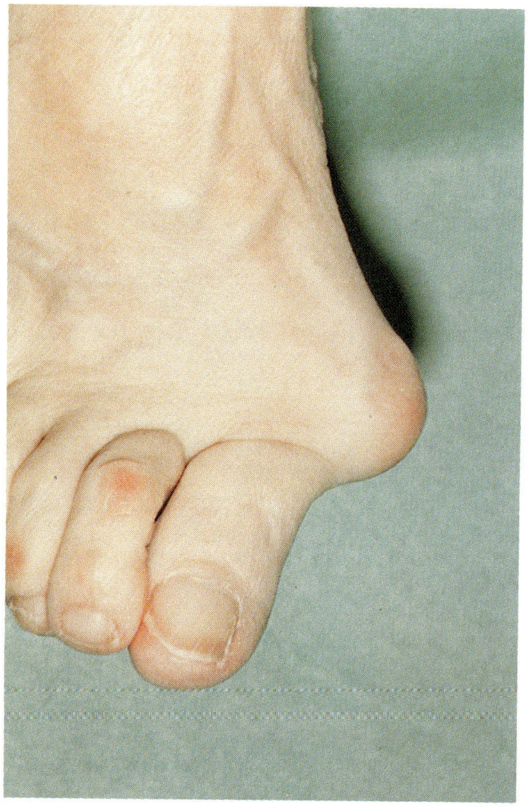

1 This patient has a hallux valgus and a bunion. There is a lateral subluxation of the big toe at the 1st metatarsophalangeal joint.

2

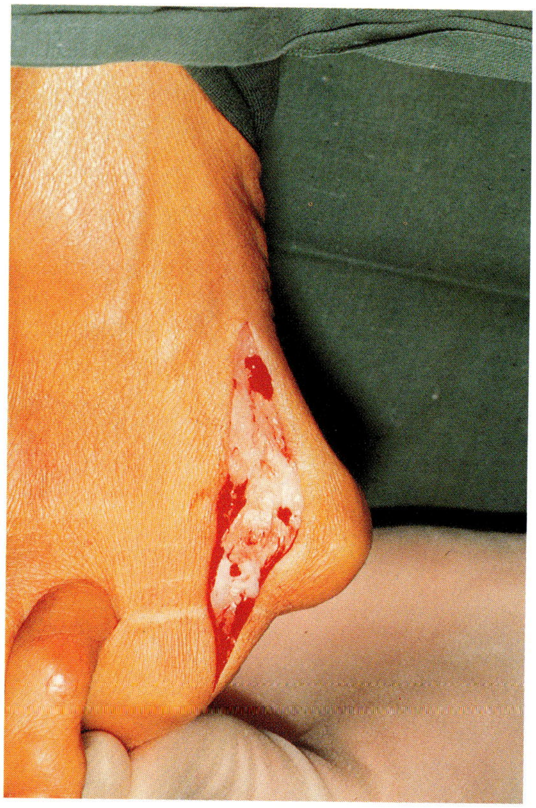

2 A tourniquet is not necessary if the anaesthetist empties the leg vein by tipping the patient slightly head down. A dorsomedial incision minimises pressure pain from shoes in the recovery period.

3

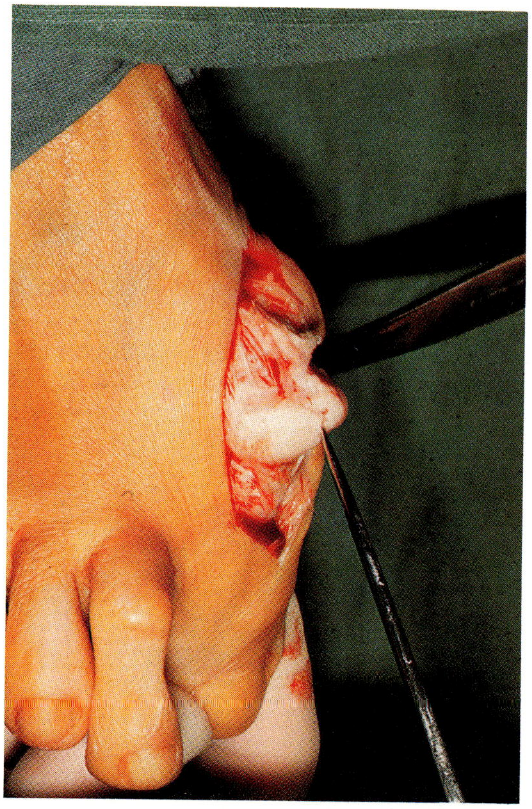

3 The tendon of extensor hallucis longus has bowstrung laterally across the deformed joint, but must be protected if seen in the course of dissection. The dorsomedial cutaneous nerve must also be preserved. The soft tissues are stripped from the 1st metatarsal head as one layer.

4

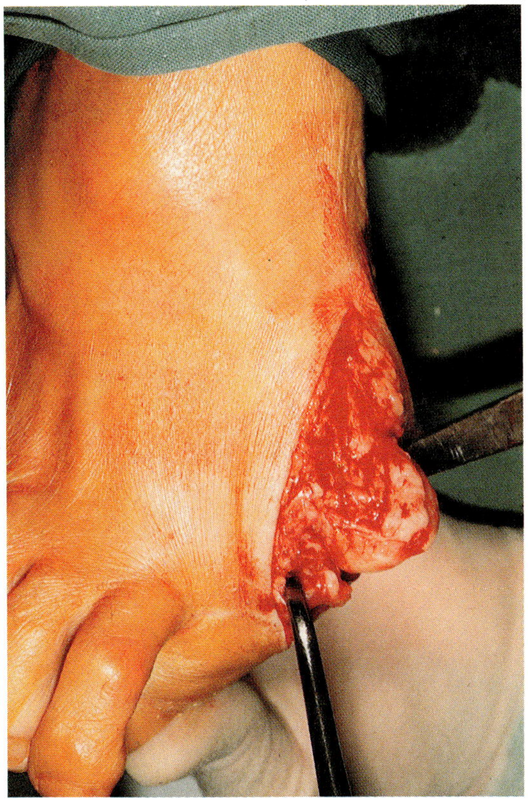

5

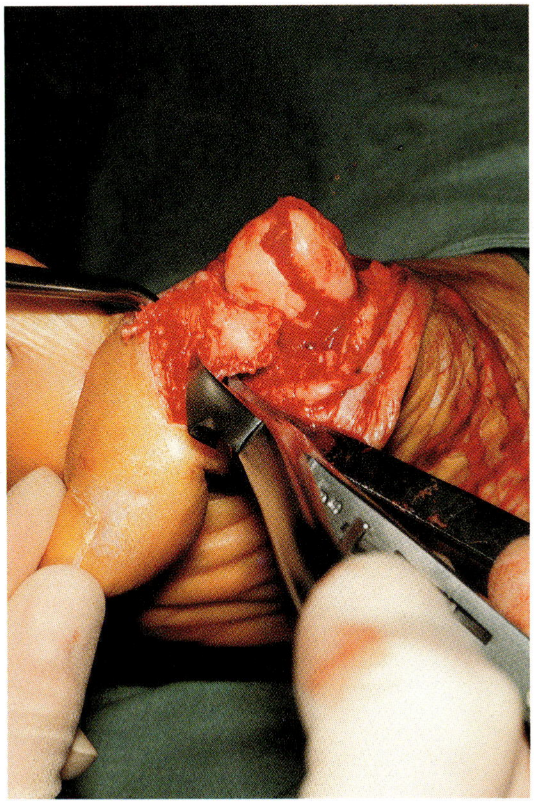

6

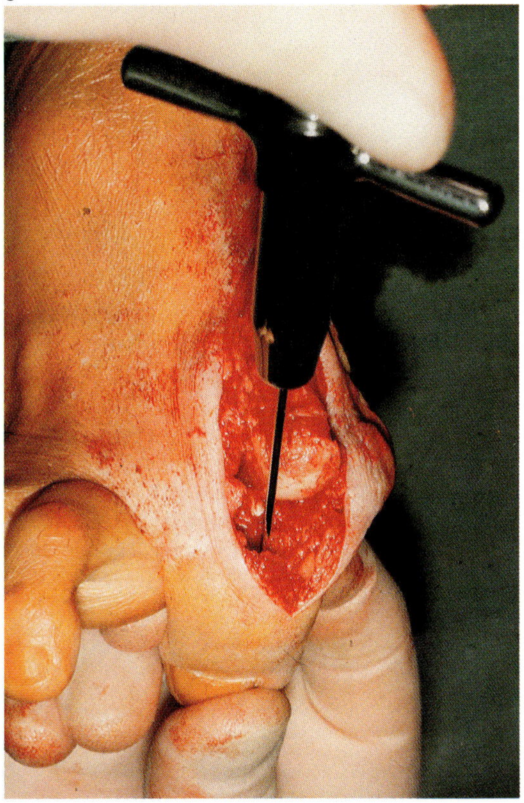

7

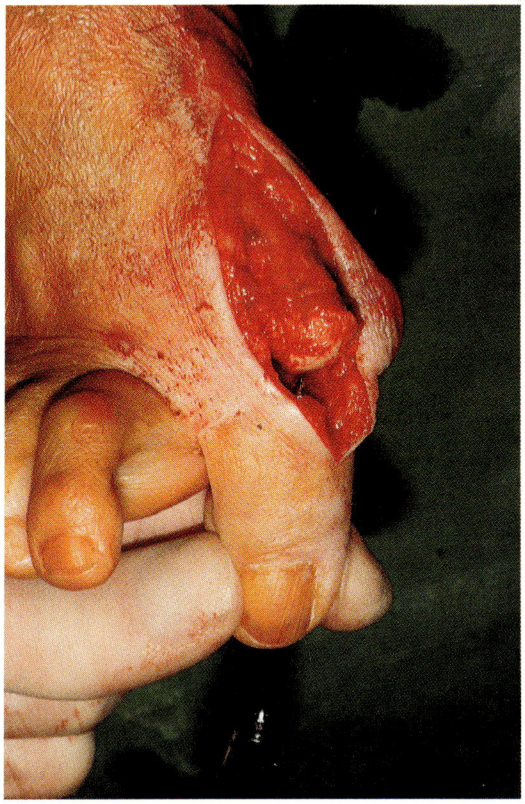

4 The exostosis of the 1st metatarsal head is removed by an osteotome. The sharp edges left on the superomedial and inferomedial margins are smoothed off.

5 The base of the proximal phalanx is stripped of the flexor and extensor tendons by sharp dissection close to the bone. By forcible flexion from the assistant the base of the proximal phalanx is elevated into the wound and can be severed by a saw or bone cutter. One third or two thirds of the proximal phalanx is removed and the sharp edges smoothed.

6 A short stout wire is used as a splint for two weeks to allow the soft tissues to heal with the big toe in a straight position. The wire is introduced into the centre of the proximal phalanx by pushing it distally from the freshly cut surface through the interphalangeal joint and through the terminal phalanx.

7 The wire holder is changed to the protruding distal tip of the wire which is then thrust proximally into the head of the first metatarsal with the big toe held in an anatomical position.

8

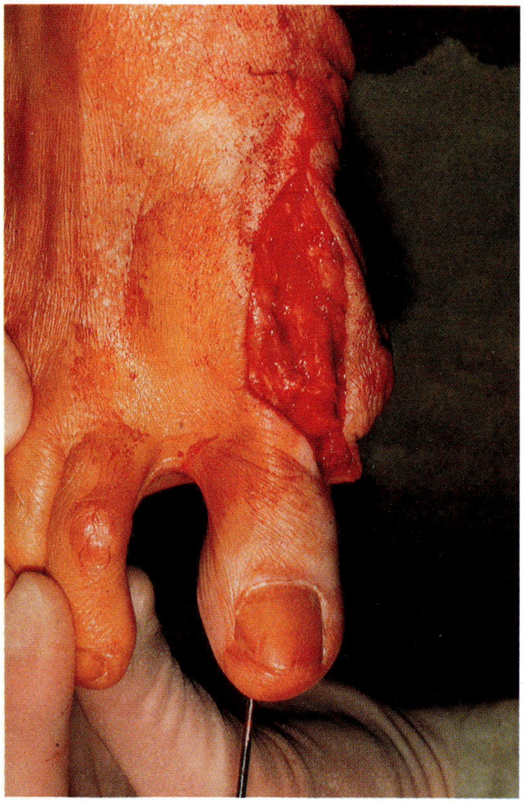

8 The big toe is telescoped on the wire to close the gap created by the removal of the proximal phalanx.

9

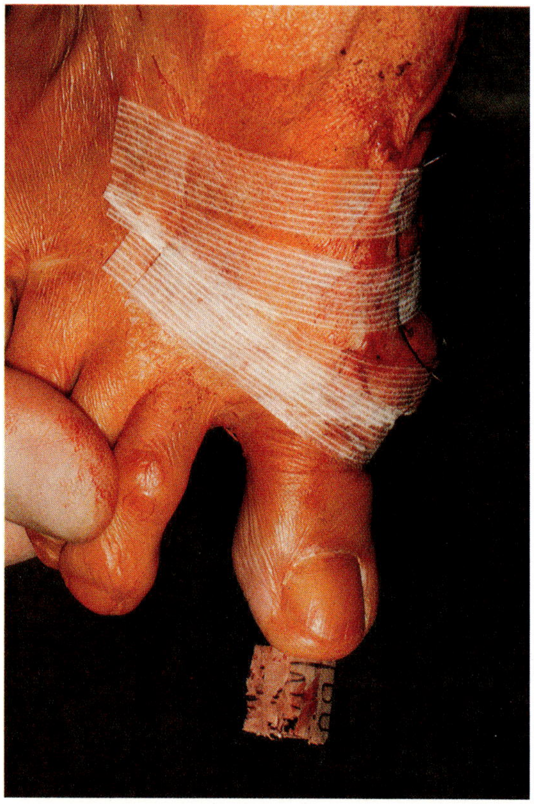

9 The soft tissues are closed by catgut and the skin by silk sutures with or without sterile adhesive tapes. The protruding tip of the wire at the end of the terminal phalanx is covered by a piece of cork or rubber.

10

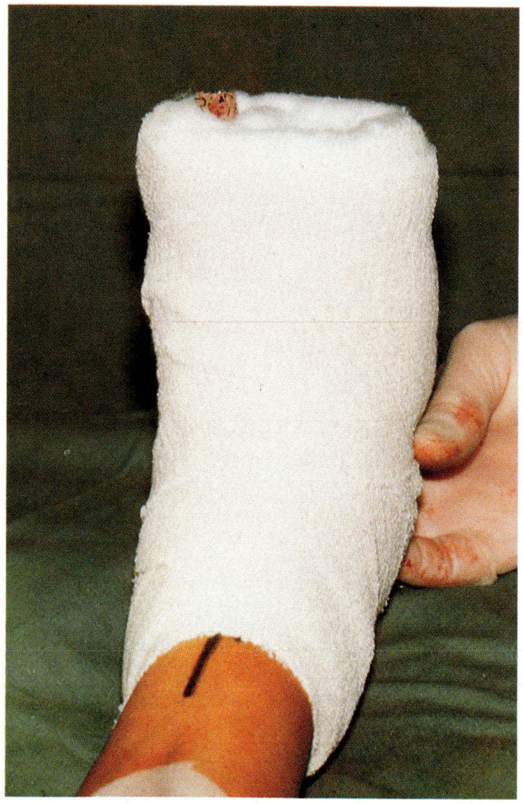

10 The foot is protected by a thick dressing of gauze, wool and crepe. The skin stitches can be removed at 10 or 12 days and the dressings reduced. The central wire can be removed two to four weeks after operation and the patient allowed to regain passive and active movement at the metatarsophalangeal joint.

Wide shoes or slippers are required for up to four weeks postoperatively.

Ingrowing toe nail

This can be a very troublesome problem in young people. Various techniques have been employed with variable success. These vary from wedge excision of the nail plus excision of granulation tissue, to excision of whole nail and nail bed or phenolisation of the latter. Local anaesthetic is satisfactory.

1

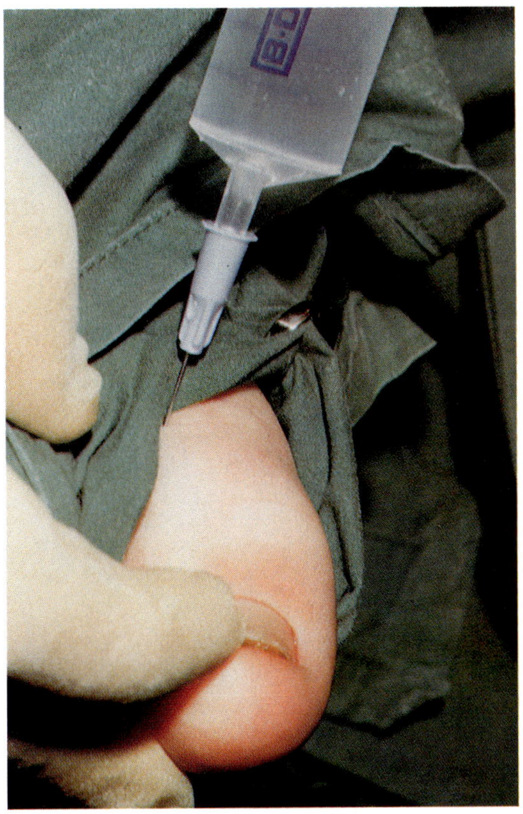

1 Excision of nail and nail bed – Zadik. Local anaesthetic using 1 per cent lignocaine is injected into the base of the toe on either side, aiming for the nerves running along the middle of the side of the toe. **Local anaesthetic should also be injected across the dorsum of the toe as a few branches pass along the top of the digit and anaesthesia will otherwise be incomplete. No adrenaline should be used as it may cause ischaemia of the toe.**

2

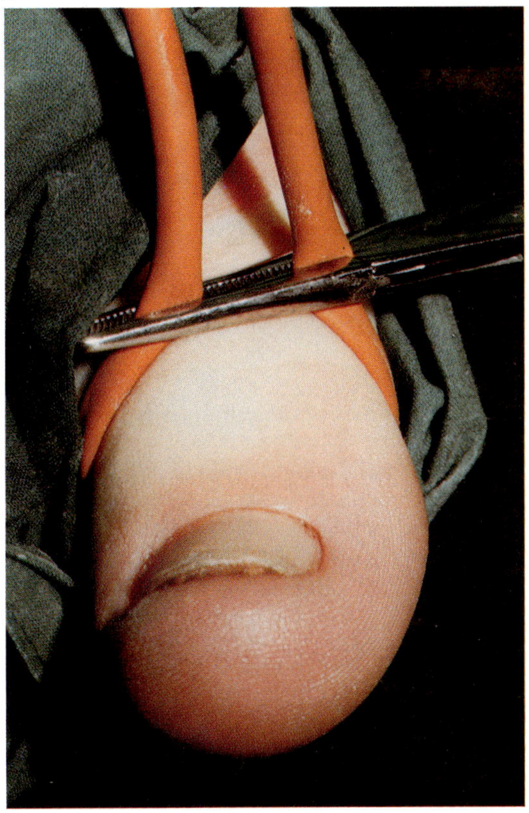

2 A simple tourniquet will allow a clear dissection of the distal tissues.

3

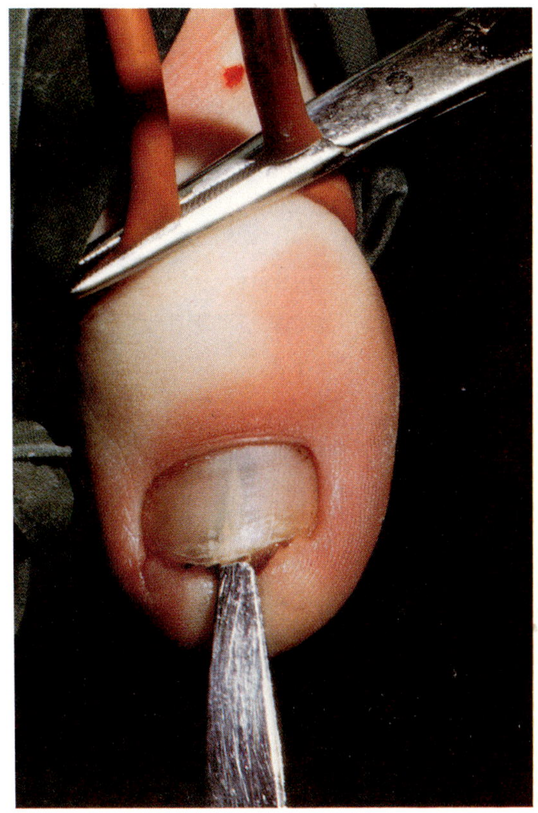

3 The nail is separated from the nail bed by the blade of scissors or flat instrument.

4

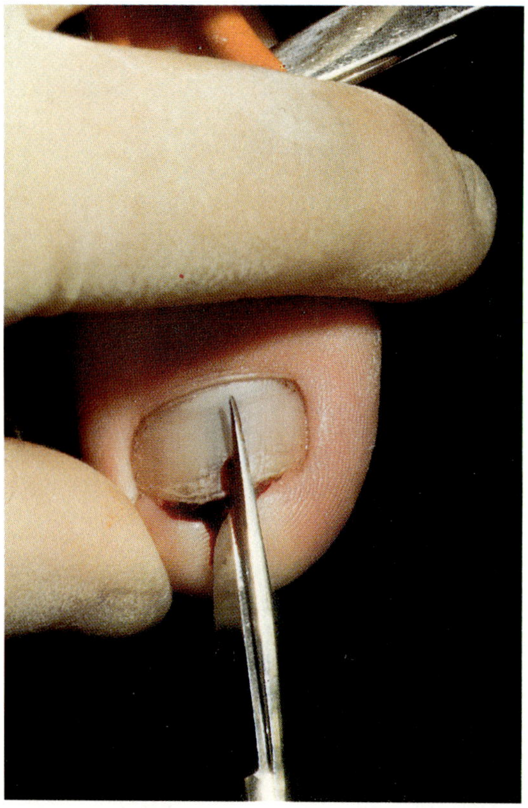

5

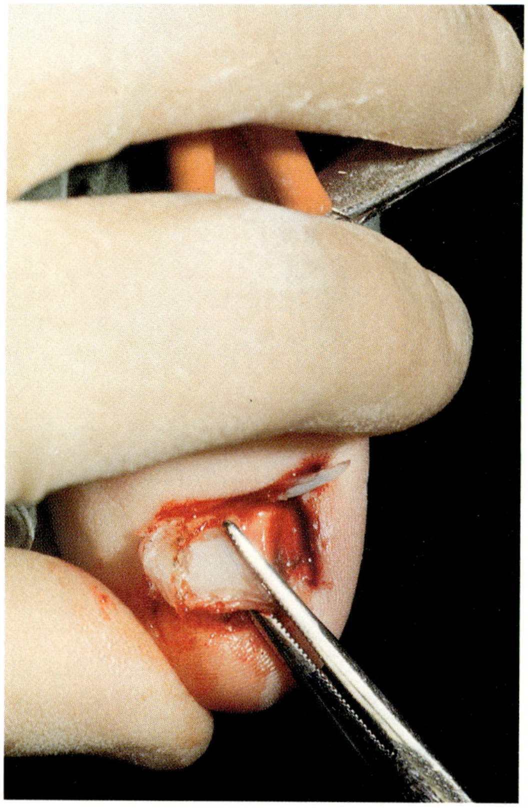

6

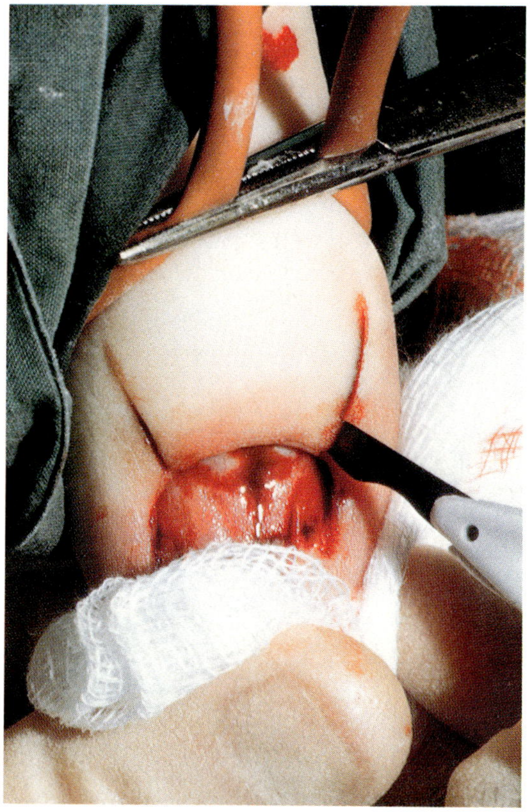

7

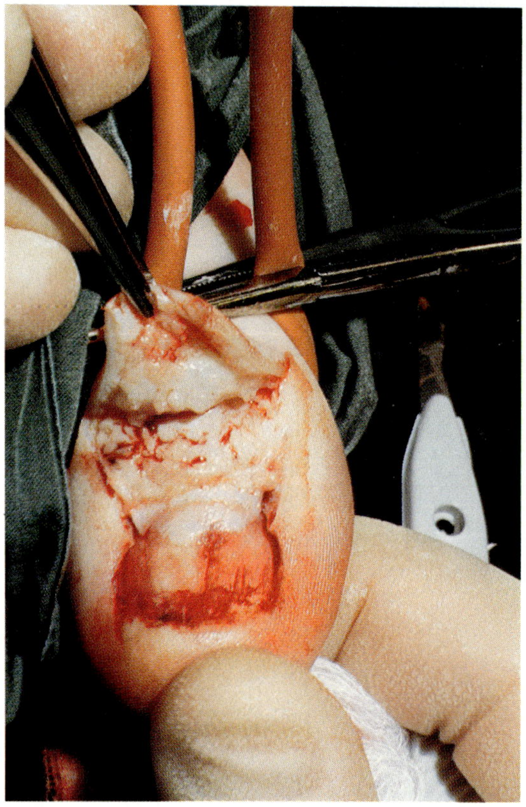

4 The nail may then be split and removed in separate halves or lifted off as a whole.

5 The second half of the nail being removed.

6 When the nail has been removed the skin is cut back at an angle towards the base of the phalanx but stopping about 6-8 mm from the joint.

7 The skin is carefully lifted up with care not to damage the insertion of the terminal slip of the extensor tendon.

8

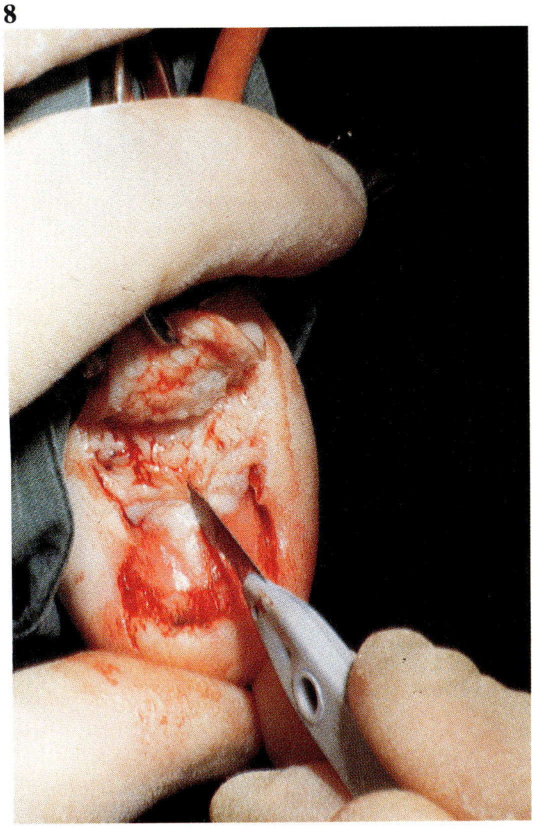

9

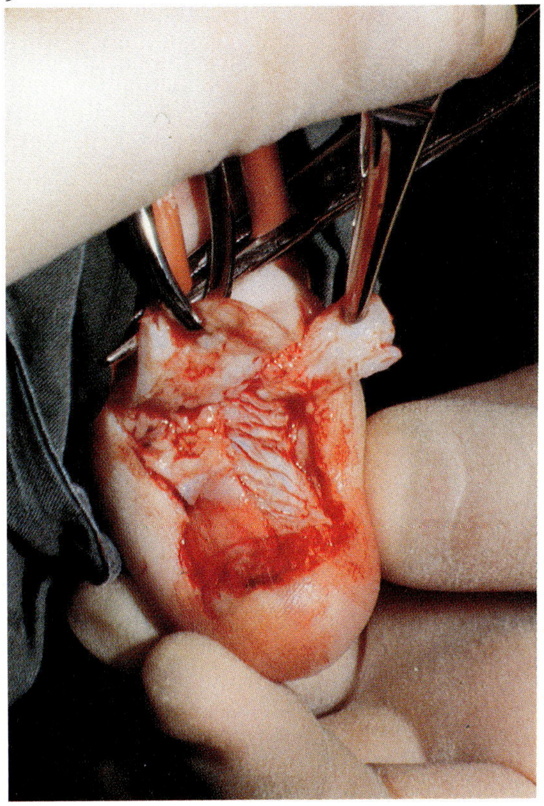

10

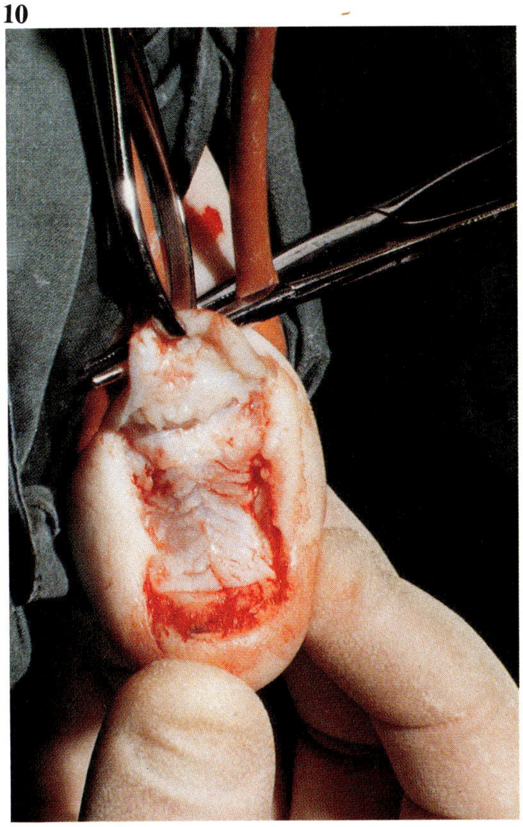

11

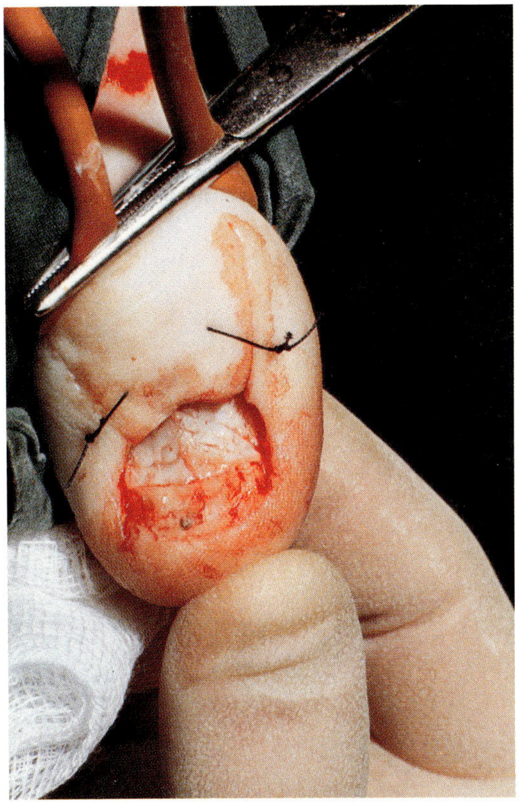

8 The nail bed is divided from just distal to the tendon to the distal third of the nail bed. The germinal layer is the proximal part of the nail bed and should be carefully excised to prevent regrowth.

9 The lateral side of the nail bed is being uplifted for excision.

10 The whole of the nail bed has been excised down to the tendon insertion. The nail bed can be alternatively destroyed by phenol left for 3 minutes and washed off.

11 The flap of skin can be stitched down with simple sutures, and dressings applied.

Note: Removal of a wedge of the nail may be accompanied by excision of granulation tissue or by curettage. Recurrence after this is not uncommon but may be diminished by application of Phenol for three minutes and this is then carefully diluted by glycerine and the whole washed off.

Trigger fingers

Triggering of fingers and thumbs is caused by a nodule forming in one or both flexor tendons close to the metacarpophalangeal joint. On active flexion the nodule is drawn out of the fibrous flexor sheath, but on attempted extension the nodule becomes jammed at the entrance to the tunnel. Forcible passive extension is required to allow the digit to straighten. The patient suffers pain on extension and may be aware of a tender nodule on the flexor surface of the metacarpophalangeal joint. Several fingers may be affected simultaneously in rheumatoid arthritis. If the thumb is affected the patient may complain of 'snapping' of the interphalangeal joint. Thumbs may also be affected in neonates but may spontaneously improve without surgery.

1

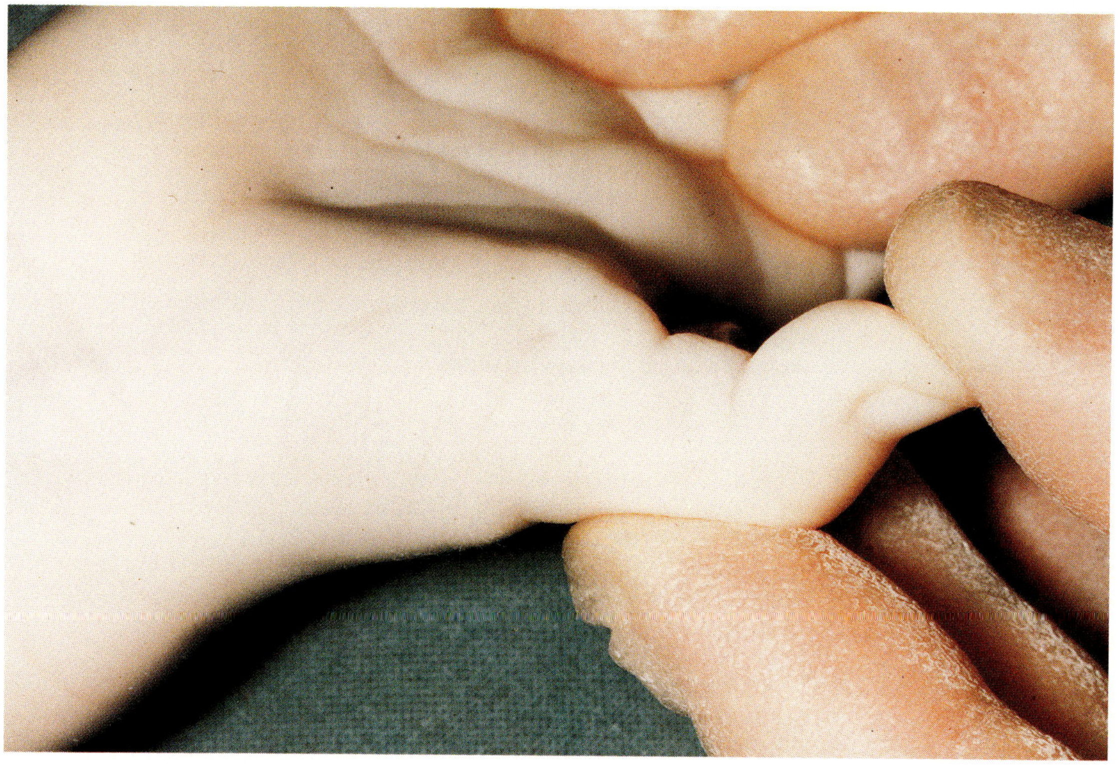

1 Surgical release of a trigger finger – in this case a thumb – is best performed under a tourniquet so that the neurovascular bundles can be seen and preserved. This usually requires a general anaesthetic. The lack of full extension of the thumb is demonstrated.

2

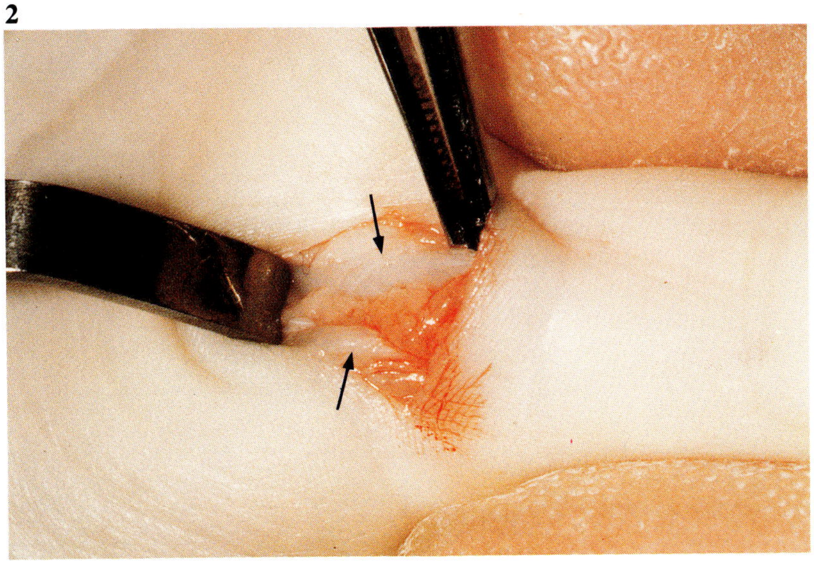

2 A transverse incision is made in the skin crease overlying the flexor surface of the metacarpophalangeal joint. Great care is required not to damage the neurovascular bundles (arrowed) – in the thumb these are particularly superficial.

The subcutaneous fat is separated from the fibrous flexor sheath beneath by blunt dissection and the neurovascular bundles are retracted.

3

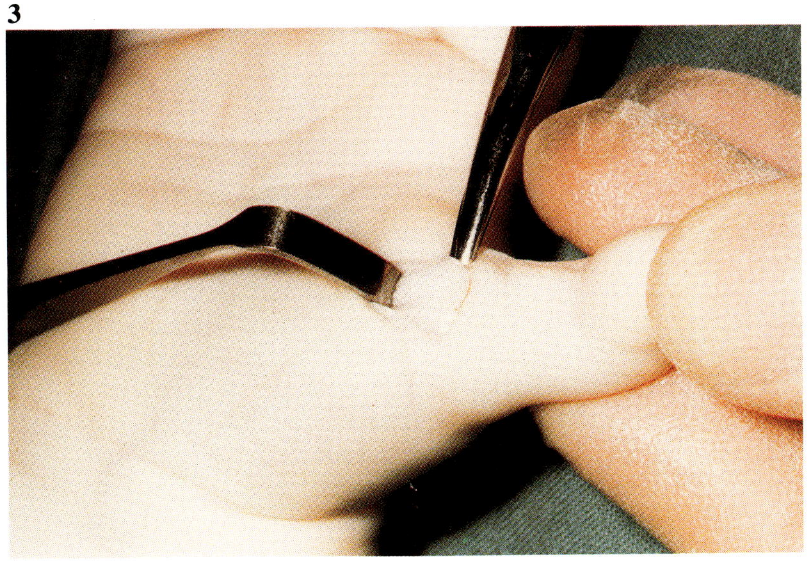

3 A longitudinal incision is made in the midline of the fibrous flexor sheath dividing the proximal 2 cm. The flexor tendons will be visible and can be lifted up on a blunt instrument to reveal the causative nodule.

4

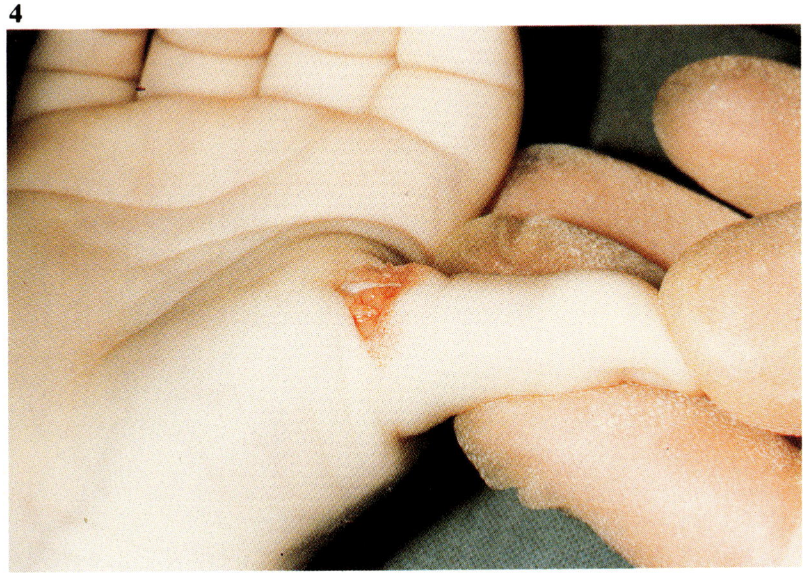

4 If the constricting sheath has been fully divided, the digit will extend fully and easily. No deep sutures are required. The skin can be closed by two or three sutures or even by sterile adhesive tape. A small dry dressing is applied. Active and passive flexion and extension movements are encouraged from the start. The dressings can be discarded at 10-12 days.

Corneal foreign bodies

Foreign bodies impacted on the surface of the eyeball constitute a common ophthalmic emergency. The most frequent history given is one in which the patient had been using a hammer and chisel, or hitting rusting metal, and immediately felt an object striking the eye. A steel foreign body can often be readily seen impacted in the cornea, usually surrounded by a rust ring. If such a history is obtained, but if there is no immediate evidence of the presence of a foreign body, every measure must be taken to locate it. It could have lodged itself beneath the upper eyelid; it is most important to exclude the possibility that the foreign body may have become retained within the eyeball. A small slit observed in the iris is pathognomonic of a retained foreign body, which may then be confirmed by ophthalmoscopic examination under full mydriasis.

A radiograph of the appropriate orbit is mandatory if such a possibility is not to be missed.

1

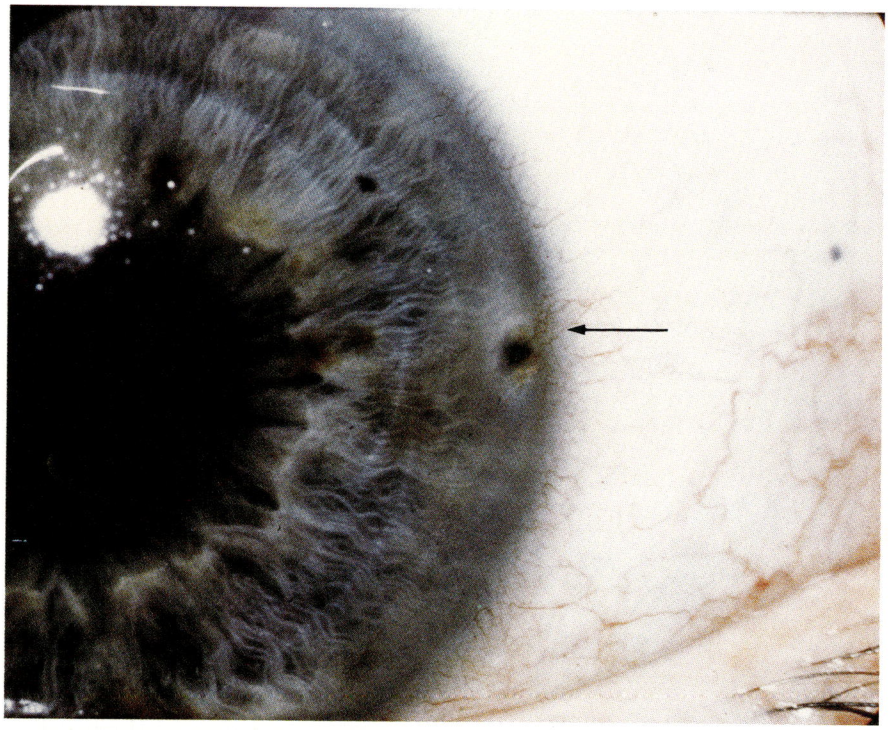

1 An embedded foreign body may be lifted by means of 19G hypodermic needle. Adequate topical anaesthesia with Benoxianate drops is required. Good illumination is essential, and some magnification desirable. Chloramphenicol ointment is then instilled, and the eye patched for 24 hours.

Caution: Great care should be taken to avoid penetrating the cornea too deeply; the anterior chamber may inadvertently be entered resulting in an aqueous leak and collapse of the anterior chamber. Moreover, foreign bodies located centrally may produce deep stromal scarring with resulting loss of visual acuity. In case of difficulty, repeated attempts to remove the foreign body should be resisted, and the patient referred to an eye surgeon.

Procedures on the eyelids

1 Chalazion (also referred to as Meibomian or tarsal cyst) is a glanulomatous condition of a Meibomian gland and although termed 'a cyst' is not really so.

2 Topical anaesthetic, for example Benoxinate or Amethocaine (Minims S & N) is instilled.

3 The eyelid is anaesthetised further by infiltrating with 1 ml Lignocaine 2 per cent.

4 A chalazion clamp is engaged and the affected lid everted.

1

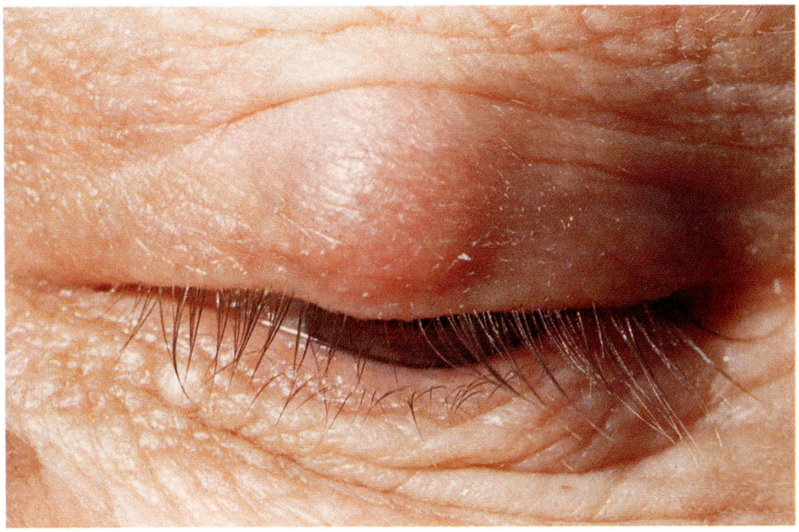

2

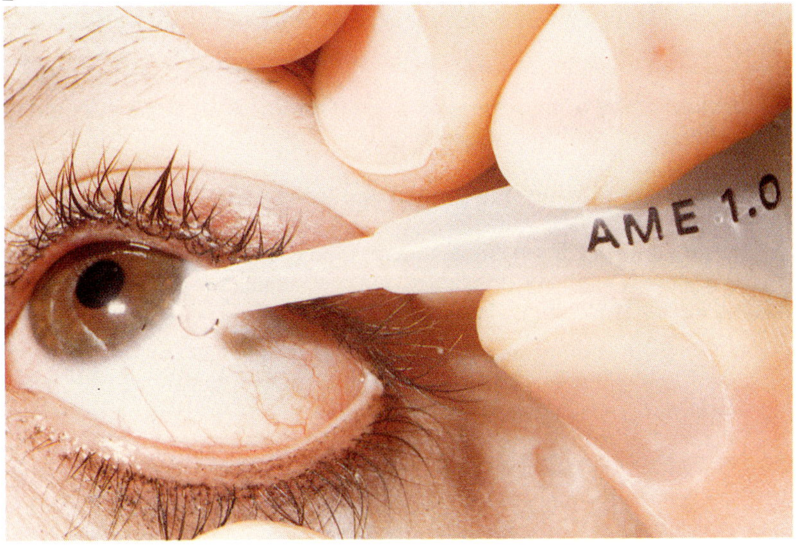

3

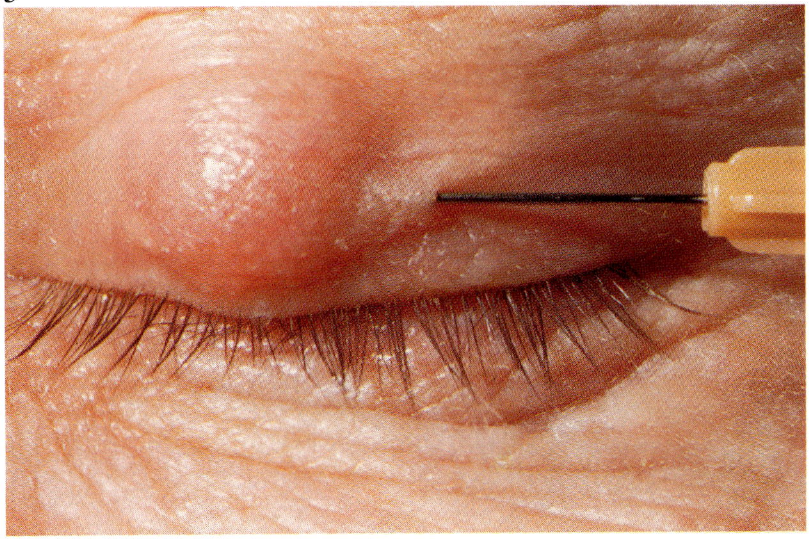

4

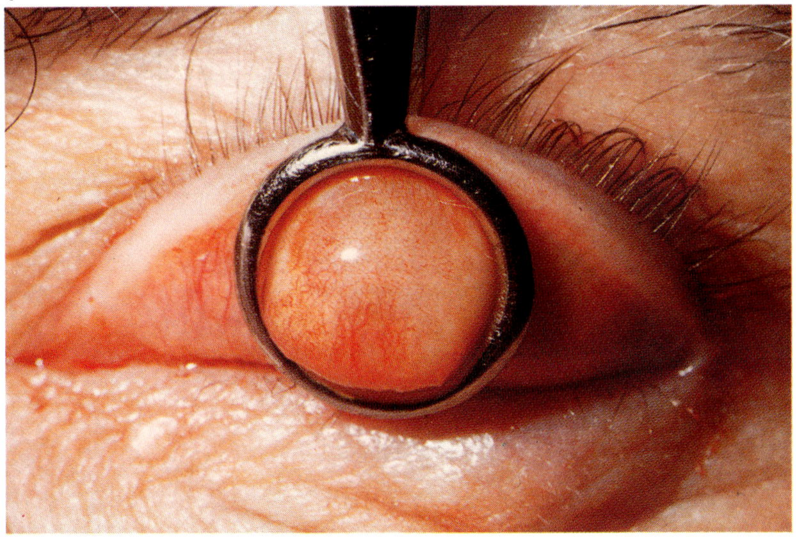

5

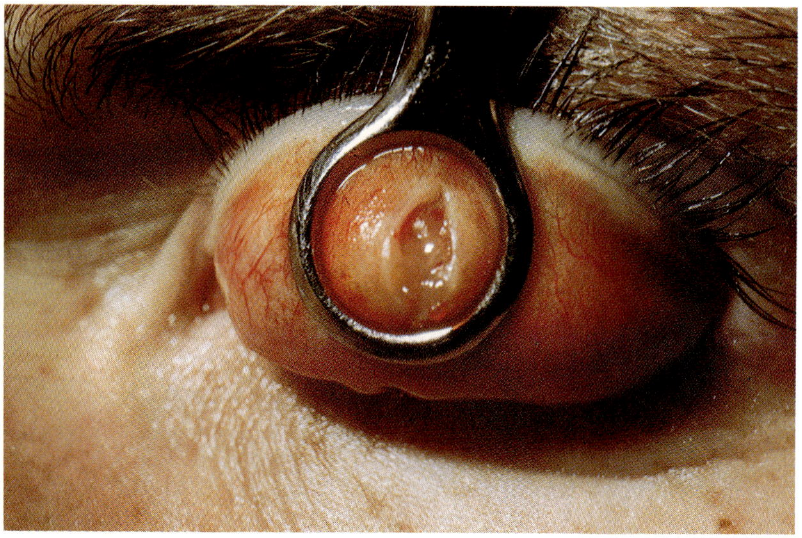

6

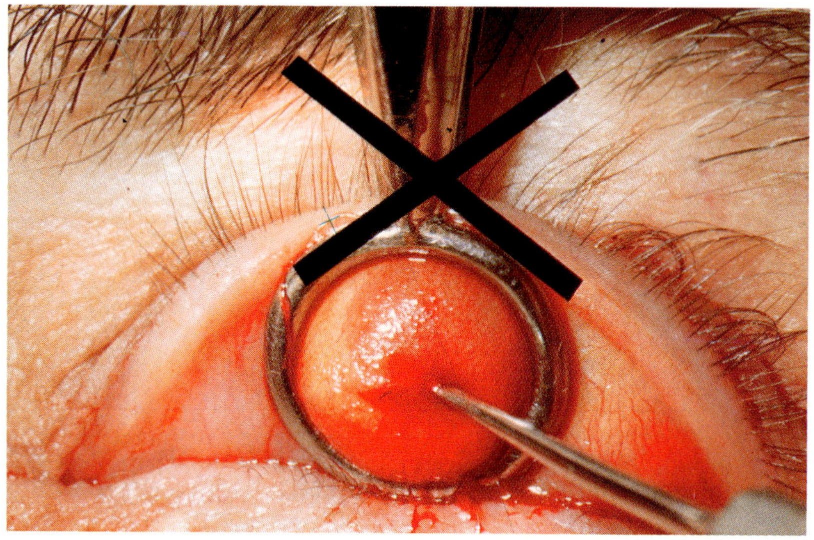

7

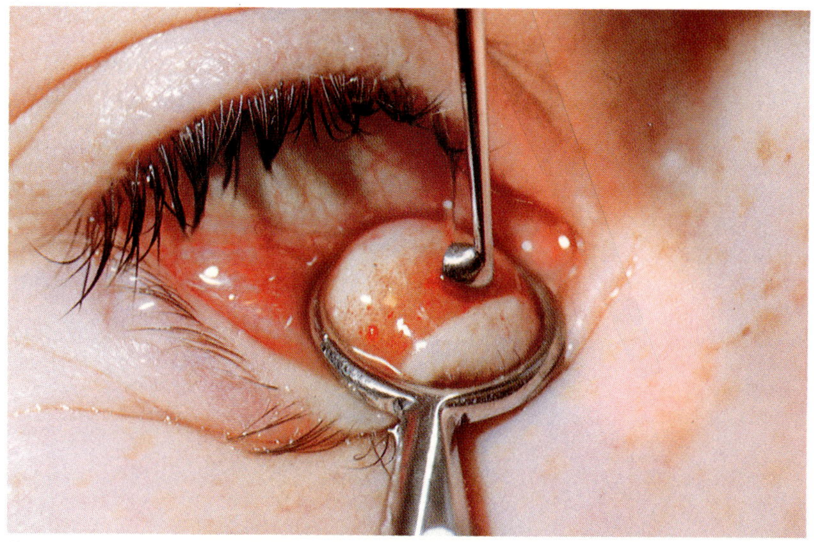

8

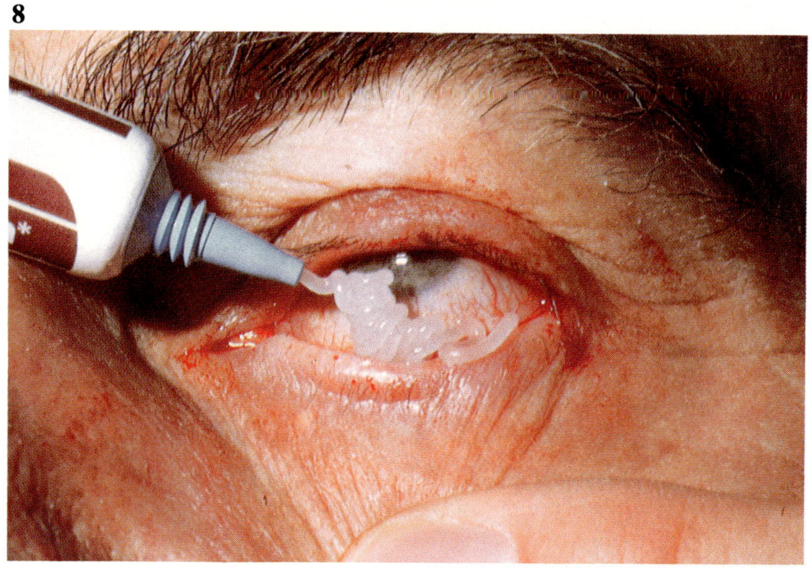

5 The cyst is incised with a No. 11 disposable blade vertically into the tarsal plate.

6 It is inadvisable to incise in a horizontal fashion as the incision would cross the line of the blood vessels.

7 The contents of the cyst are evacuated using a small curette.

8 Liberal amounts of antibiotic ointment are inserted for a few days. Firm pressure is applied to eyelids to minimise bleeding. The eyepad can usually be discarded after a few minutes.

Entropion

1

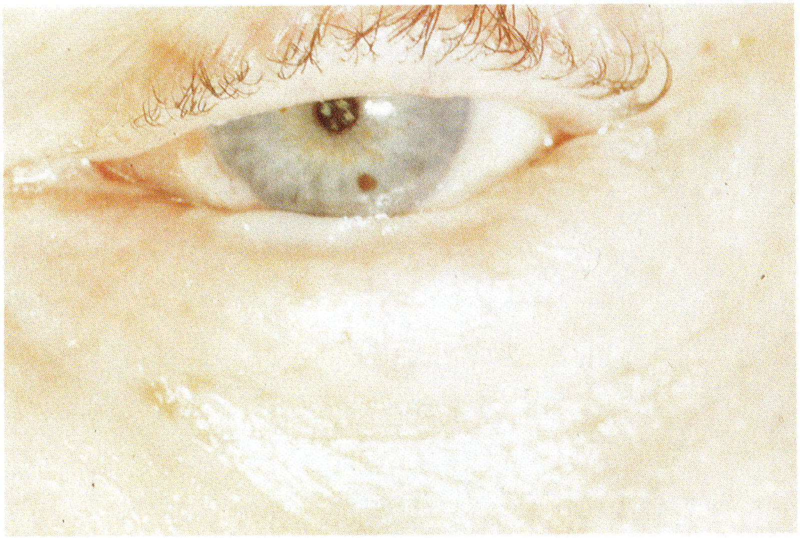

1 A senile spastic entropion. This is an inturning of the lower eyelid, causing irritation due to the eyelashes rubbing against the cornea. Several procedures are available for its correction; those in current use include: *Ffooks's modification of the Wies procedure* (Trans. Ophthal. Soc. U.K. 1965, 85, 175), and *modified Wheeler's procedure*.

Ffooks's modification of the Wies procedure

2 The lower eyelid is anaesthetised adequately by topical instillation of Benoxinate drops and local infiltration with 2.5 ml of Lignocaine two per cent with Adrenaline 1 in 200,000 (as in Figures 3 &4). A lid spatula or guard of the 'Shoehorn' type is inserted into the lower conjunctival fornix, taking care not to abrade the cornea. The lower eyelid is lifted away from the eyeball by an assistant, levering the lid guard against the patient's forehead.

2

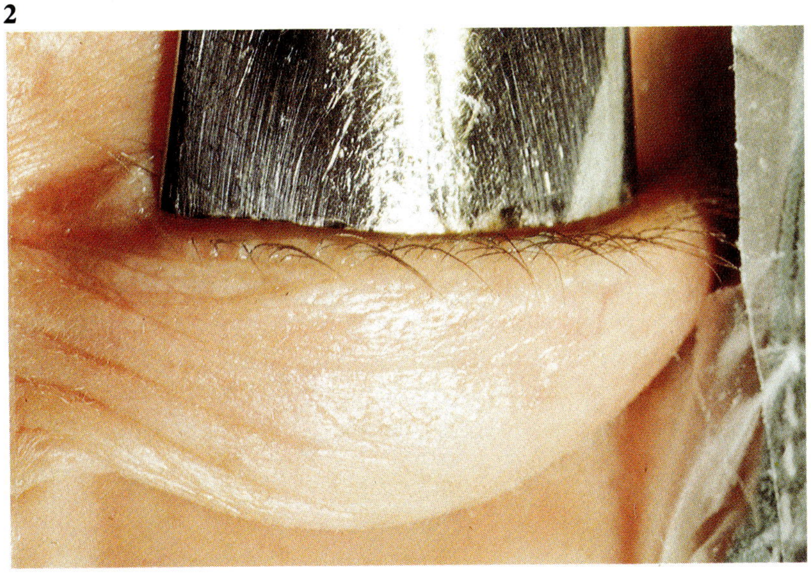

3 A horizontal incision is made into the skin of the eyelid, 4 mm below the lid margin, in the middle one-third of its extent.

3

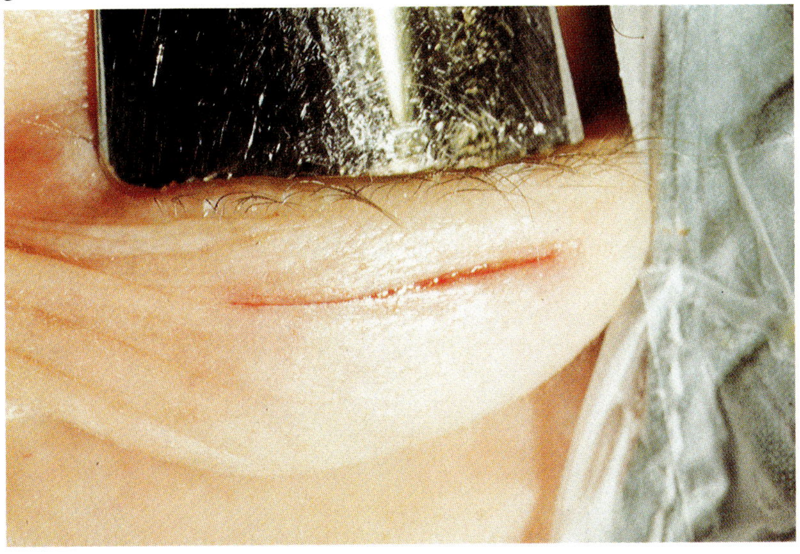

4

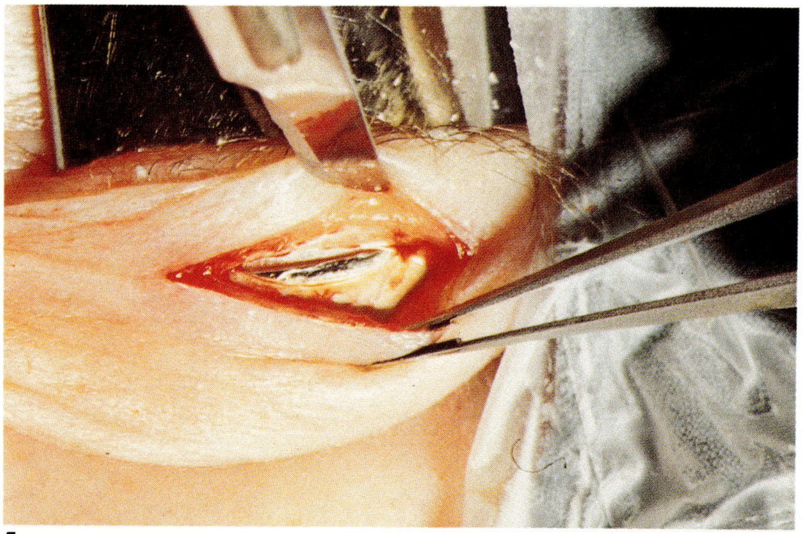

5

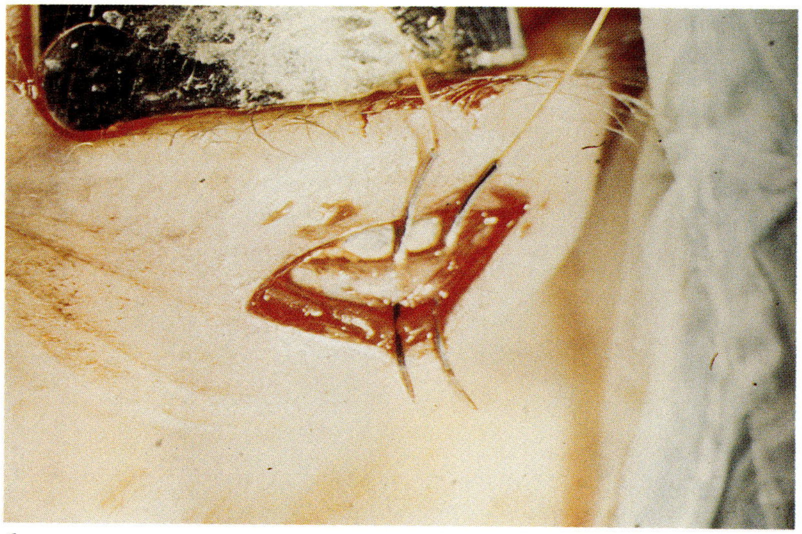

4 The incision is deepened through the orbicularis to expose the tarsal plate, which is also incised horizontally.

Caution: It is important to avoid placing the incision below the lower edge of the tarsal plate. The latter is identified by its white colour; the grating sensation encountered on its division is unmistakable.

5 Two double armed 4/0 catgut sutures are inserted backhand into the divided lower end of the tarsal plate.

6 These sutures are then passed along the plane between the orbicularis and the skin to emerge just below the eyelash margin. They are secured in a tight knot in order to permit the partial transposition of the lower end of the tarsal plate. The orbicularis muscle is not sutured.

7 The skin edges are sutured with 7/0 Prolene or silk. The sutures are removed on the fifth day.

6

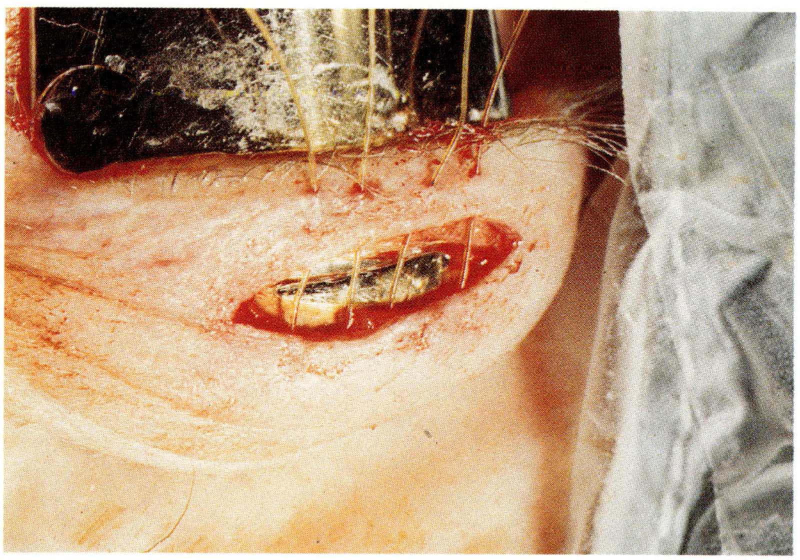

7

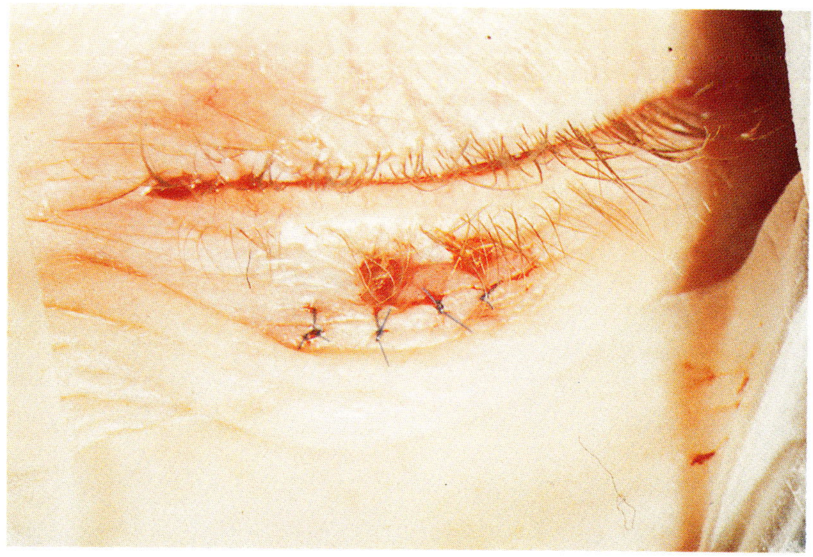

Modified Wheeler's procedure

1

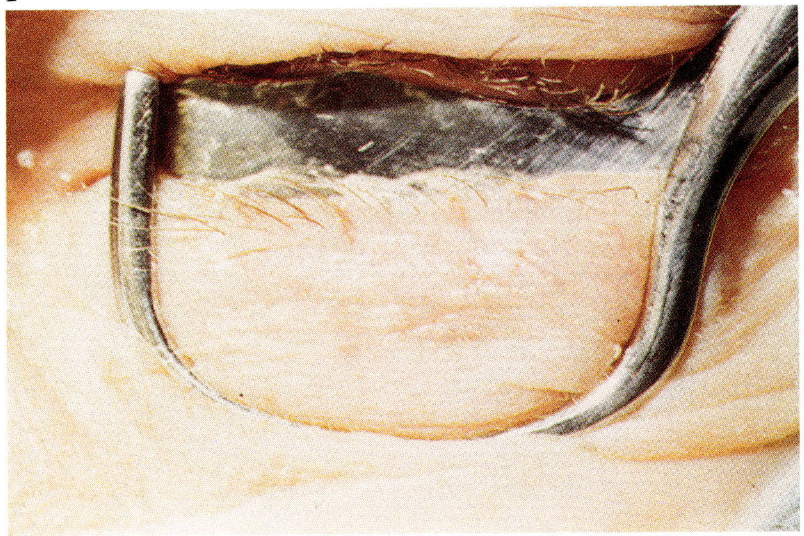

1 After anaesthetising the eyelid (as in Figures 3 and 4) a lid clamp is inserted.

2

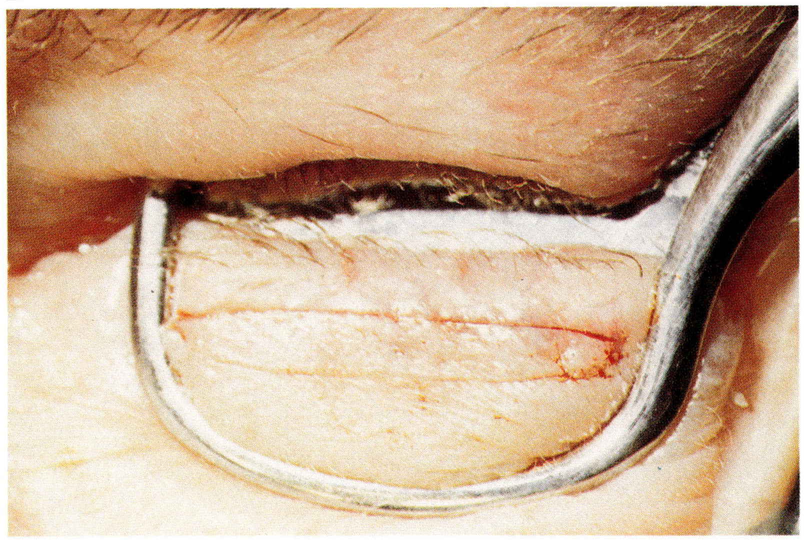

2 An incision is made 3 mm below and parallel to the lower lid margin for the entire length of the clamp.

3

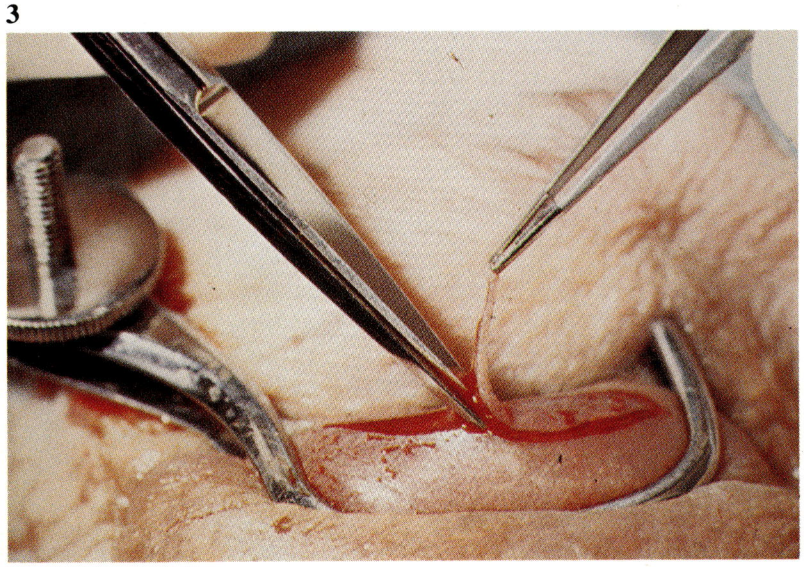

3 If superfluous lid folds are present in the lower lid, a skin ellipse is excised.

4

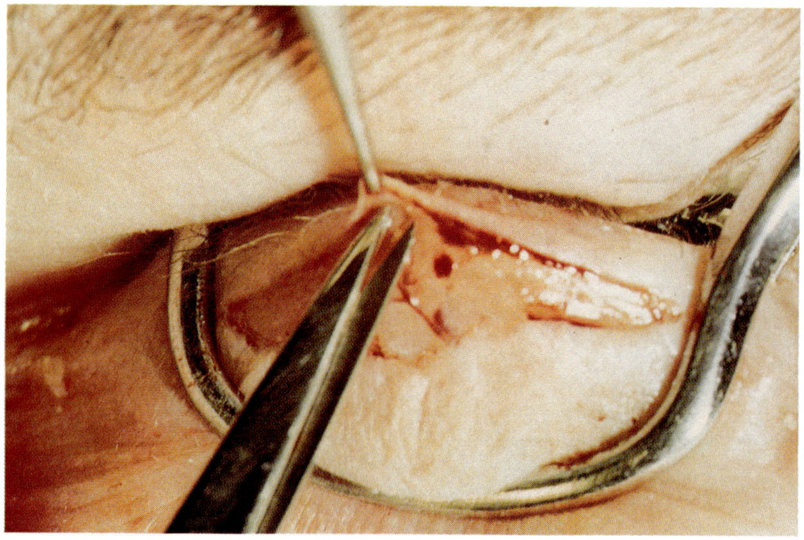

5

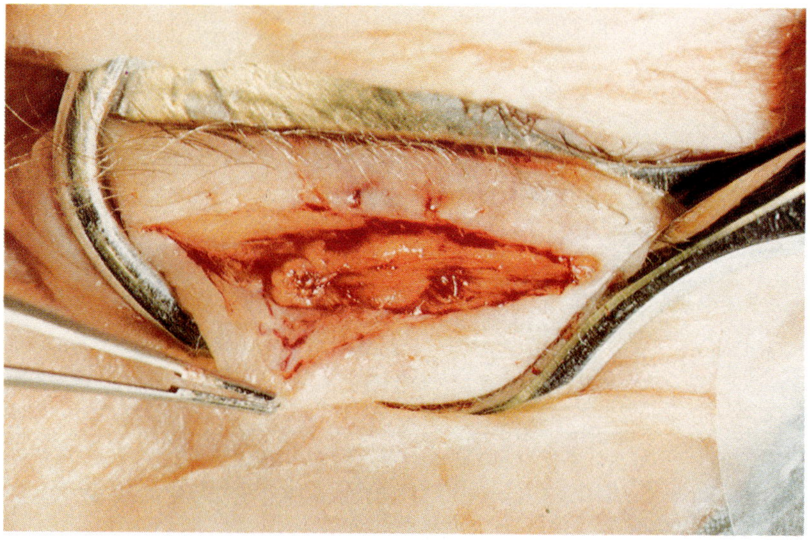

4 & 5 The skin is undermined above to expose the orbicularis muscle. The lower edge is also undermined.

6

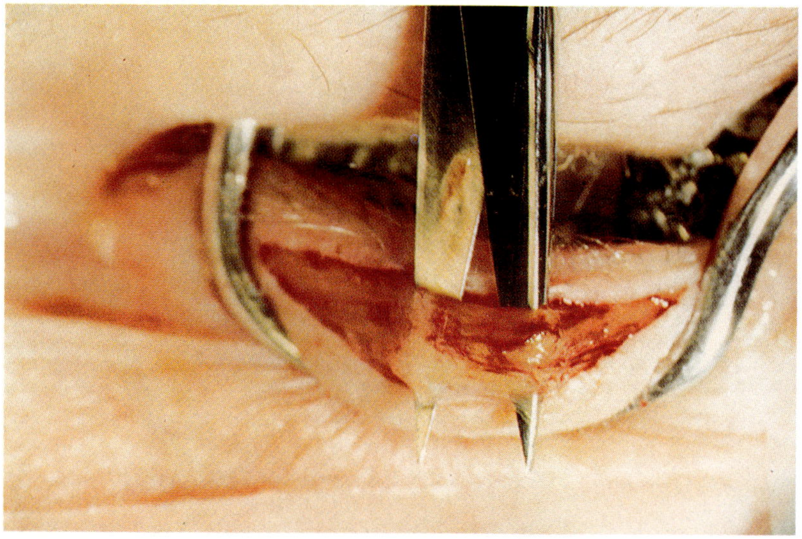

6 A 4 mm band of this muscle is defined by making horizontal incisions 3 mm and 7 mm below the lid margin, and spreading with scissors.

7

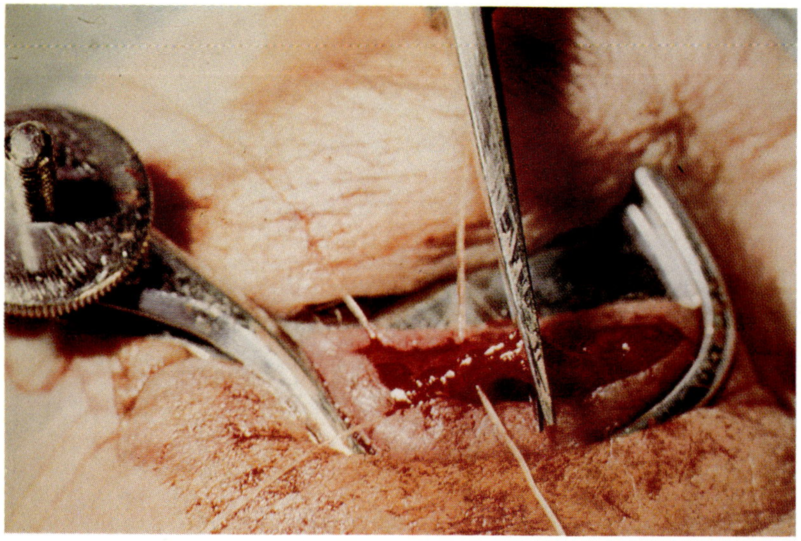

7 This band of orbicularis is divided vertically. Two mattress 4/0 catgut sutures are inserted at 2 mm and 5 mm respectively from one end of the cut muscle.

8

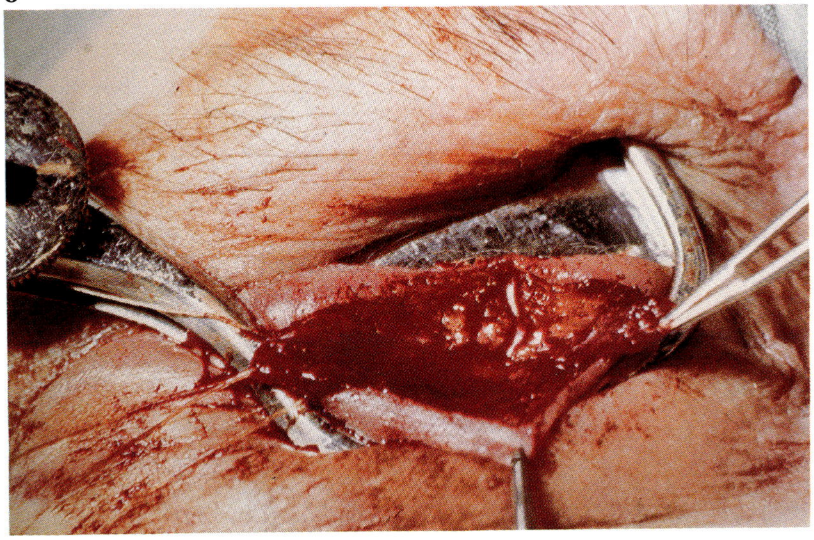

9

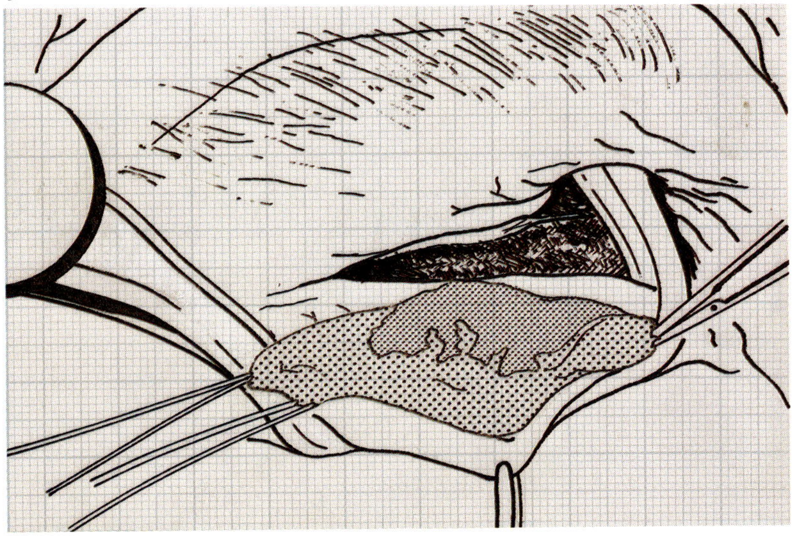

10

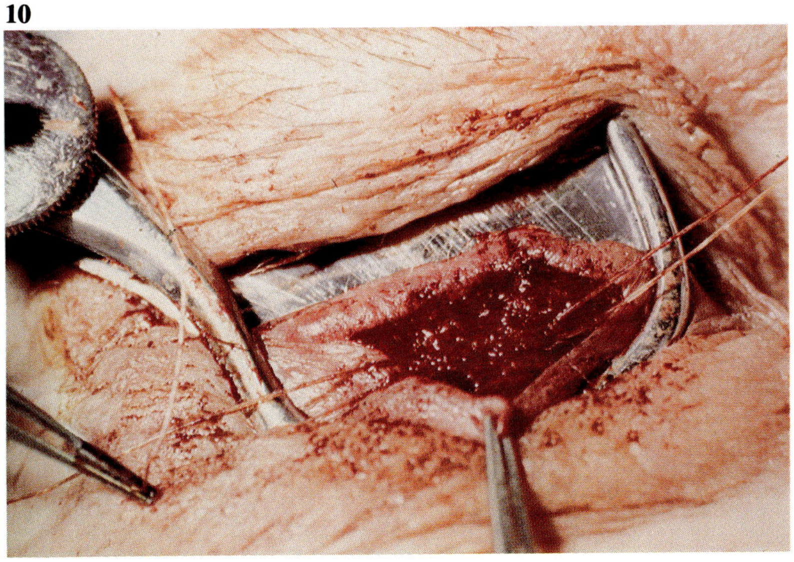

11

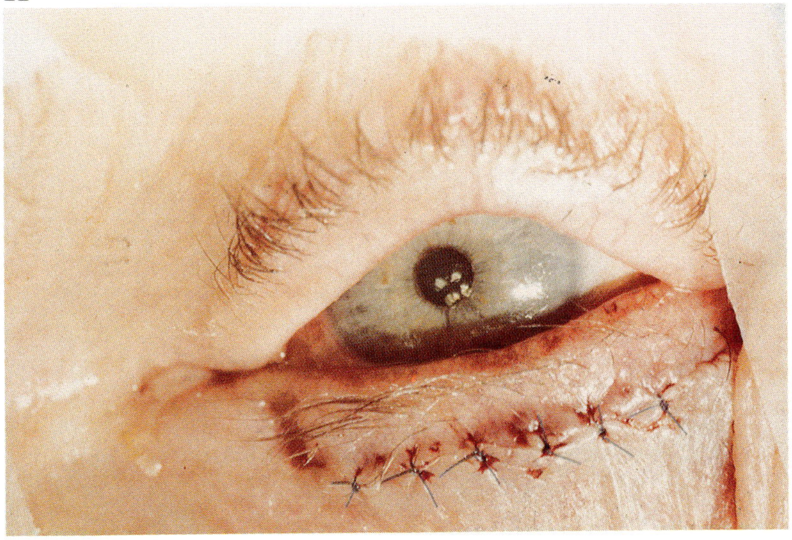

8 A partial tarsectomy is performed by making a triangular incision in the tarsal plate with its apex just below the lid margin. This is deepened down to the palpebral conjunctiva from which it is dissected. The edges of the tarsus are approximated by three interrupted 5/0 collagen sutures.

9 Diagram to illustrate the partial tarsectomy in Figure 24.

10 The two bands of orbicularis are overlapped. The mattress sutures transfix the overlying band, and one needle of each suture is carried through the lower border of the tarsus, where it is secured.

11 The skin is closed with interrupted 7/0 Prolene. Sutures are removed on the fifth day.

Ectropion

Cautery

1
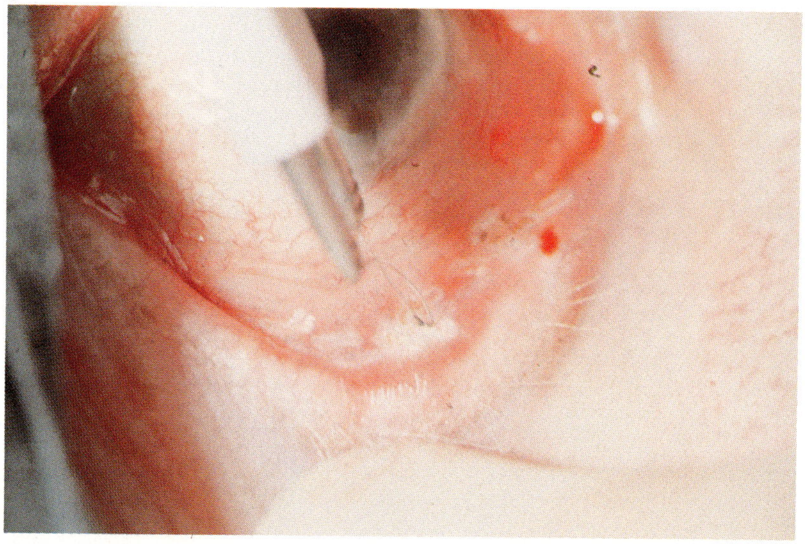

1 The eyelid is anaesthetised by local infiltration with Lignocaine 2 per cent and topical Benoxinate drops. For mild forms of ectropion all that may be required to correct a slightly lax lower eyelid is the application of a row of cautery burns on the conjunctival aspect, 2 mm below the lid margin.

2
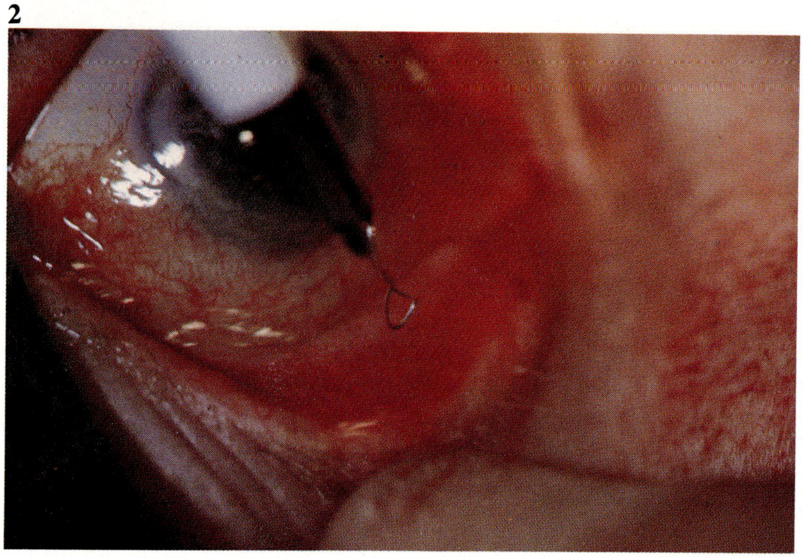

2 Cautery applied behind the lacrimal punctum restores the apposition of the punctum to the eyeball. The punctum may require dilatation to enable the tears to flow into the lacrimal passages.

Caution: Care should be taken to avoid contact between the red hot cautery point and the eyeball, particularly the cornea. It is helpful to instruct the patient to look upwards and pull the lower lid away from the globe.

Wedge resection

1

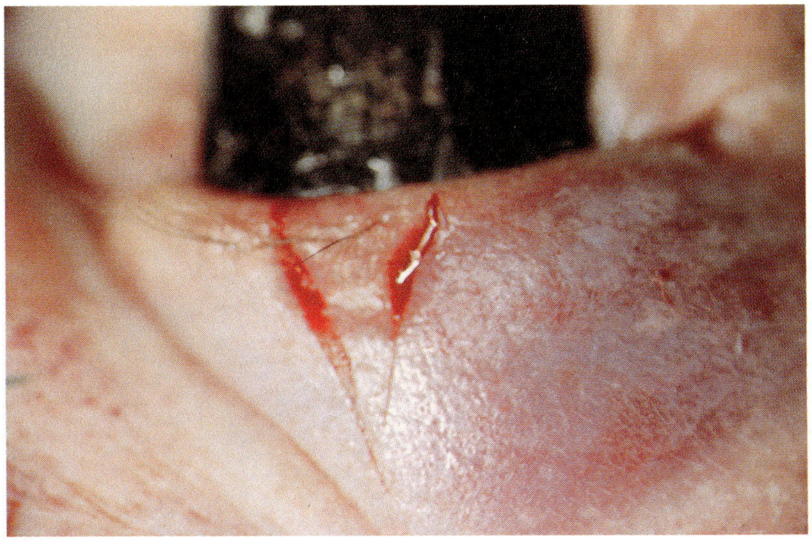

1 For severe forms of ectropion of the lower eyelid, the lid is shortened by the excision of a triangle of full-thickness lid, base up, as outlined.

2

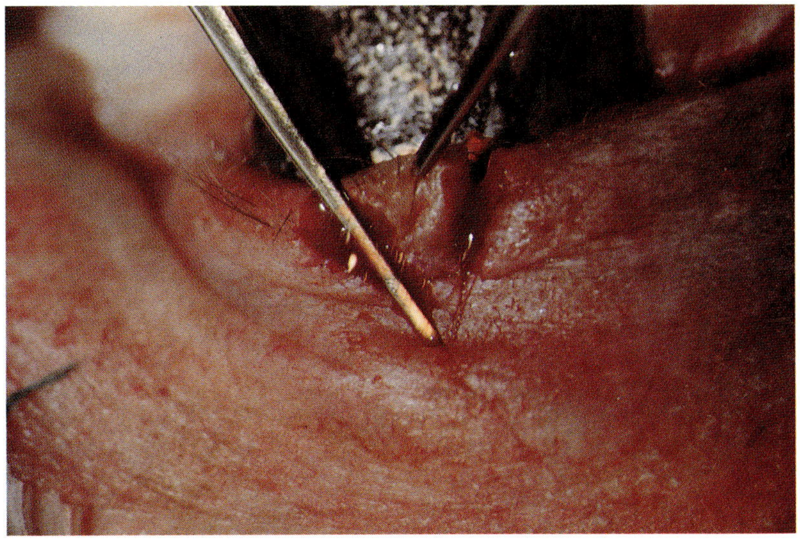

2 The triangle is excised. Note the protective shield for the eye.

3

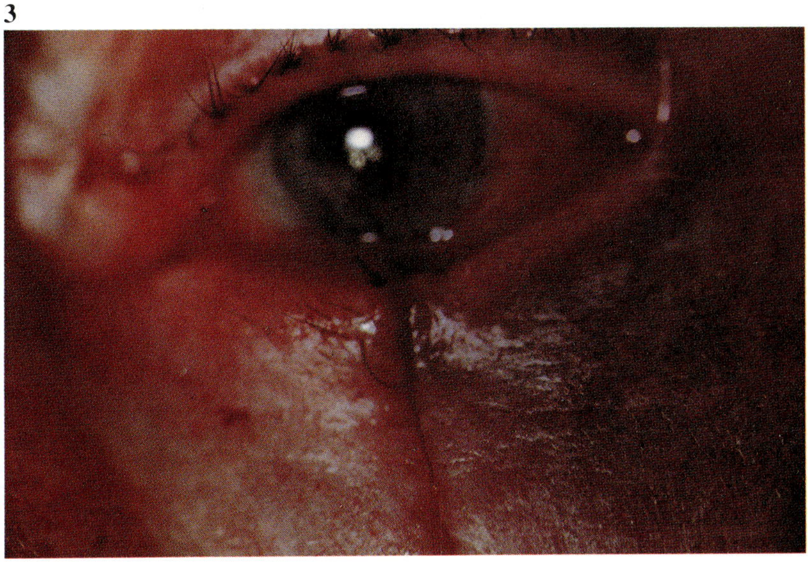

3 The divided ends are brought together in layers. 5/0 catgut is utilised for the tarsal plate and orbicularis muscle. The skin is closed by 7/0 Prolene.

4

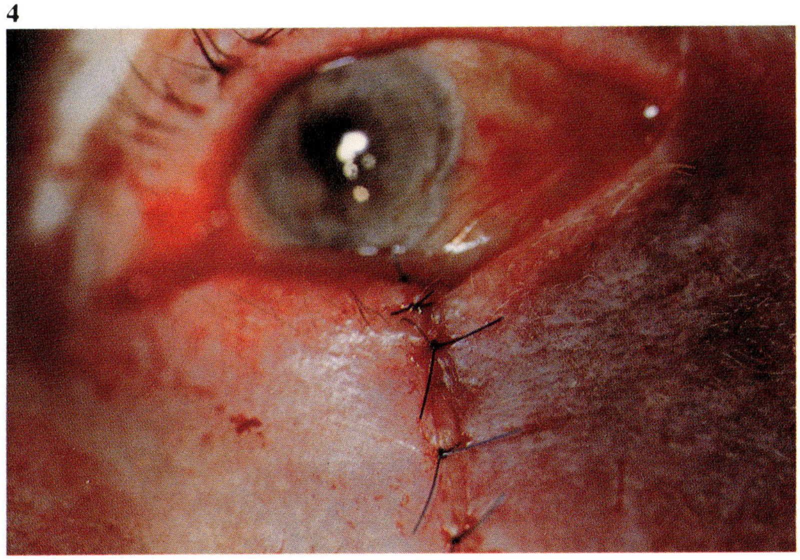

4 Caution: Care should be taken to avoid obtaining a 'step' on the lid margin.

Procedures on the tear ducts

Syringing (lacrimal sac washout)

1

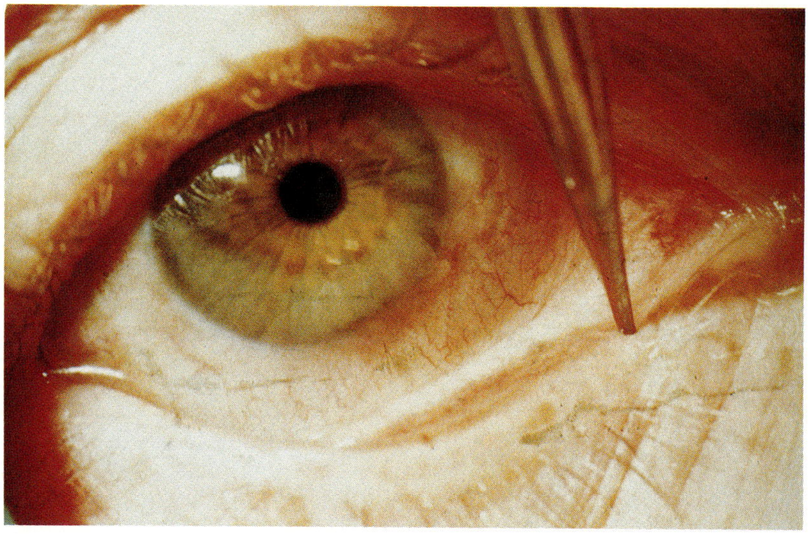

1 The lower lacrimal punctum is identified and stretched vertically by the tip of a Nettleship dilator.

2

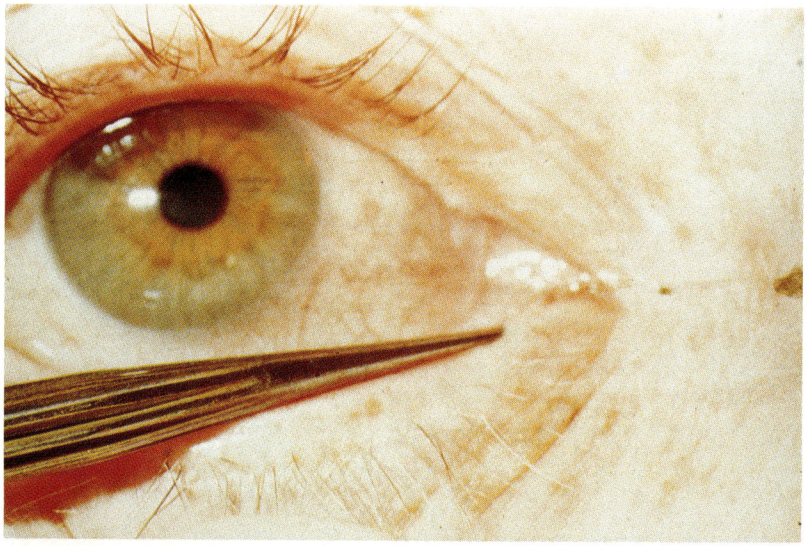

2 The dilator is introduced horizontally for a distance of 2 mm along the canaliculus.

3

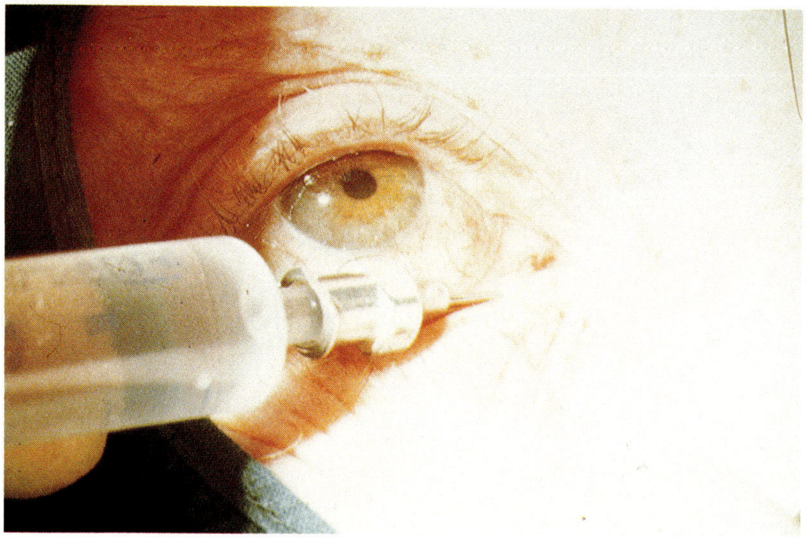

3 A lacrimal cannula attached to a 2 ml syringe containing saline is introduced along the inferior canaliculus until the lacrimal sac is entered, and the tip of the cannula rests against the lacrimal bone. The plunger of the syringe is depressed; if the nasolacrimal duct is patent, the patient experiences fluid trickling to the back of the throat. Regurgitation from the upper punctum points to an obstruction in the nasolacrimal duct, which may require probing. The upper punctum may be occluded by means of a punctum dilator, and the procedure repeated to determine freedom of flow under pressure. If no access into the tear sac is permitted, this is an indication that the site of obstruction lies in the lower canaliculus.

Probing

1

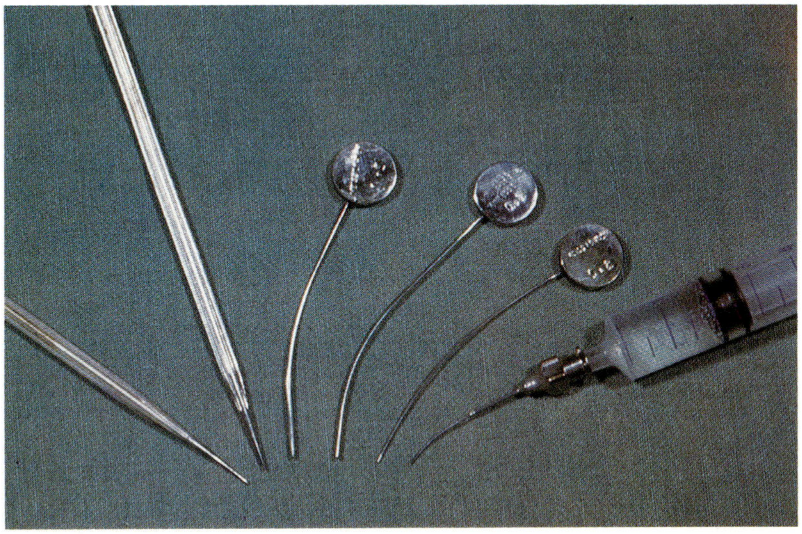

1 The instruments required – a punctum dilator, lacrimal cannula, a set of probes of various diameters and a syringe.

2

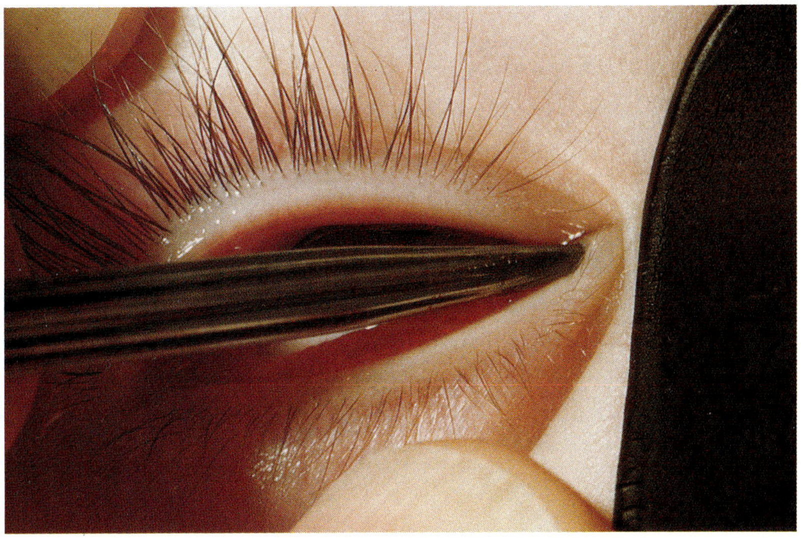

2 In the case of congenital obstruction in infants, probing should be carried out under general anaesthesia given by an experienced anaesthetist.

Caution: Injecting large amounts of saline is to be avoided since this may produce laryngeal spasm.

3

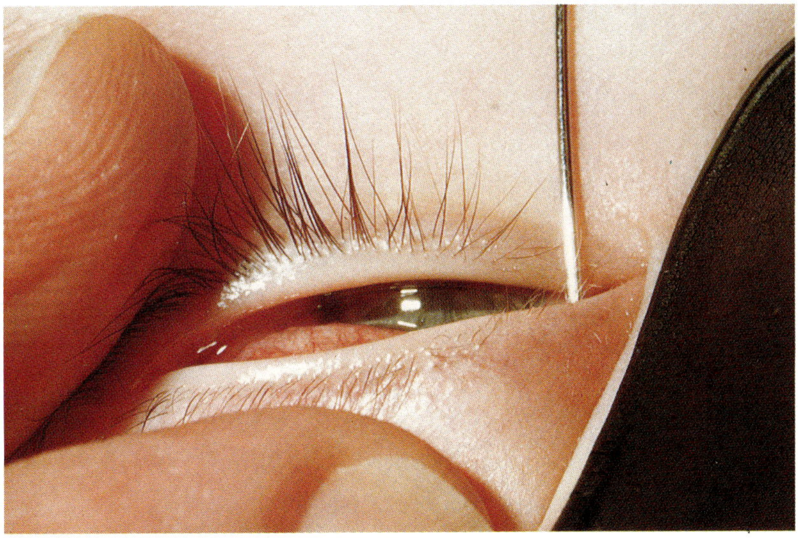

3 A Foster probe 0.8 mm diameter size is introduced first vertically for 1.5 mm.

4

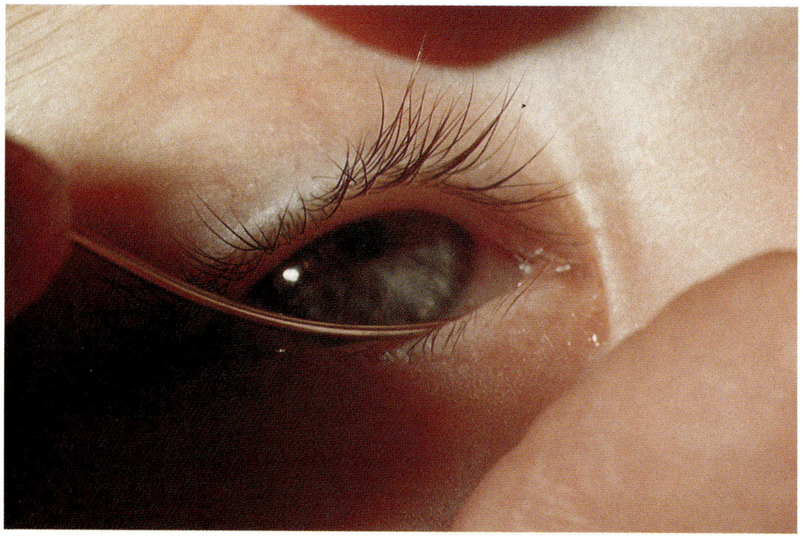

4 The probe is then directed horizontally, and gently advanced into the lacrimal sac until the lacrimal bone is felt.

5

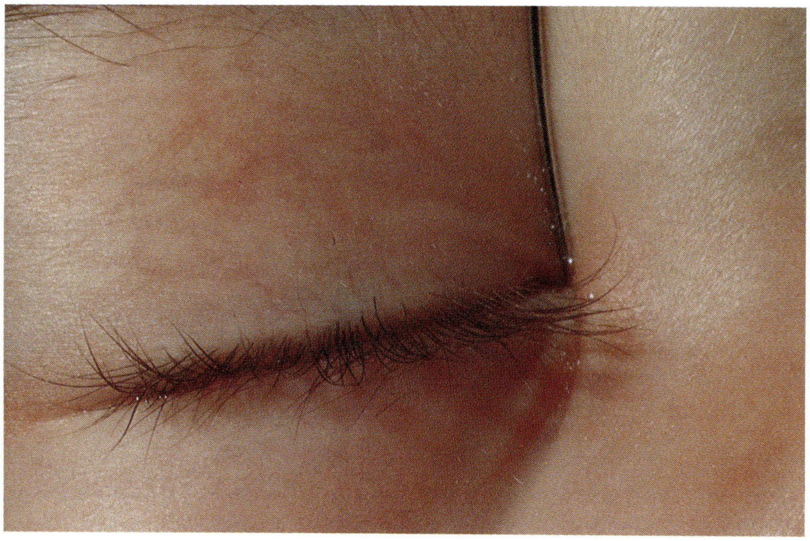

5 By using the lacrimal bone as a fulcrum, the probe is then rotated to a vertical position and gently pushed downwards, slightly backwards and laterally until its end is engaged into the nasolacrimal duct. This procedure may be repeated with a probe of a larger diameter.

Caution: No force should be necessary; overcoming of a membranous obstruction is often accompanied by an audible click. Probing in infants should be delayed for as long as possible as there is often some spontaneous improvement; it is seldom necessary to intervene before the first birthday unless the lacrimal sac is distended into a mucocele by purulent material.

Three snip procedure for spastic occlusion of the lower lacrimal punctum

1

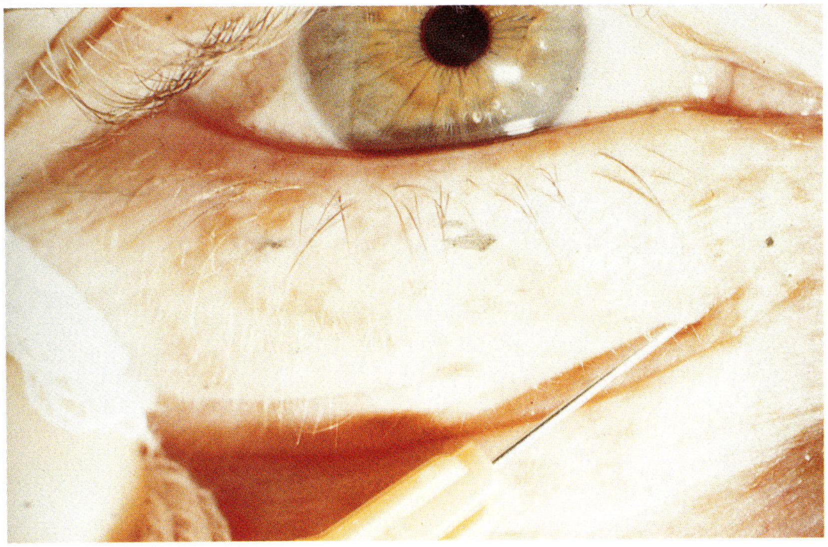

1 The medial aspect of the lower lid and canaliculus are anaesthetised. The lower punctum is usually identified with some difficulty; this is dilated (as in Figures 1 and 3 in probing section page 132) sufficiently to admit the tip of a pair of fine pointed scissors.

2 One blade of the scissors is introduced vertically from the punctum to the ampulla, with the other blade on the conjunctival aspect. The first snip, about 1.5 mm in length, is made through this vertical part of the canaliculus.

3 Tweedy's canaliculus knife is then introduced into the horizontal part of the canaliculus for a distance of about 5 mm, with the cutting edge facing upwards and backwards. The handle of the knife is then raised, thereby obtaining a 3 mm incision. The point of junction of the first and second cuts is at the ampulla. The third cut is completed across the base of the flap, by joining the beginning of the first incision with the end of the second.

A punctum dilator is introduced postoperatively on alternate days for two weeks to maintain patency.

2

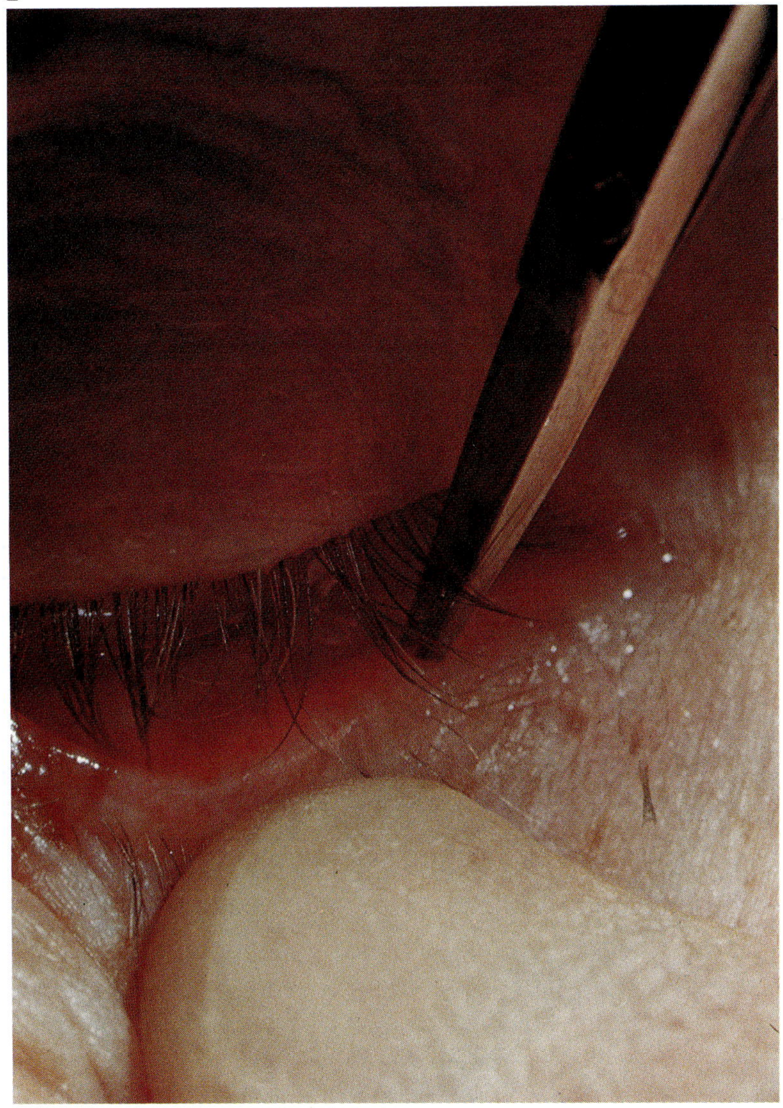

3

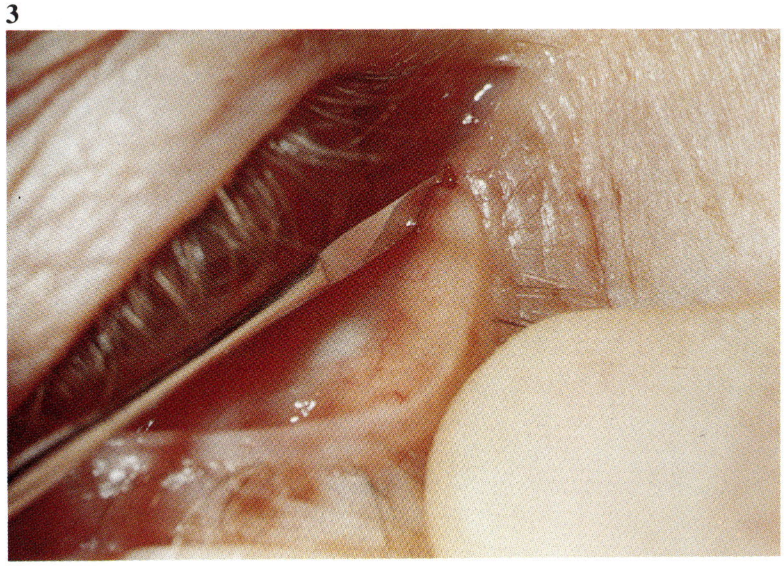

Plastic surgery

Basic principles

Placing the scar
A scar is the inevitable result of any full thickness incision in the skin. To obtain the best possible results with a minimum amount of visible scarring accurate placing of the incision is essential in elective operations. **The most pleasing site for a scar is in the skin-crease lines.** These can be seen easily in older people particularly on the face, for example the oblique nasolabial fold or the transverse forehead creases. On the limbs and trunk they are not as easily seen, especially in children. To elicit the creases the skin is moved either by the patient grimacing or the surgeon pinching the skin. The creases are then marked and plotted near the lesion so that the best excision line can be selected. Marking must be made prior to infiltration with local anaesthetic as this may distort the local anatomy.

Sutures
Any suture inserted into the skin makes an additional wound and therefore leaves a potential scar. To minimise this scarring the needle and suture material selected should be as fine as possible while strong enough to hold the wound together. The suture bites should be as small and few in number as possible, knotted accurately without undue tension and removed as early as possible.

Subcuticular sutures, absorbable or non-absorbable, can be used to strengthen the closure without surface skin marks and permit wound closure with a smaller number of skin sutures, which can be removed earlier. **Fat sutures should not be used for strength of closure; they tend to cut out or cause fat necrosis.** Fine fat sutures can help to eliminate a small dead space. Where there is a large potential cavity suction drainage is required.

The suture material employed will vary greatly depending on the circumstances. Braided silk is easier to knot and may be best for the beginner. It is also useful in the mouth or near the eye where monofilament synthetic sutures could be painful. However, silk can cause local tissue reaction and should not be used for buried sutures near the skin surface as it may cause palpable irregularities especially if infection occurs and the black colour may be visible through the skin.

Monofilament synthetic sutures such as nylon or polypropylene cause less tissue reaction but need more careful tying of the knots. Their greater strength allows finer materials to be used. A synthetic monofilament subcuticular suture can be left in place for several weeks and is then easily removed causing minimal discomfort. Absorbable sutures of the natural or synthetic variety are best for subcutaneous use. Also in children, fine absorbable sutures placed in the skin eliminate the need to remove the sutures later.

Tape sutures applied across the wound to relieve the skin tension have several advantages. They can allow earlier removal of sutures and in some cases avoid the need for skin sutures entirely. This is a particular advantage in children.

The shape of the excision
When the defect resulting from removal of an oval or circular lesion is closed by direct suture the resulting scar becomes longer and each end of the scar is liable to bunch up and form a lump in the shape of a raised cone – the 'dog ear'. This can be prevented by converting the defect into an elliptical or fusiform shape before excision. Alternatively the dog ear can be defined and trimmed after the central portion of the wound has been approximated. The amount of extra skin to be excised should be kept to a minimum as it contributes to a longer scar.

Grafts and flaps

When a defect in the skin is too great to close by direct suture tissue must be introduced to allow tension-free closure of the wound. Free grafts of split thickness or full thickness skin are the easiest and most frequently used method. Depending on the size of the defect and on the availability of suitable loose donor skin local flaps can be used for one stage closure of defects. Distant flaps, for example the cross finger flap allows skin from elsewhere to be transferred. This type of operation requires two stages, an attachment phase followed after sufficient time for the blood supply to grow in by detachment of the flap from the donor area.

Scar revision

When a scar is unsatisfactory for any reason and has to be revised the onus is on the surgeon not to make it worse. Therefore careful planning is essential. For a tattooed scar the complete pigmented part of the skin scar has to be excised. If the scar is in a good line but puckered the skin scar is excised in toto. Any deep tethering is freed but it is not essential to remove all the deep scarring. In fact it is better not to do so as the larger wound thereby created is more likely to develop haematoma and recurrent tethering. The wound is sutured carefully in layers using fine materials paying particular attention to correct alignment of tissue layers.

If there is a shortage of skin the possibility of bringing in additional skin by either a graft or flap should be considered. A linear contracture can be corrected by a Z-plasty. When the scar is not in a good direction, realignment is needed and can be accomplished sometimes by a Z-plasty or the scar can be disguised by a W-plasty.

Placing the scar

1

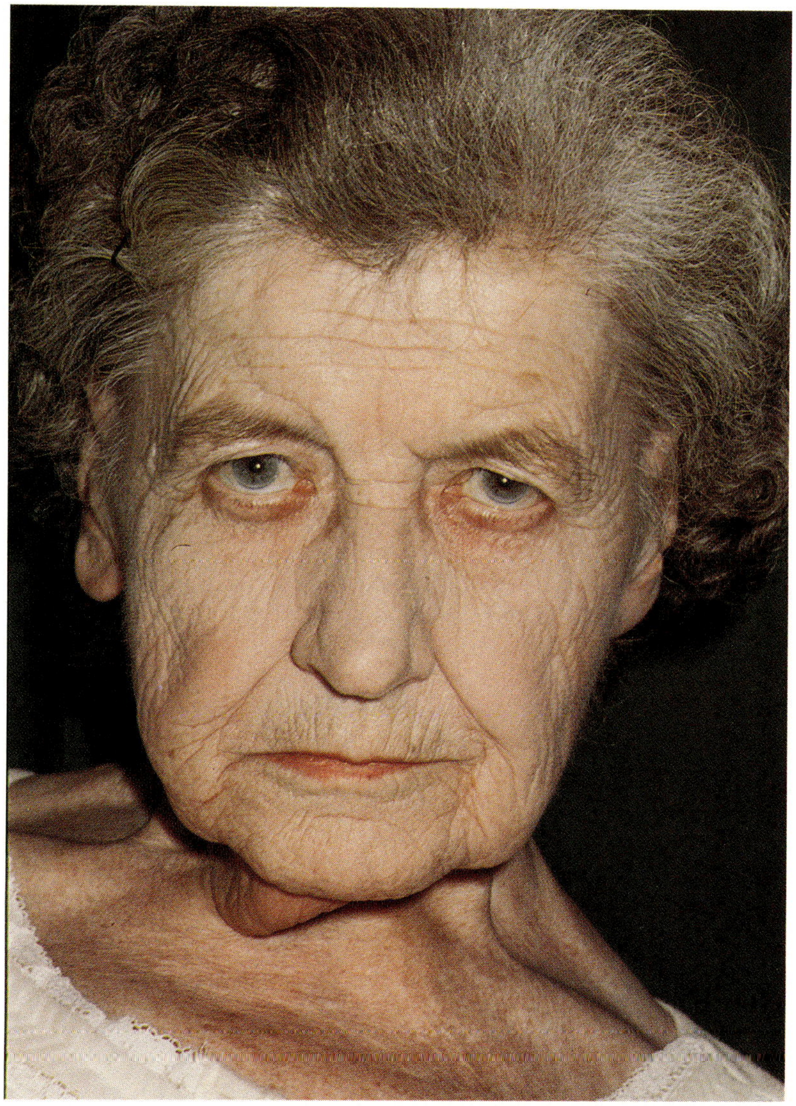

1 **Face skin creases.** In the elderly the skin crease lines are readily visible. In a young person they can be elicited by pinching the skin or observing facial grimaces.

2

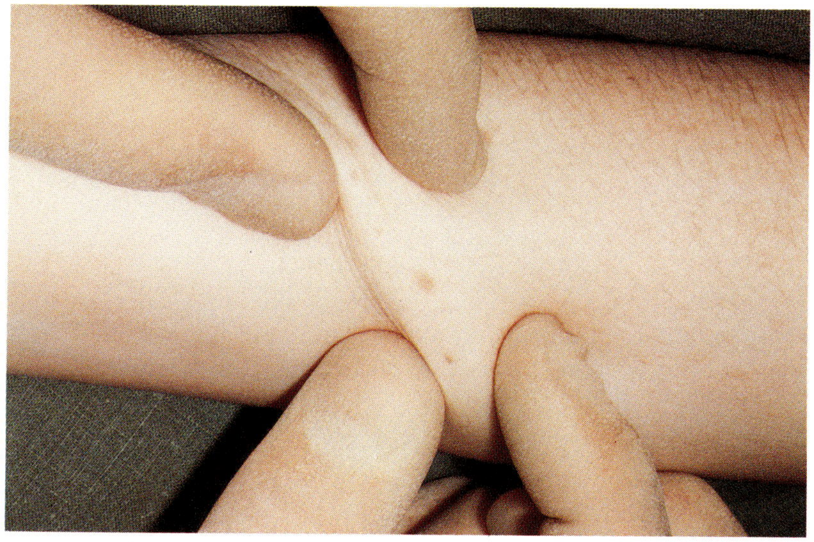

2 **Limb skin creases.** On the arm gentle pinching of the skin in various directions shows the skin crease direction.

3

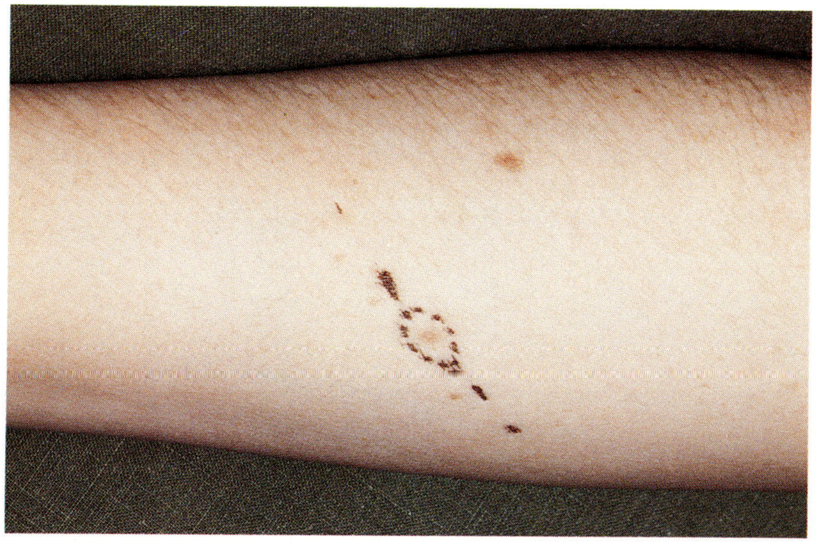

3 **Marking skin crease lines.** The ellipse for excision of a small mole is marked with the long axis in the direction of the skin crease line.

4

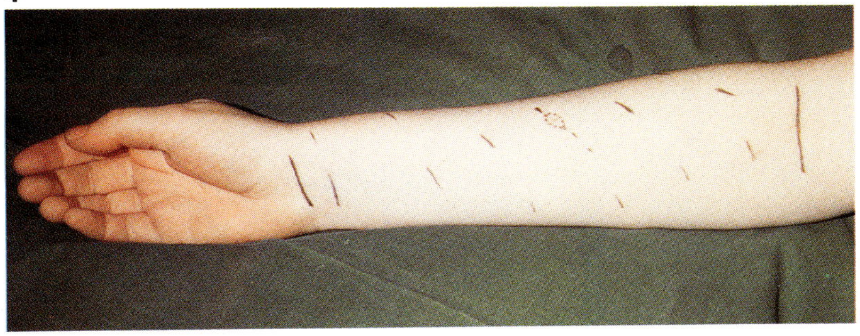

4 Pattern of skin crease lines in the forearm. The oblique direction of the lines becomes transverse at the joints.

5

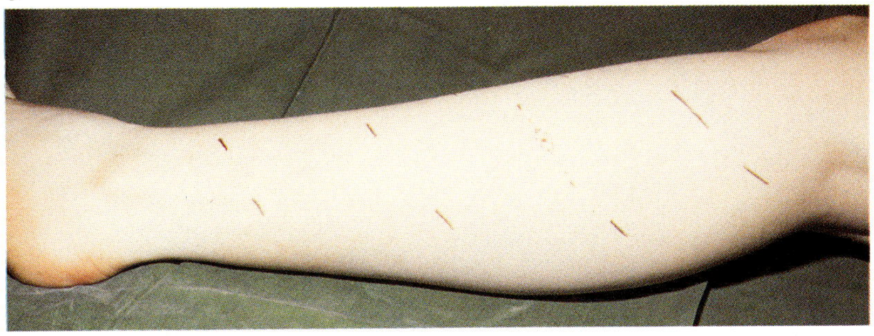

5 Pattern of skin crease lines on the lower limb.

Suture removal and wound healing

In all sutured wounds there is a fine balance which has to be resolved. Sutures left in give wound security but the longer they are in, after 48 hours, the greater the chance of permanent marks being left by the skin sutures. Buried sutures of absorbable synthetic suture should be inserted to give added strength and act as a longer term support for the wound after removal of the skin sutures. Support by skin tape can be applied after surgery and replaced after suture removal to splint the wound and decrease the tension.

Sutures of the face and neck can be removed after five to seven days, even earlier in the eyelids. Arm wounds are slower to heal and sutures should be left for about seven to ten days. On the lower limb or back, wound healing is very slow and some sutures should therefore be left in for about 14 days. If the wound closure has great tension then sutures should be left in place proportionally longer and the closure should be reinforced with subcuticular sutures.

Excision biopsy of a lesion on the leg

1

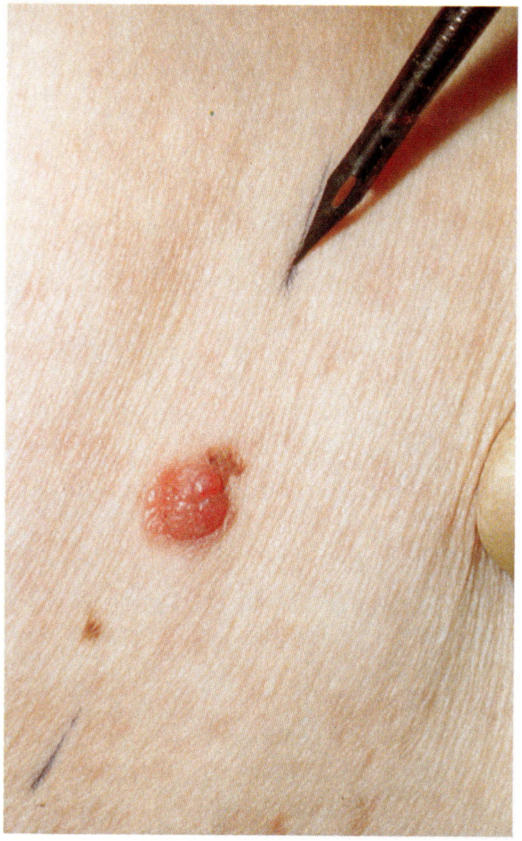

1 The skin creases are found by gentle pinching pressure on the skin and marked with pen and ink.

2

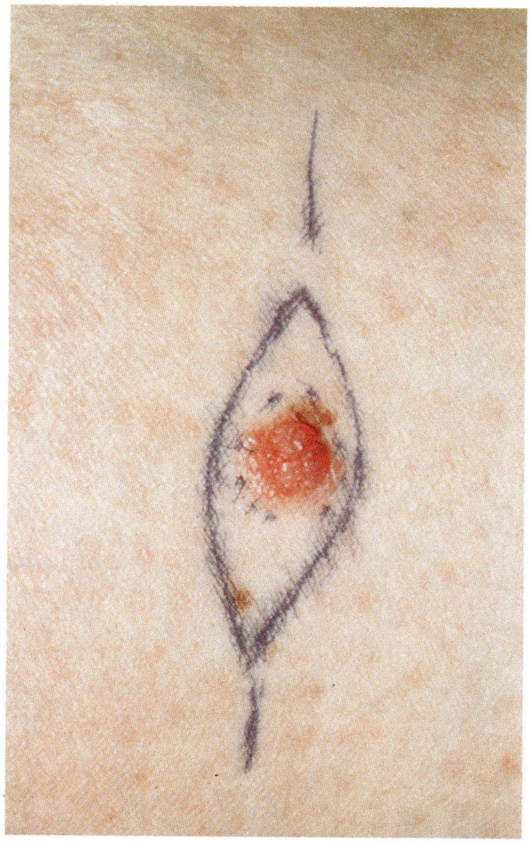

2 The ellipse for excision is placed in the direction of the skin-crease line. A small clear margin of normal skin is removed also.

3

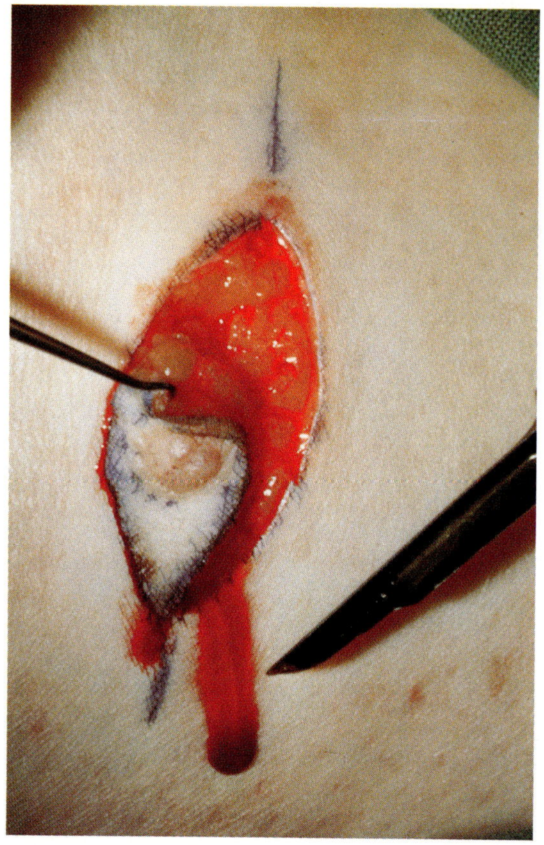

3 The biopsy is handled gently using a skin hook in the edge of the specimen. The lesion itself is not touched.

4 The depth of excision should include a small clear margin of subcutaneous fat. The specimen must be sent for histological examination.

5 The wound is closed by small interrupted sutures of monofilament Prolene. In order to gain even closure the first suture can be placed at the centre to halve the wound.

4

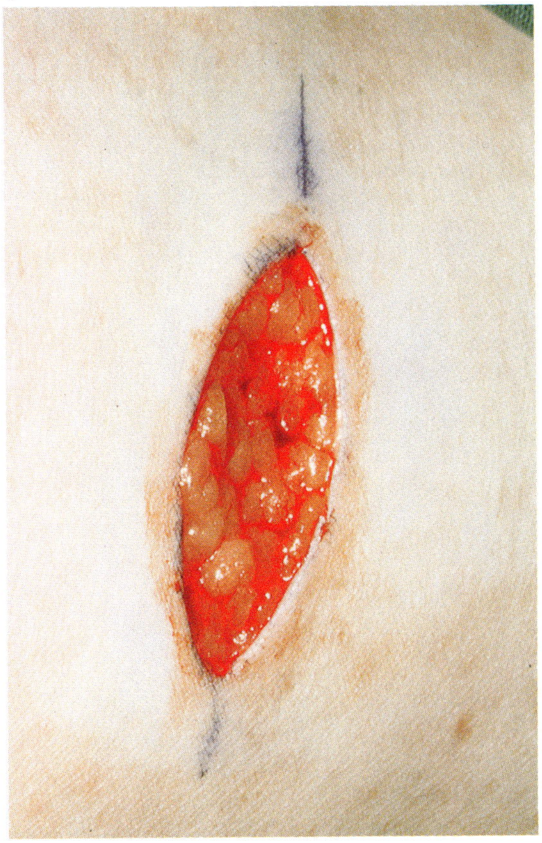

5

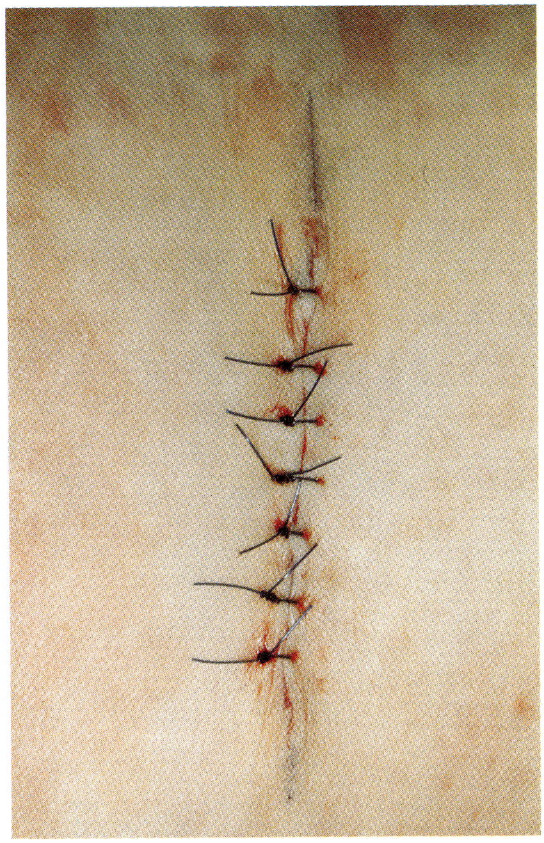

Excision biopsy of a mole of the face

1

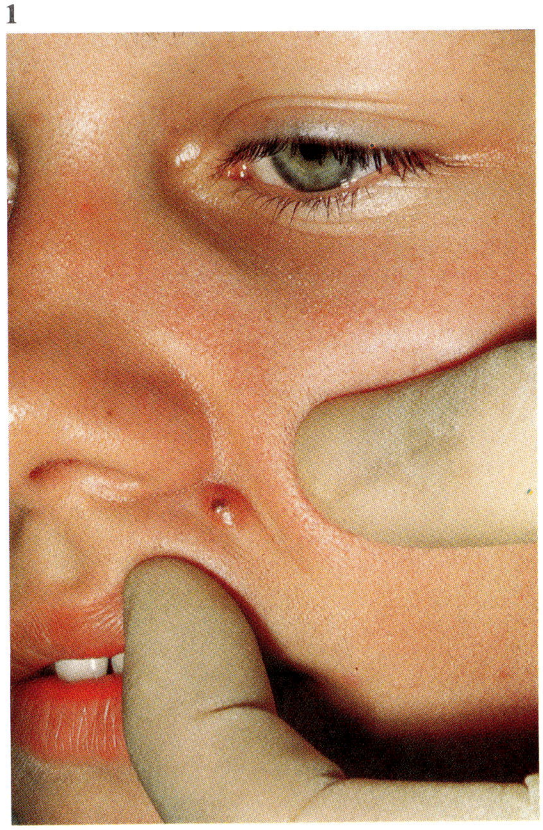

1 The direction of skin crease lines is found by asking the patient to smile or by pinching the skin.

2 The crease lines are marked and an ellipse of excision drawn with a small clear margin.

3 The lesion is excised holding the scalpel at right angles to the skin making sure that the edge of the excision is perpendicular to the skin surface. The specimen must be sent for histological examination.

2

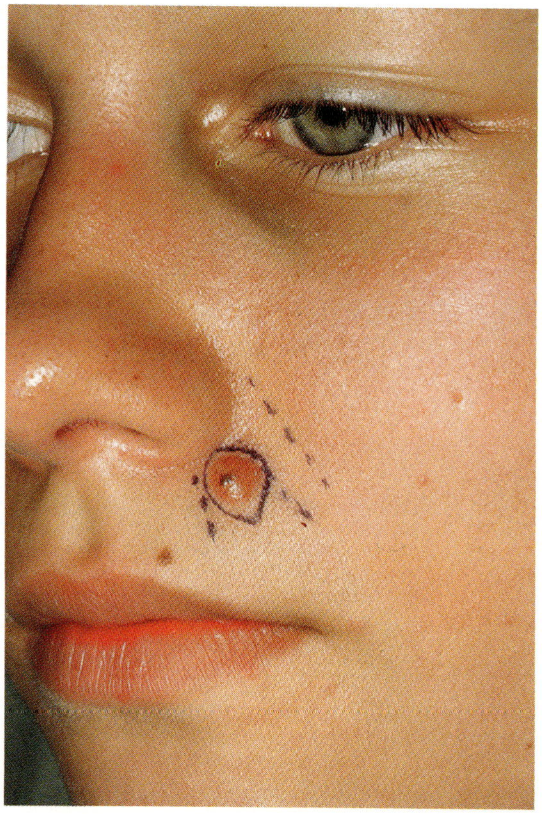

3

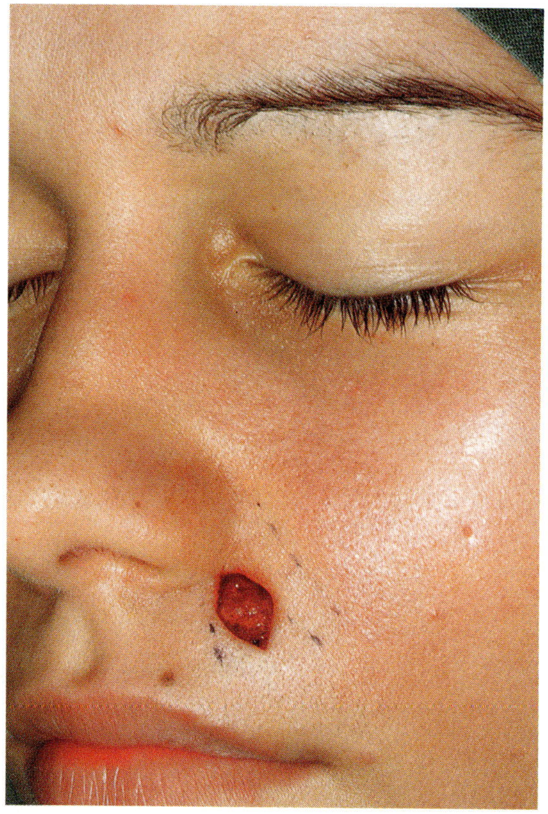

4 Interrupted skin sutures of fine monofilament Prolene are inserted. The needle is seen entering the skin at right angles to the surface. The skin margin is held by a skin hook or fine forceps in order not to traumatise the wound margin unnecessarily.

5 The needle leaves the other side of the skin at right angles, the skin hook acting as a counter pressure. It is not usually necessary to pick up the skin with an instrument.

4

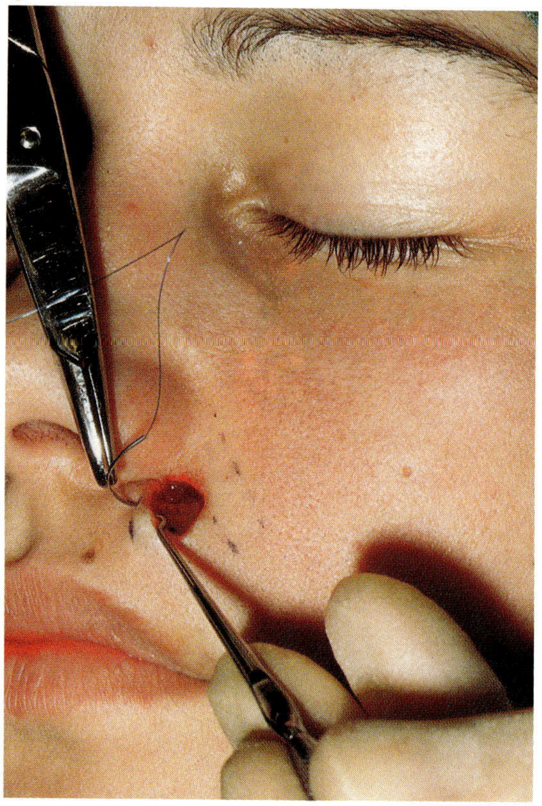

5

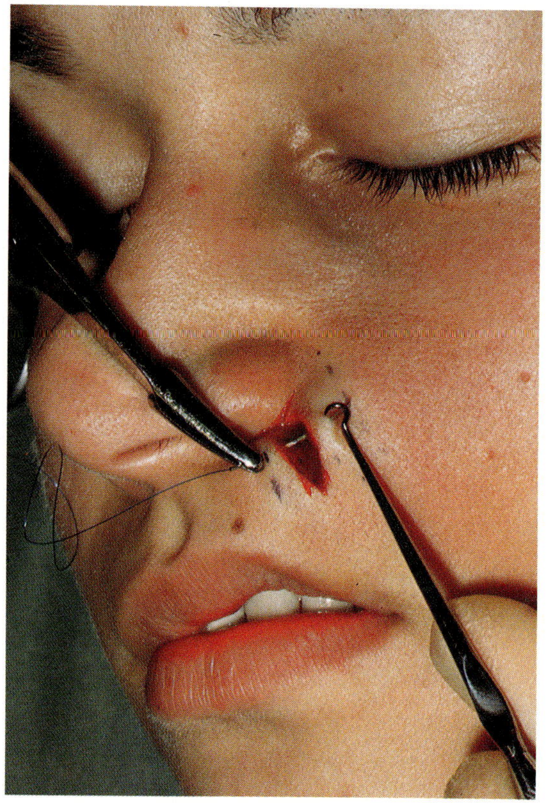

6 The finished wound with a neat row of fine interrupted sutures. The wound should be slightly everted throughout.

6

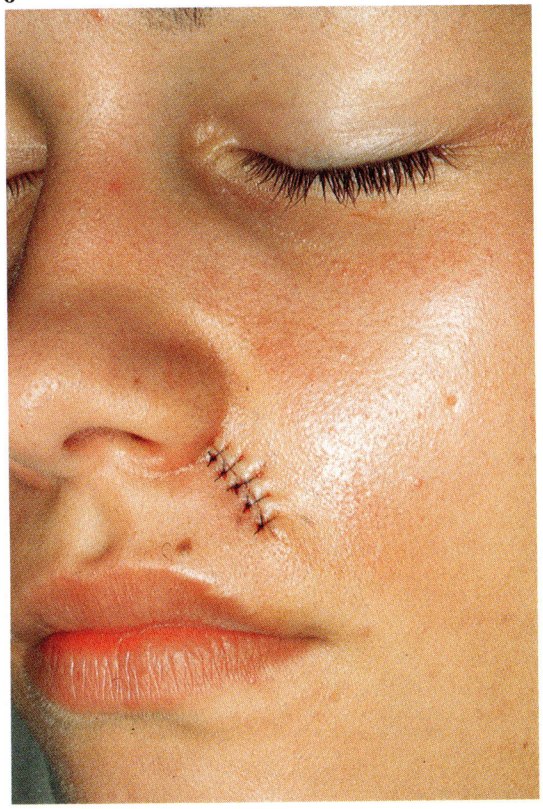

Excision biopsy of a larger lesion on the face leaving a curved scar

1

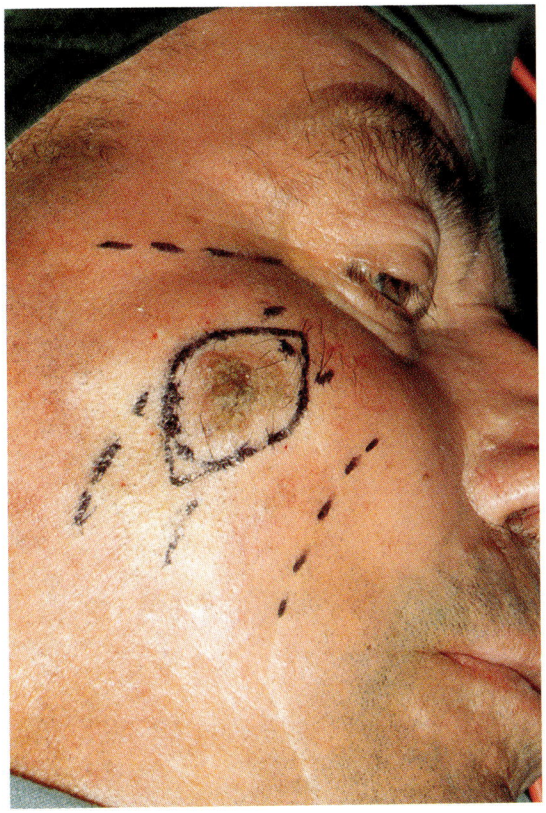

2

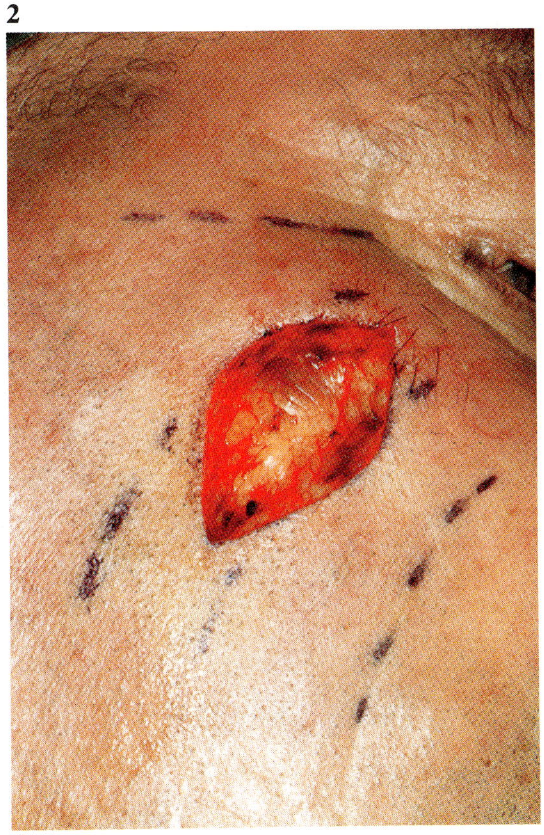

1 Where the skin-crease lines are curved, the resulting scar should be in a curve. The axis of the ellipse for excision is roughly parallel to the lines drawn but is more curved on the convex side of the lesion.

2 In the face, biopsy of a superficial lesion should not be carried deeper than the level of the facial muscles or the facial nerve will be put at risk. Fibres of the zygomaticus muscle can be seen in the depth of the wound.

3

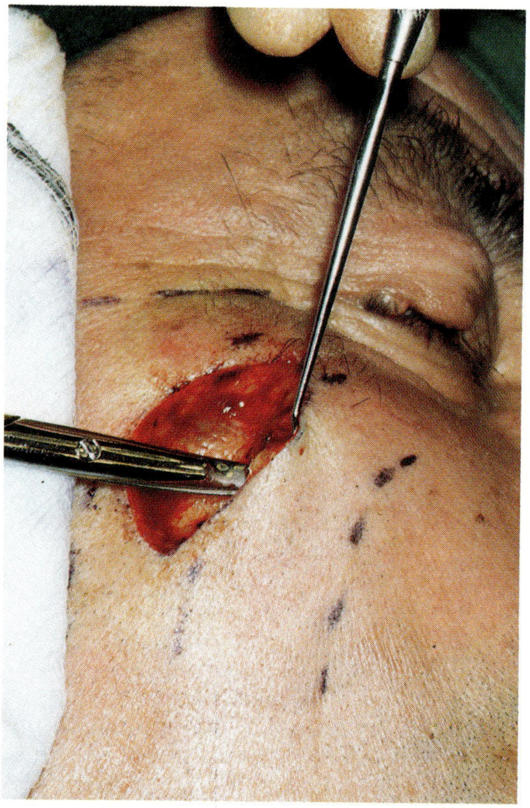

4

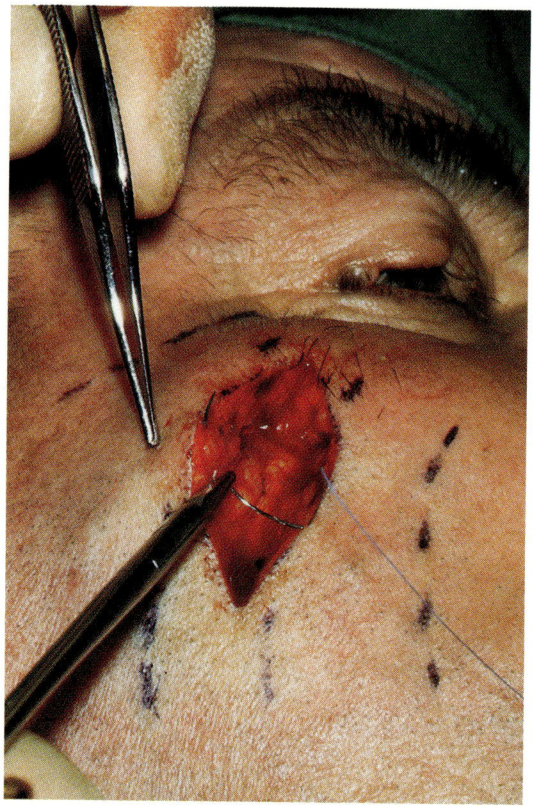

5

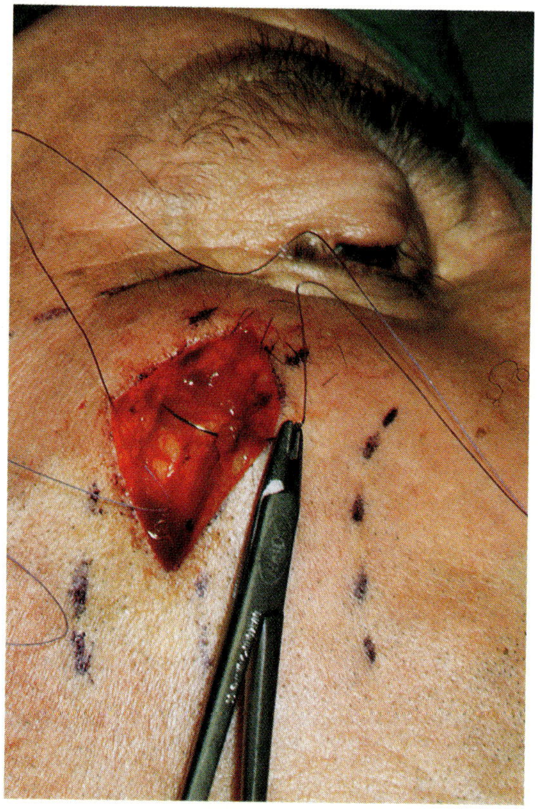

6

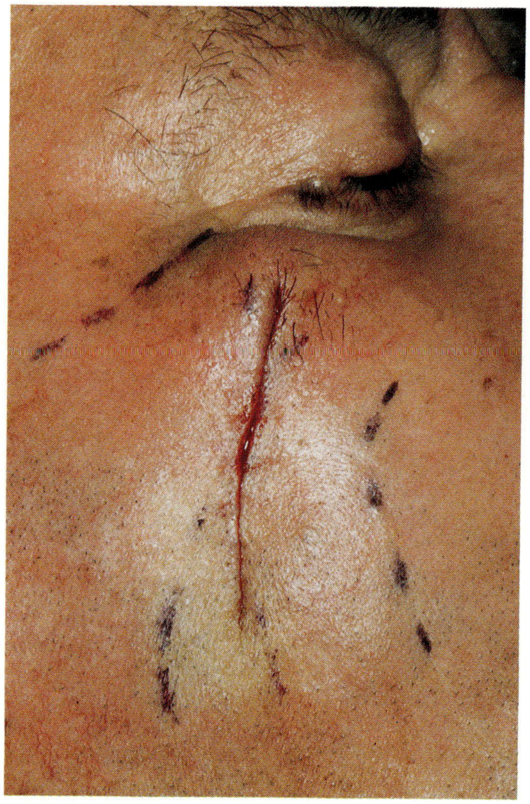

3 Undermining is carried out in the level of the subcutaneous fat. There should be more undermining on the concave side of the wound.

4 A subcuticular suture of Vicryl absorbable synthetic suture or catgut is inserted at the centre of the wound to halve it.

5 The subcuticular suture is completed taking a small bite of deep dermis on each side of the wound and tied to leave the knot buried at the subcutaneous surface.

6 By repeated halving of the wound with subcuticular interrupted sutures the problem of closing a wound where the sides are unequal is overcome without asymmetry or bunching.

7

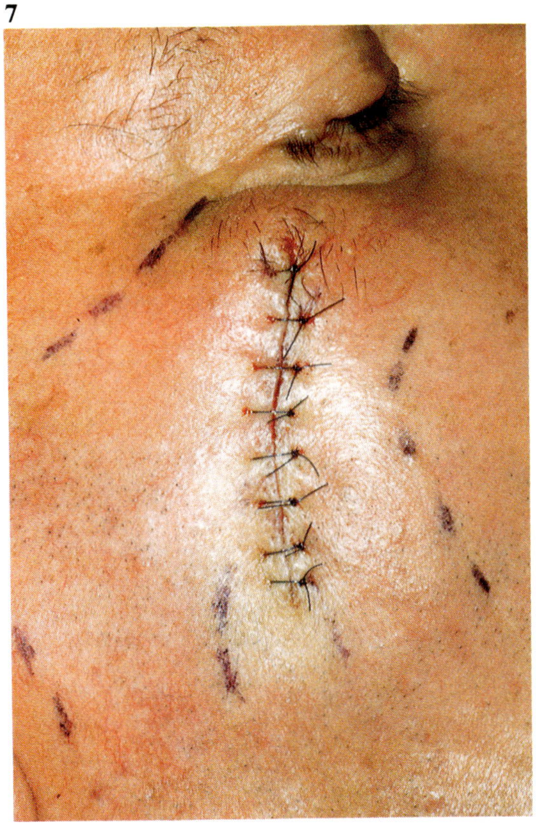

8

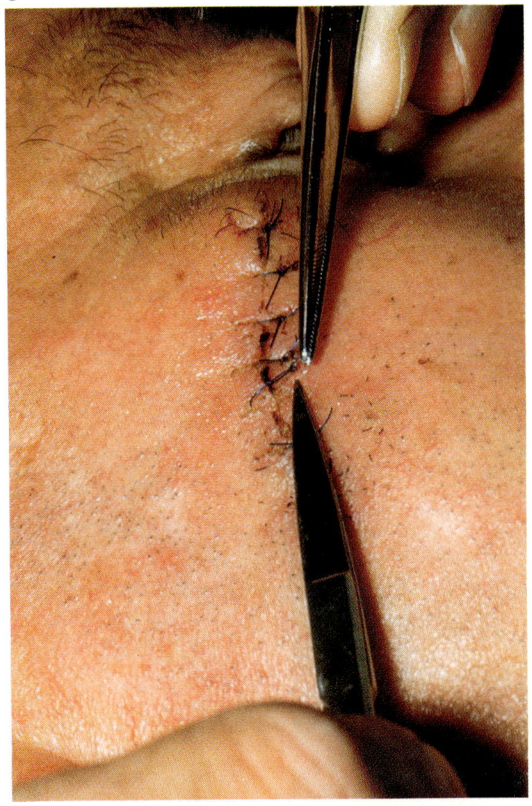

9

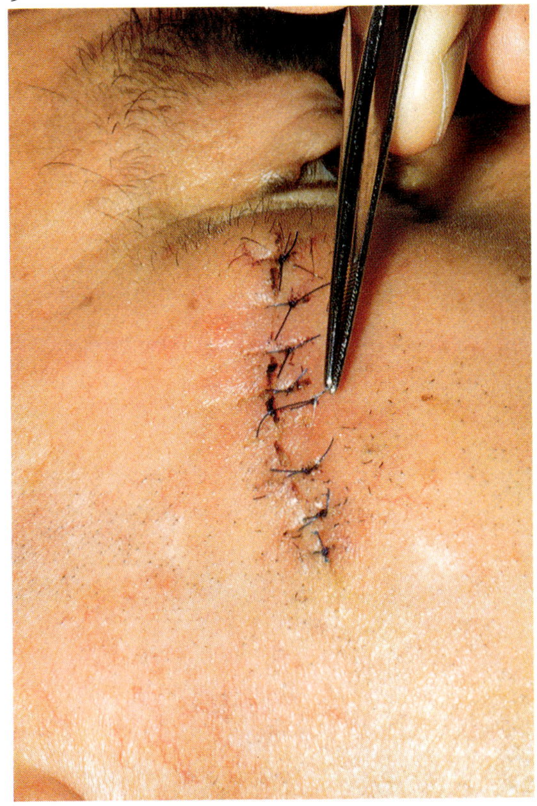

7 Interrupted sutures of fine Prolene are then inserted.

8 One week later the sutures are removed. The suture is lifted with forceps and cut.

9 The suture is then removed by pulling out the suture towards the cut side. This is to prevent any distraction of the wound if there should be any resistance to removal of the suture.

10 As there is considerable wound tension, the centre sutures are removed and adhesive tape is applied before the remaining sutures are removed.

10

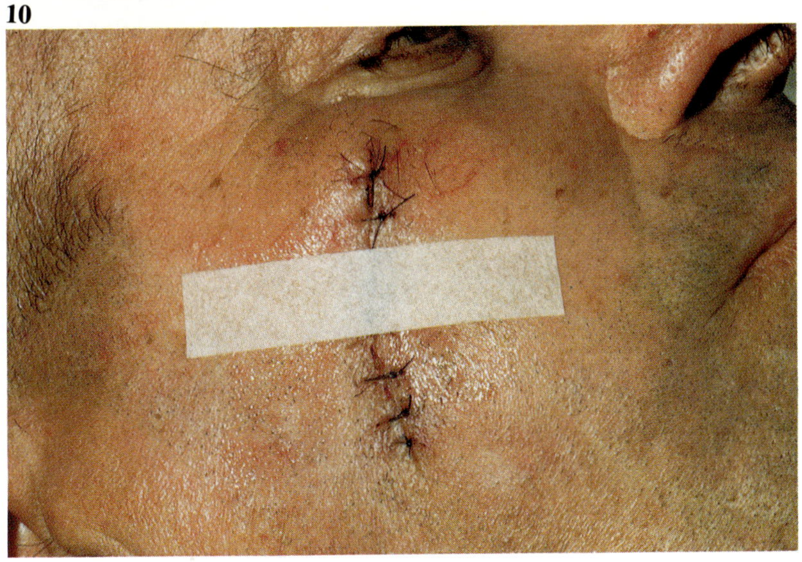

Shaping the excision, removal of 'dog ears'

Excision biopsy of larger lesion of back, possible malignant melanoma.

1

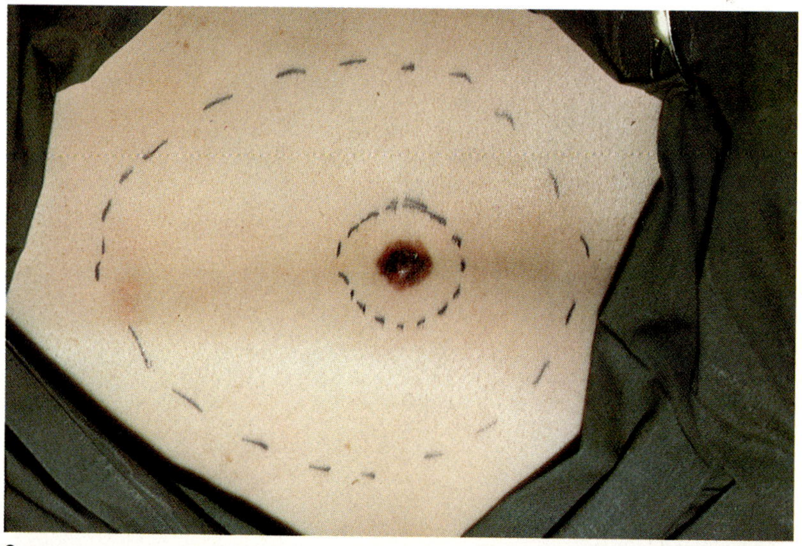

1 Excision biopsy margin is marked. The outer circle is the margin for wide excision such as would be necessary if it were a malignant melanoma.

2 After excision, frozen section biopsy was performed. It showed a pigmented basal cell carcinoma and excision was therefore adequate. The wound has become an oval showing that wound closure with a transverse scar would have the least tension.

3 The wound edges are undermined above and below after checking by traction on skin hooks that the wound will close without undue tension.

2

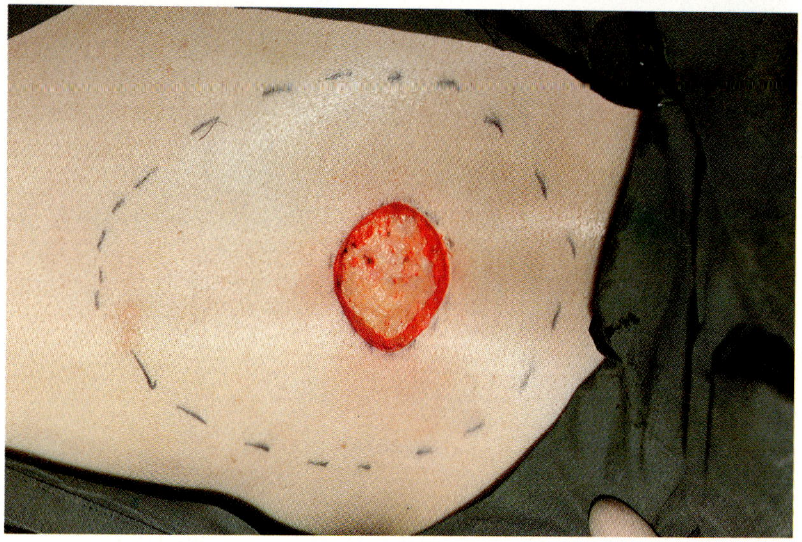

3

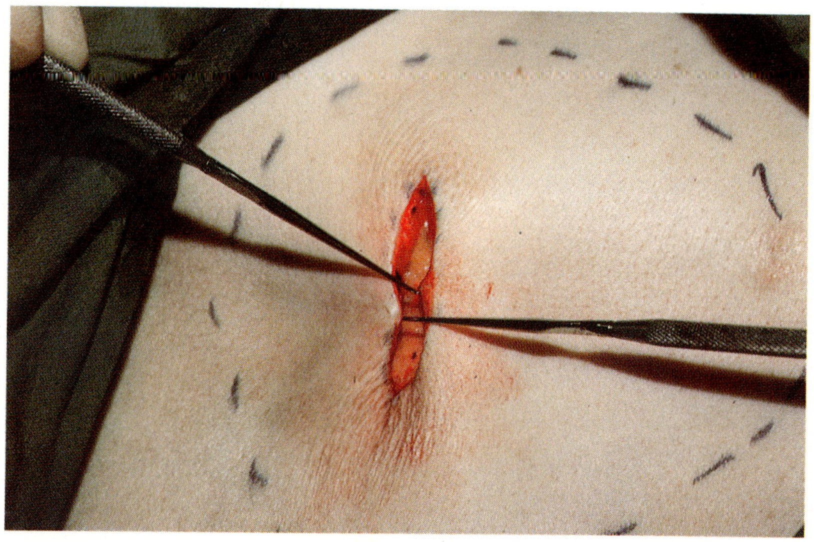

4 Subcuticular sutures are inserted and the ends of the wound bunch up into standing cones ('dog ears').

4

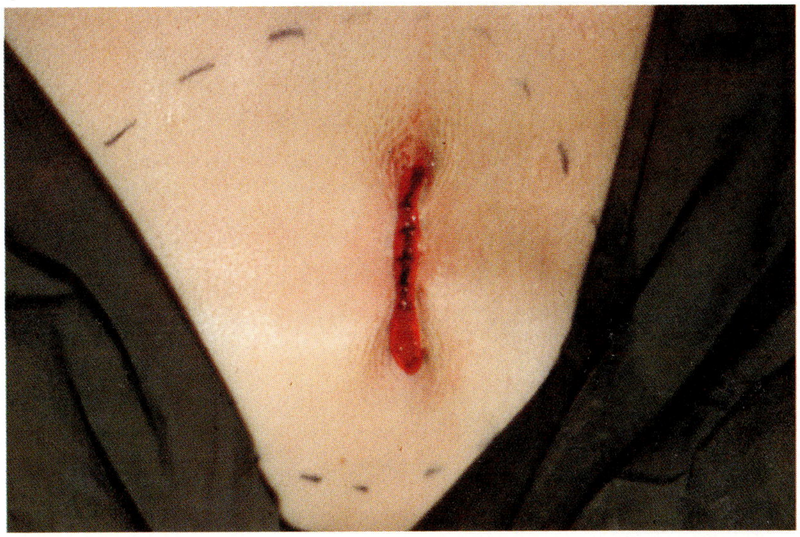

5 To remove the excess skin careful marking is required. A skin hook is inserted into the apex of the cone to draw it out slightly. The skin margin to be excised is shown marked in a continuous blue line, which is a continuation of the edge of the wound.

5

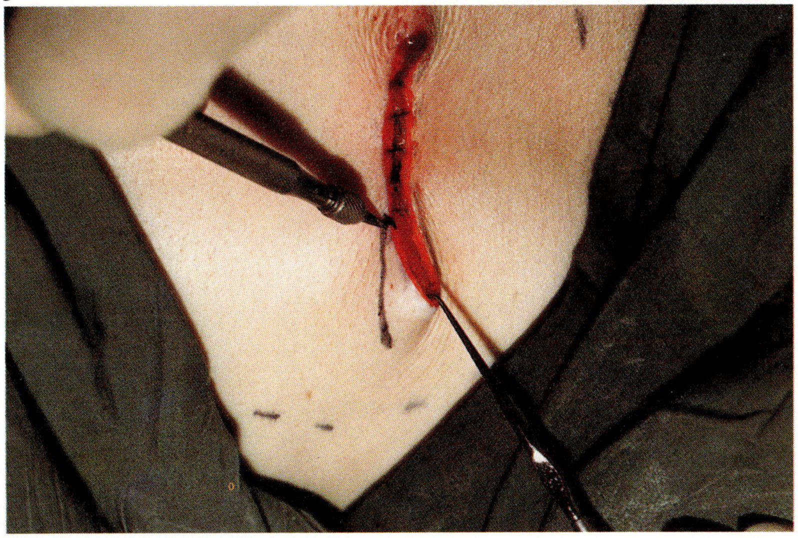

6 The skin is then incised along this line, and the skin hook transferred to the distal edge of the triangle of skin, which is pulled up to the opposite side. The next incision line is then shown drawn in a dotted line which is a continuation of the other wound edge meeting the first line. This dog ear is then excised. The dog ear at the opposite end of the wound has already been excised.

7 The wound is closed with a continuous subcuticular monofilament suture and the wound reinforced by skin tapes. The ends of the subcuticular suture can be secured by tying them together (see Wound Repair, **6**).

6

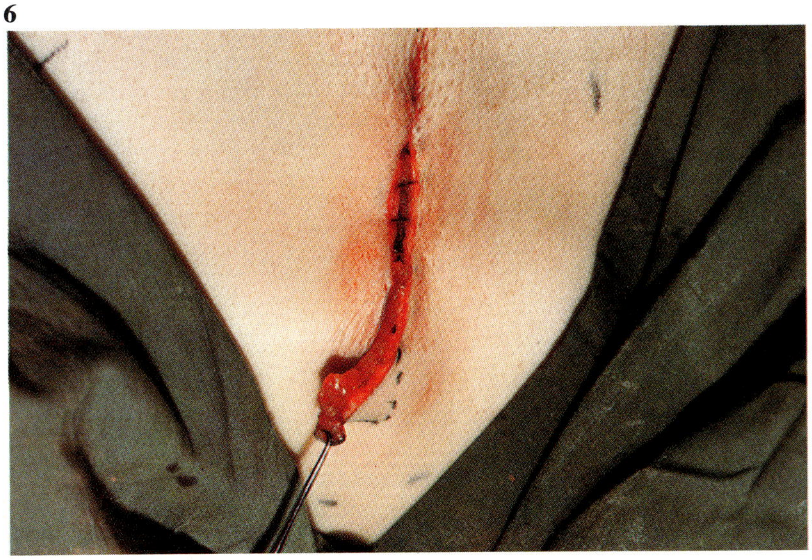

7

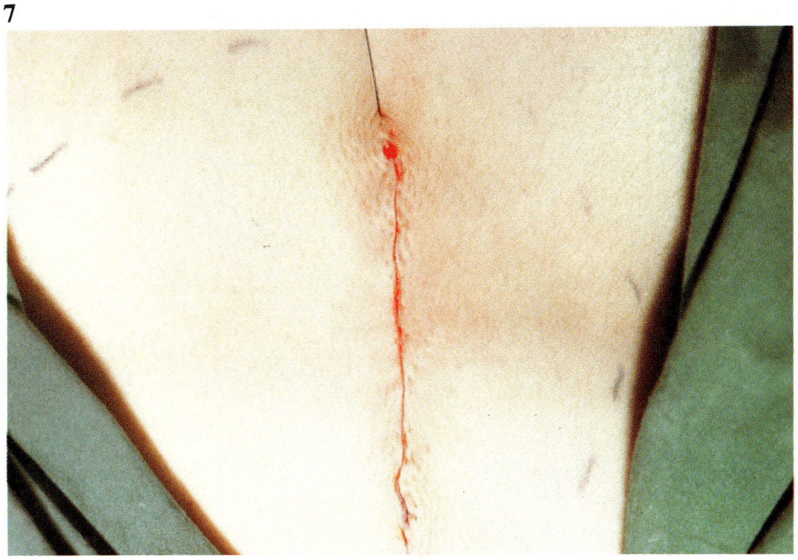

Wound repair

1

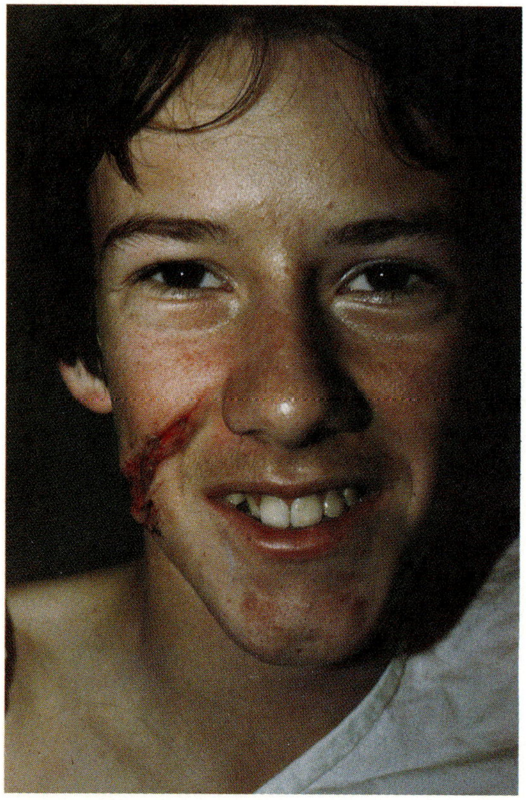

1 **Chainsaw laceration of the right cheek.** Full examination pre-operatively to exclude facial nerve damage is essential. Note the relatively symmetrical smile.

2

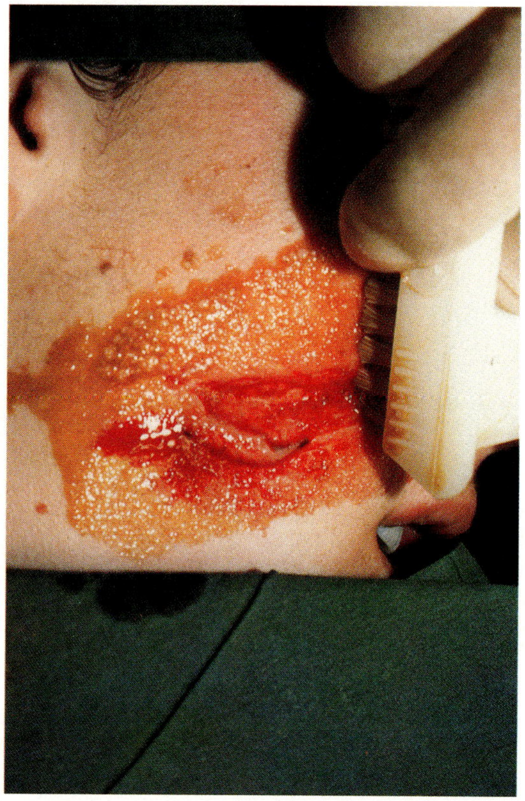

2 **Thorough cleaning is performed** by scrubbing the skin with a sterile brush or toothbrush, under adequate anaesthetic – local or general.

3

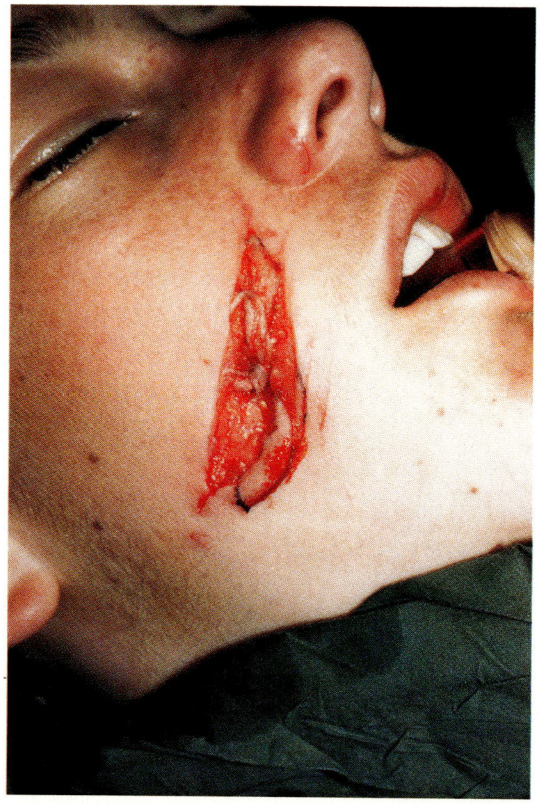

3 **Areas to be trimmed are marked with pen and ink.** Trimming of the wound is kept to an absolute minimum in clean cut wounds. Ragged areas only are trimmed. Routine excision of the wound edge is not necessary on the face.

4

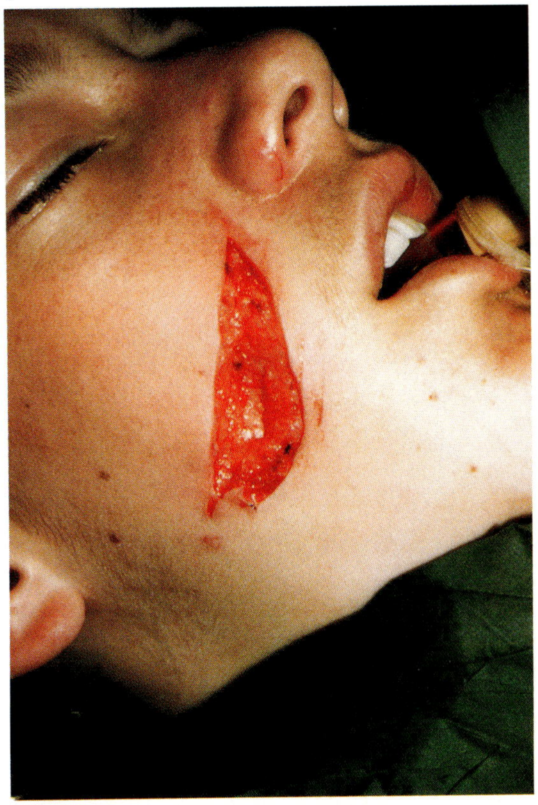

4 The wound has been trimmed prior to suturing.

5

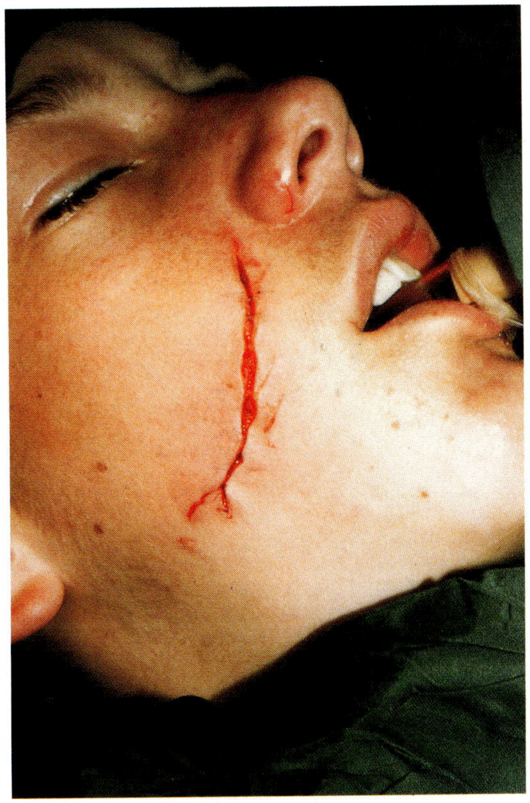

5 The basic principle in suturing is to approximate the tissues into the correct anatomical relationship. Repair should start by repairing features such as the red margin of the lip or the alar of the nose. In this case ink marks are placed to help alignment of the cheek tissues. A subcuticular interrupted absorbable layer of sutures is then inserted.

6

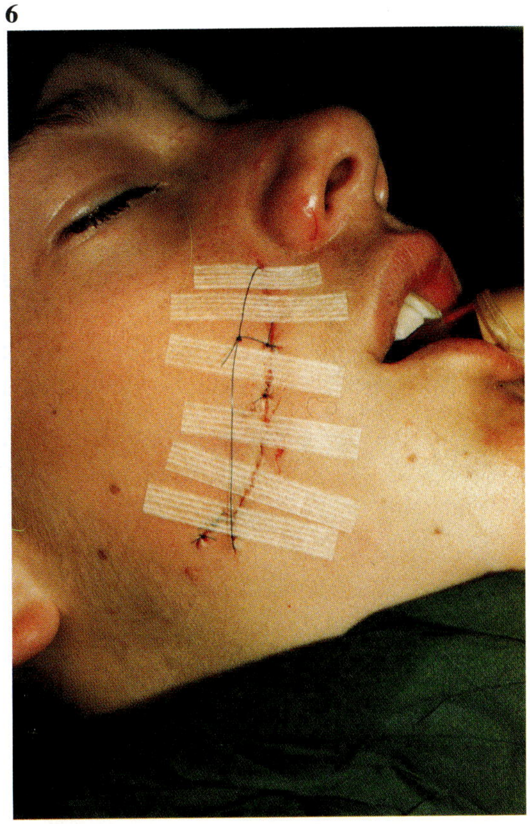

6 Wound repair is completed by a continuous subcuticular suture, a few interrupted skin sutures and steristrips.

Biopsy of pyogenic granuloma

1

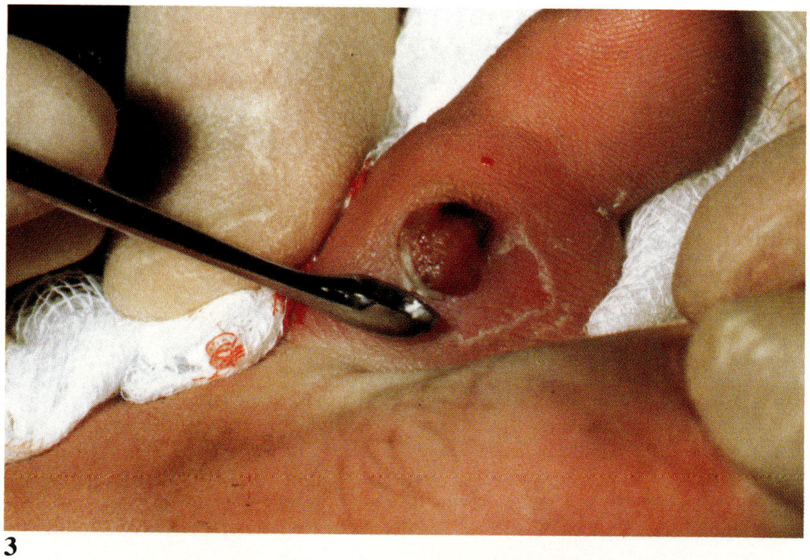

1 Under local or general anaesthetic the granuloma is removed using a Volkman's spoon. A pneumatic tourniquet has been applied without exsanguination of the limb in case it is a malignant tumour which might be disseminated.

2

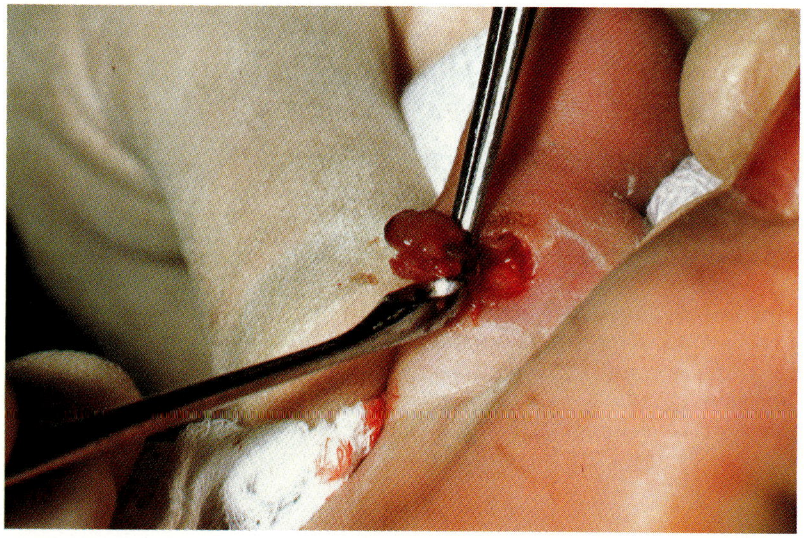

2 It is essential that the specimen of tissue is sent for histological examination. It should not be handled roughly but be picked up with fine forceps or skin hook in order not to destroy the specimen. The base of the wound is carefully inspected for the presence of any foreign body.

3

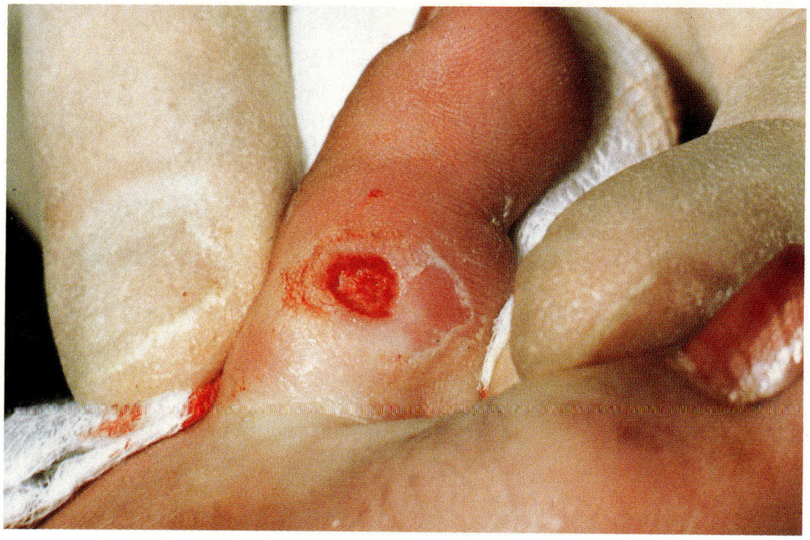

3 Curettage is carried down until a clean fibrous base is obtained and a non-adherent dressing is then applied.

Tattoo excision

1

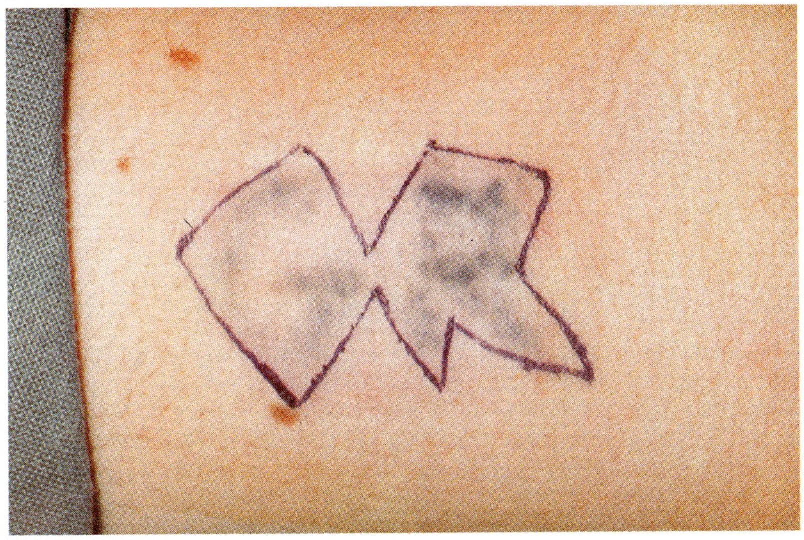

1 To disguise the nature of the scar, the excision is planned and marked in an irregular pattern. If the letters alone are excised the resulting scar can still be 'read'.

2

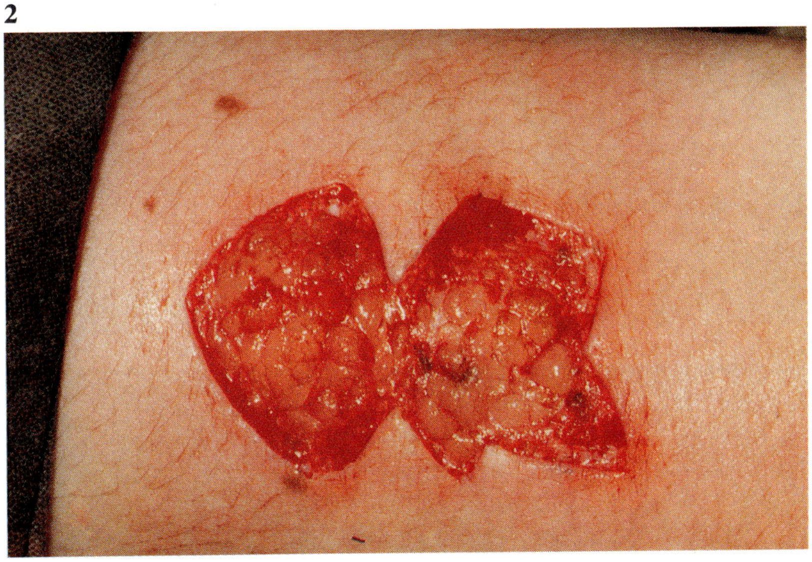

2 After haemostasis the undermining of the wound edge is performed.

3

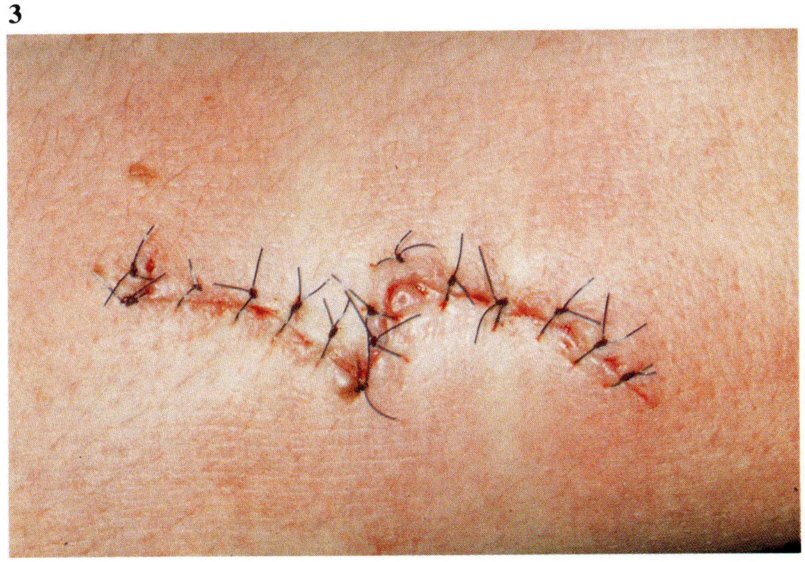

3 Sutures are inserted to approximate the wound edge. If possible a zigzag closure is obtained by interdigitating flaps from opposite sides. If it proves impossible to close the wound by direct suture a skin graft can be applied. See following section.

Cutting and preparing a split thickness skin graft

1 The correct set-up is essential. The first assistant who holds the donor site is the key person in cutting a good skin graft. The thigh is supported by the flat of each palm and the finger tips and heel of the palm grip the skin, putting it under slight tension to prevent rotating movement. The skin graft knife is placed flat on the greased skin. The surgeon holds a greased flat board in front of the knife to flatten the donor site. The second assistant – if available – exerts a pull away from the knife to complete the tensioning of the donor site. It is important to set the knife correctly. The thickness of the skin varies according to donor's site, age of patient, presence of rheumatoid disorder. In patients being treated with steroids, the skin can be particularly thin.

1

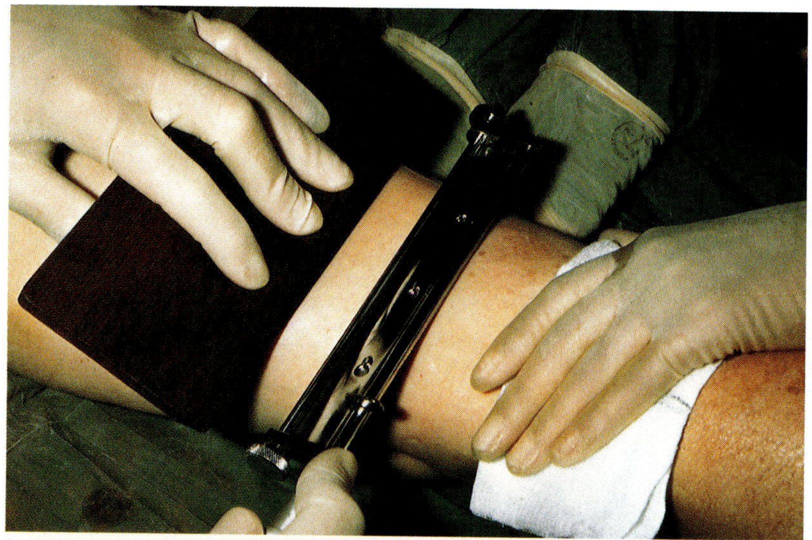

2 Using a steady, rhythmic, slicing action the graft is cut, pressing slightly down on the leading edge of the skin graft knife. To increase the thickness of the graft firmer pressure can be applied. A good guide to the setting of the knife for a moderate thickness split skin graft is to use a disposable scalpel blade as a template between the guard and the cutting edge. If fat is seen protruding through, the level is too deep and the graft must be replaced on the donor site. A new skin graft can be cut at another site using a thinner setting.

2

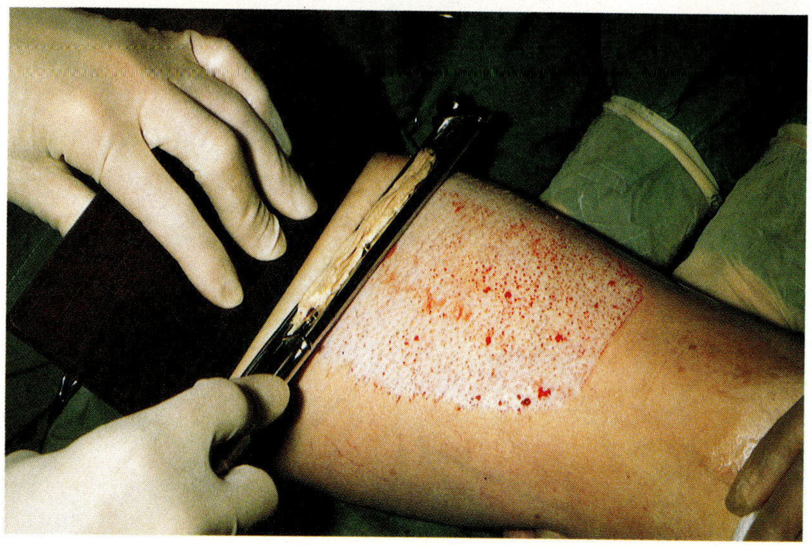

3 The graft can be removed by turning the blade up at the end of the required size or the knife can be pulled backwards leaving the graft on the donor site.

3

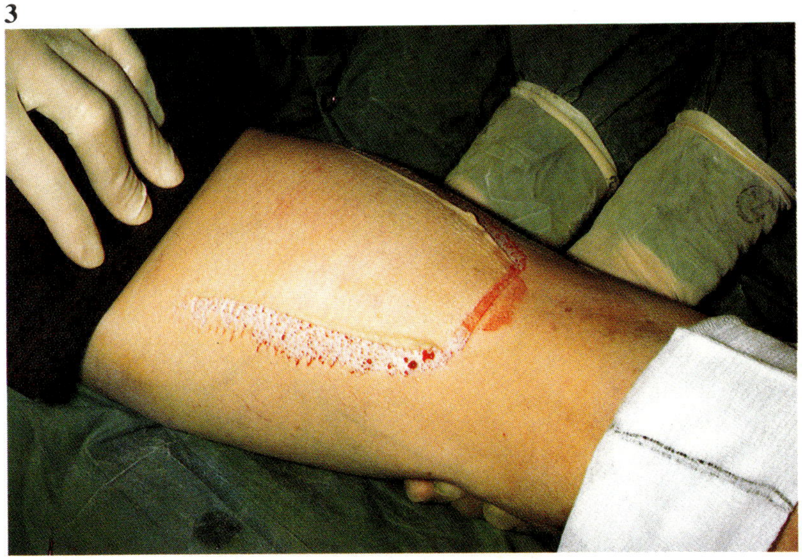

4 The graft is then removed by trimming it with fine scissors. The graft must be kept moist in damp isotonic saline gauze to prevent its desiccation and death.

4

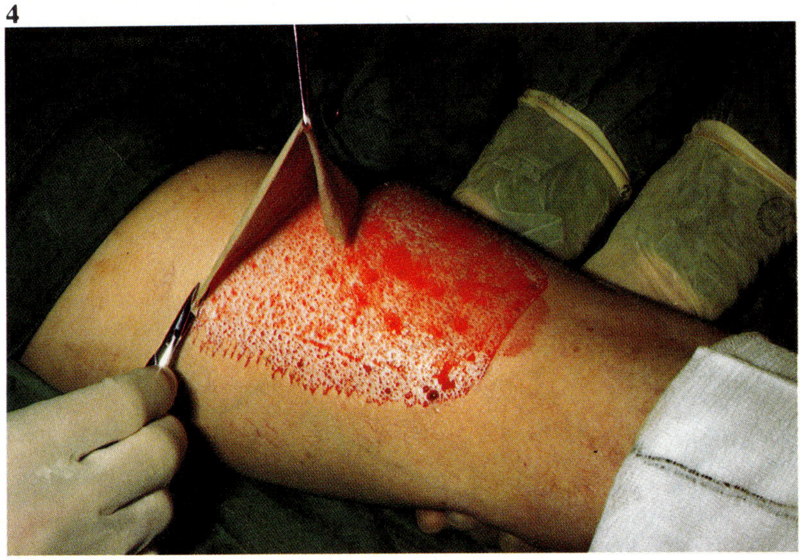

5 A donor site dressing is applied using Vaseline gauze for the inner layer.

6 A gauze layer and a generous layer of absorbent wool is then applied.

5

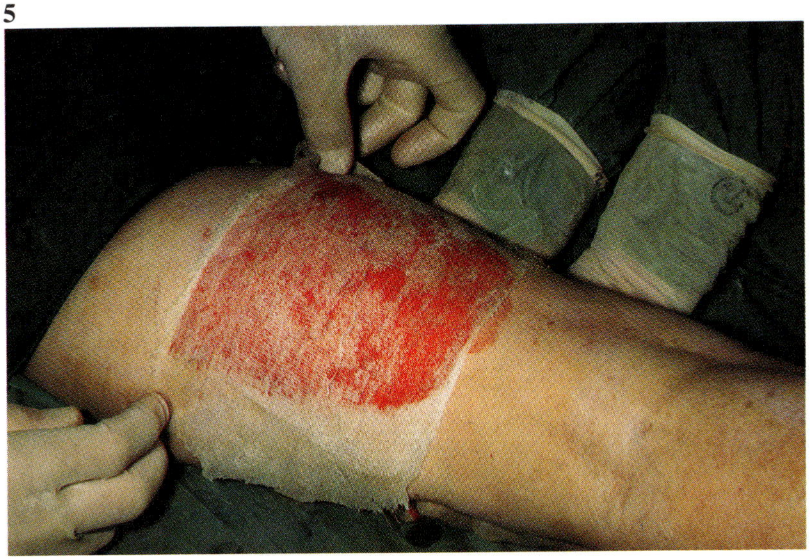

6

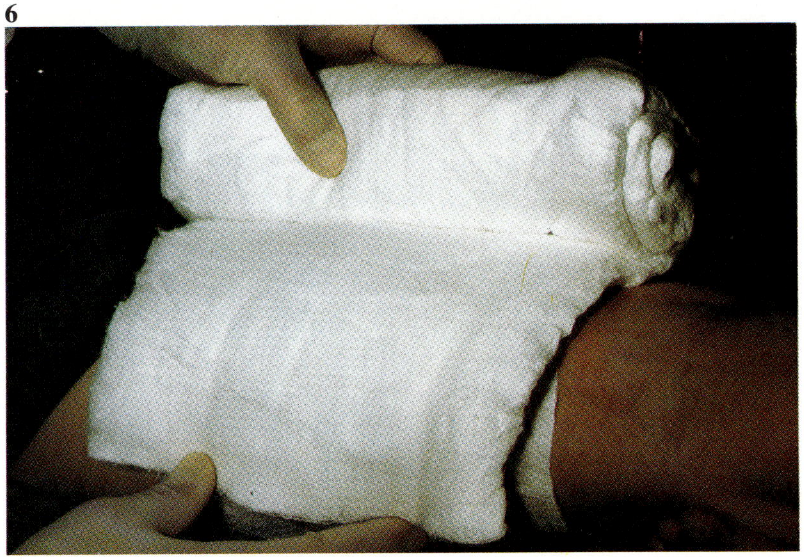

7

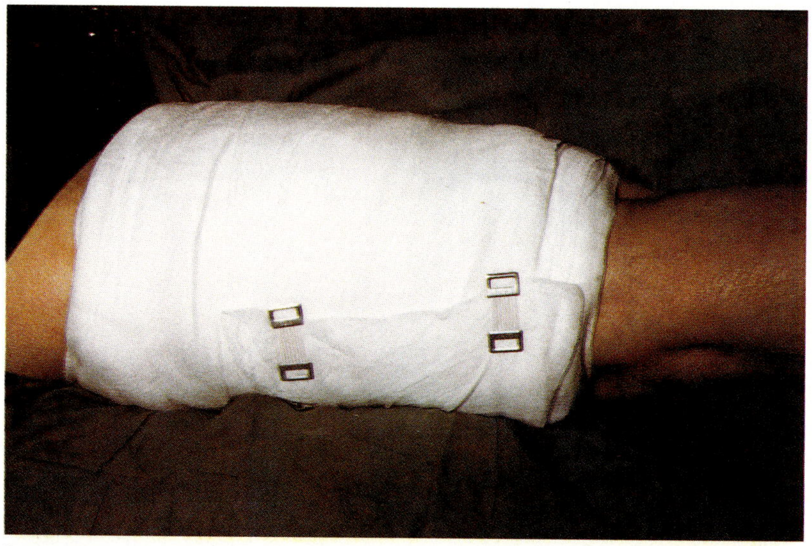

7 The dressing is firmed up with a circumferential bandage and is left undisturbed for a week to ten days by which time healing should have taken place.

8

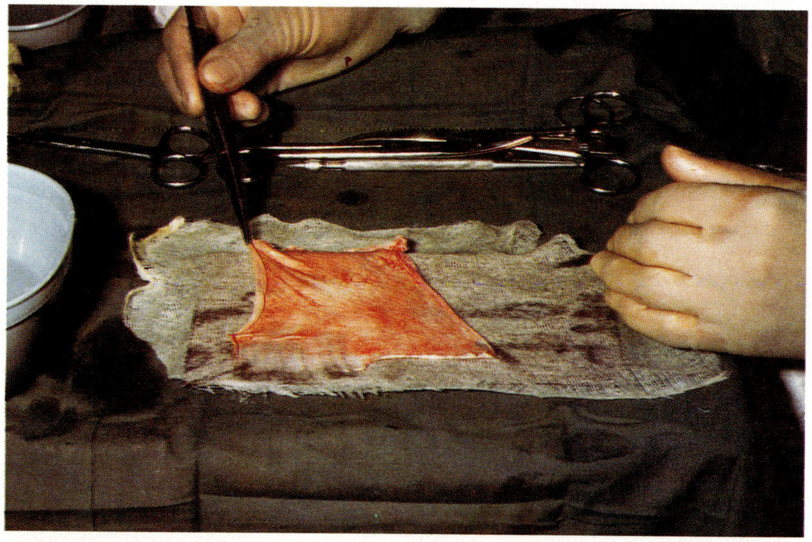

8 The graft is spread on a layer of Vaseline gauze shiny side up as a backing to make it easier to handle. A bowl of isotonic saline nearby is used to moisten the graft.

9

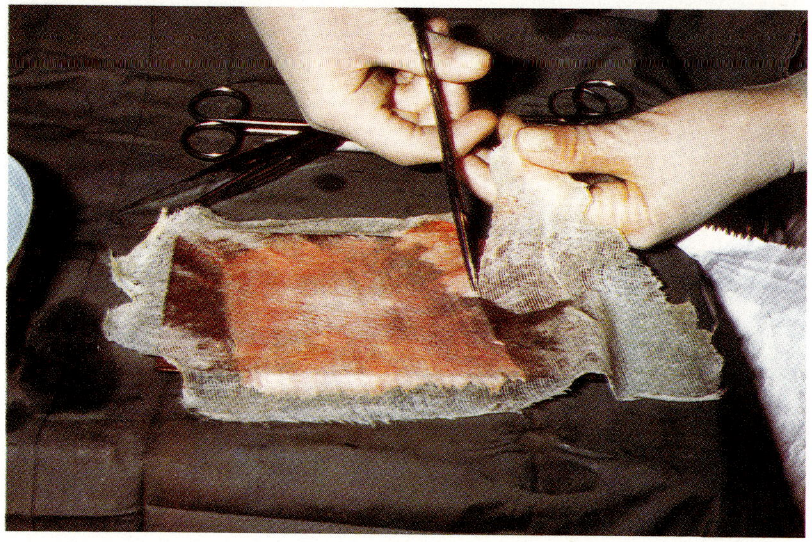

9 Once the graft is spread, the edge of the gauze is trimmed and the graft is then covered with a saline gauze until it is required.

Application of a split skin graft. Tie over (bolus) dressing

1

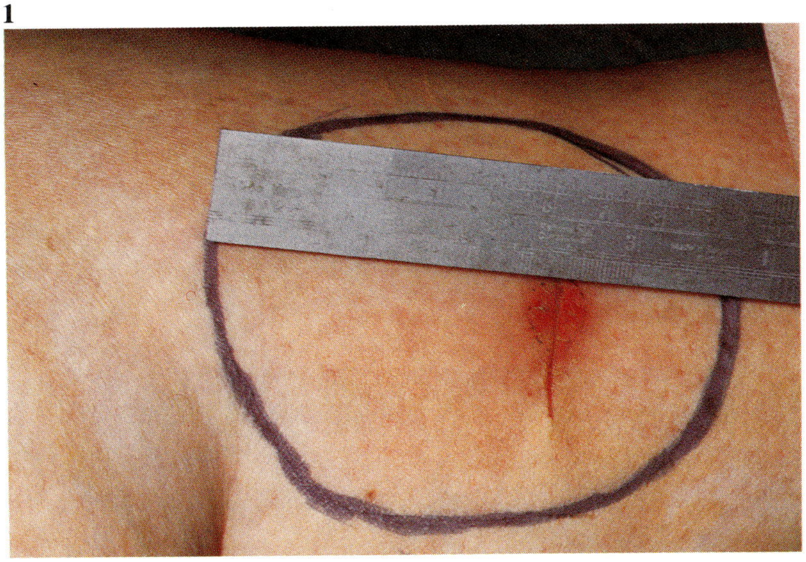

1 Wide excision of a malignant melanoma following a biopsy. The width of the excision depends on several factors including the Breslow thickness measured by the pathologist on a fixed specimen.

2

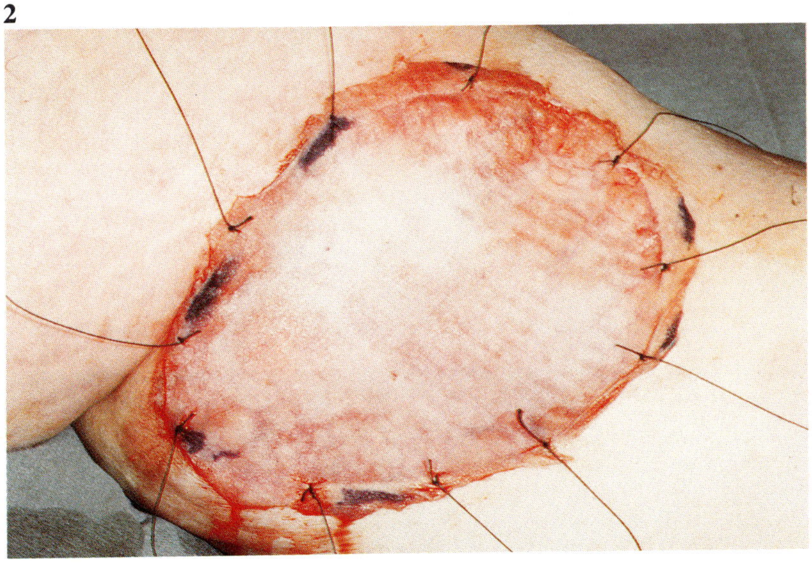

2 The split skin graft is applied to a defect on the calf, cut side down, with an overlapping edge all round. The backing gauze is removed and sutures are placed at the wound margin. For ease of insertion the needle is passed from graft outwards taking a double bite on the graft. The suture end is left long.

3

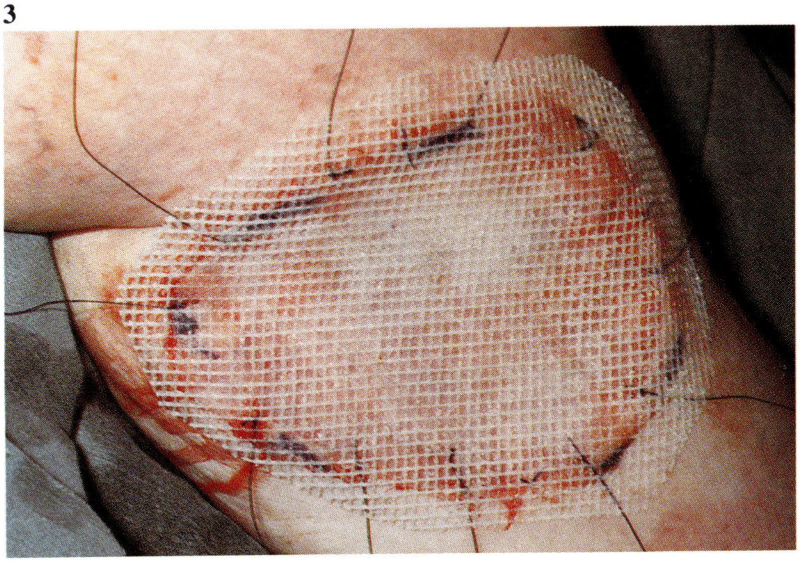

3 Vaseline gauze is applied to the graft.

4

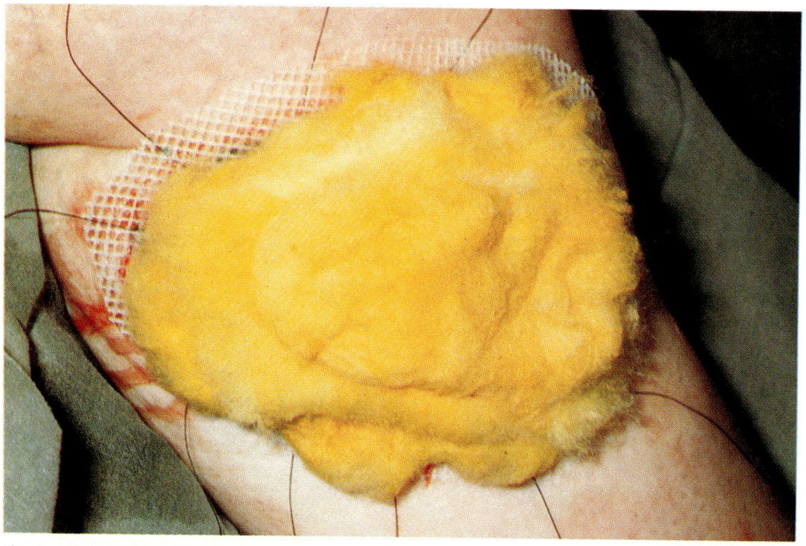

5

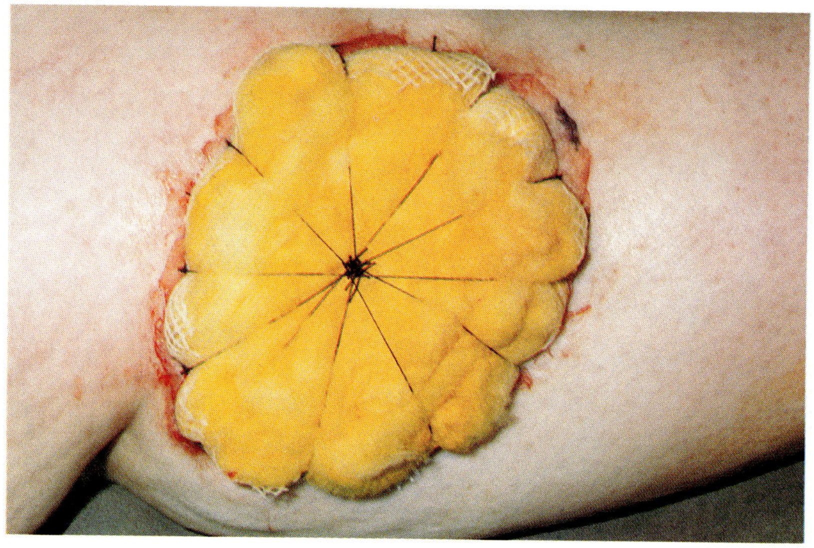

6

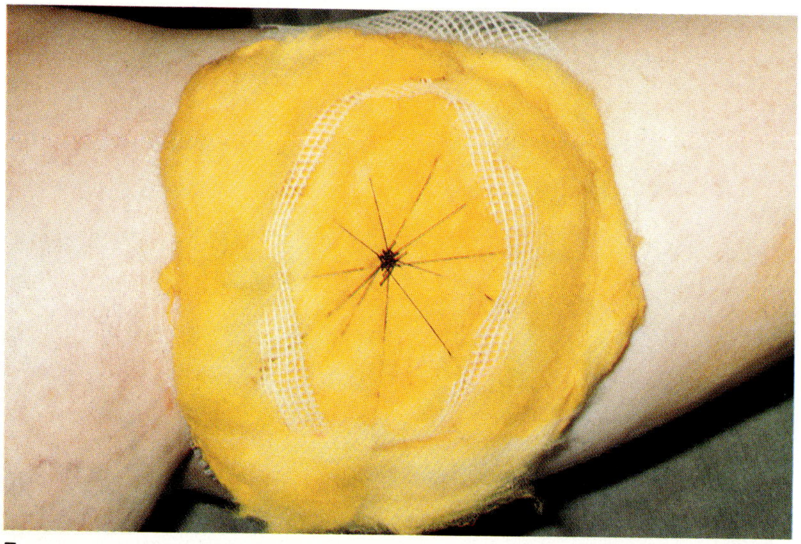

4 A loose padding of flavine wool is applied as a bolus to fill the defect.

5 The long suture ends are tied over neatly to exert even pressure over the graft.

6 The periphery of the bolus is padded with a feathered wool dressing to distribute pressure evenly.

7 A gauze and wool dressing is applied.

8 Firm crêpe bandage is applied to cover the graft and immobilise the joint below and the joint above. If necessary a Plaster of Paris back slab can be applied. The tie over dressing is usually left in place for one week.

7

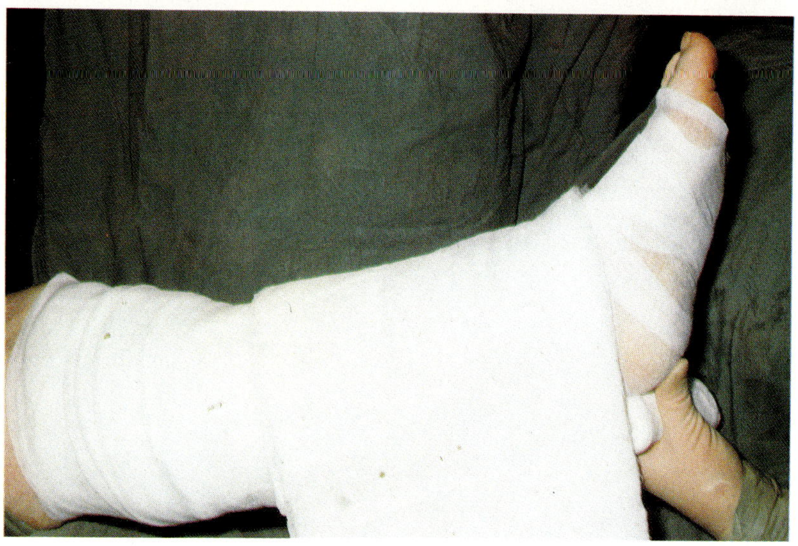

8

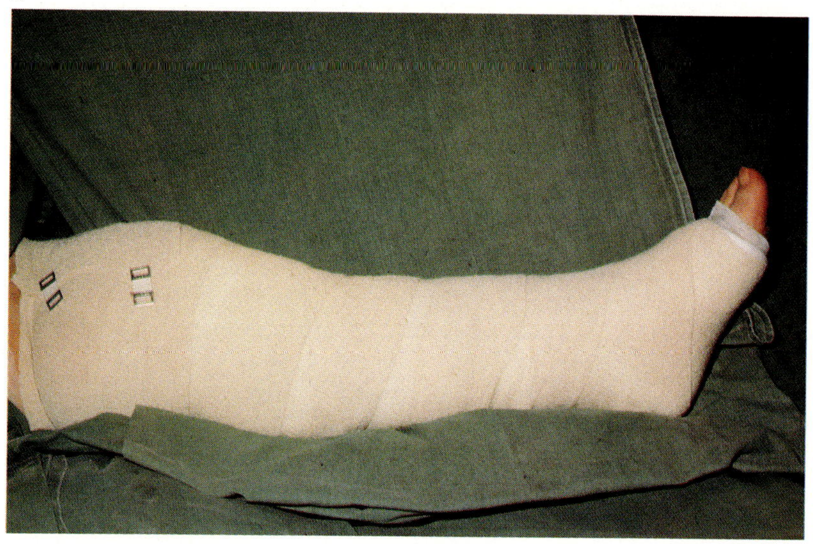

Application of a split thickness graft by staples or sutures

1

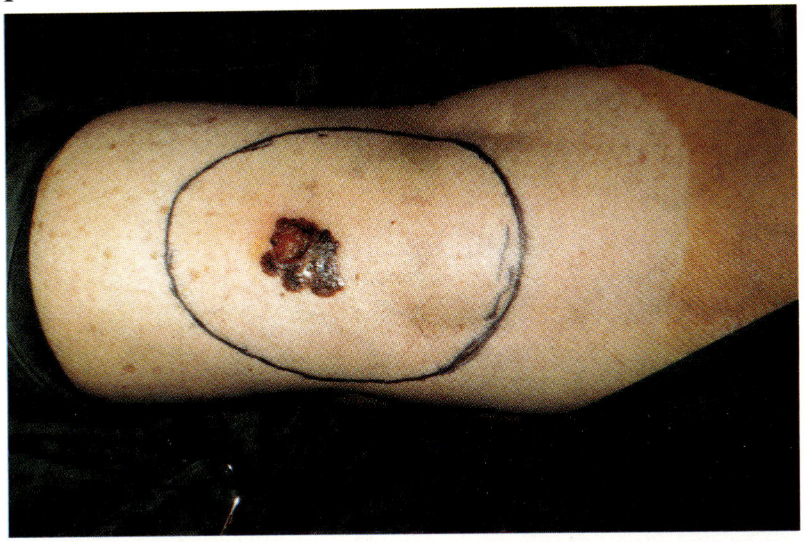

1 A malignant melanoma of the popliteal fossa marked out for wide excision. The wider margin of 7.5 centimetres clear is placed proximally.

2

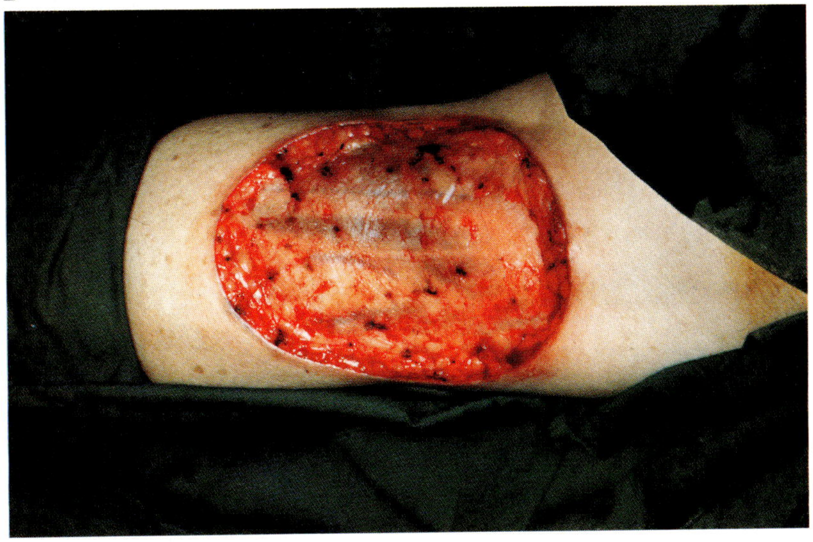

2 The excision is carried out down to but not including the deep fascia.

3

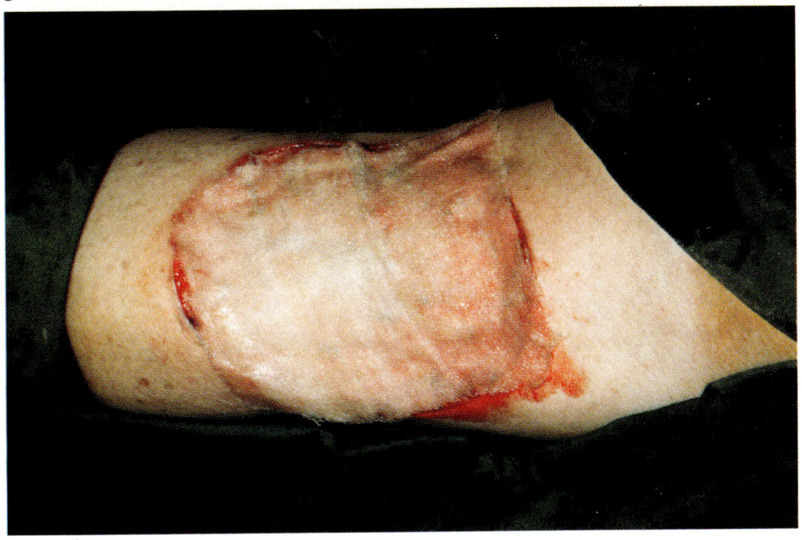

3 A graft cut before the excision is placed over the defect.

4

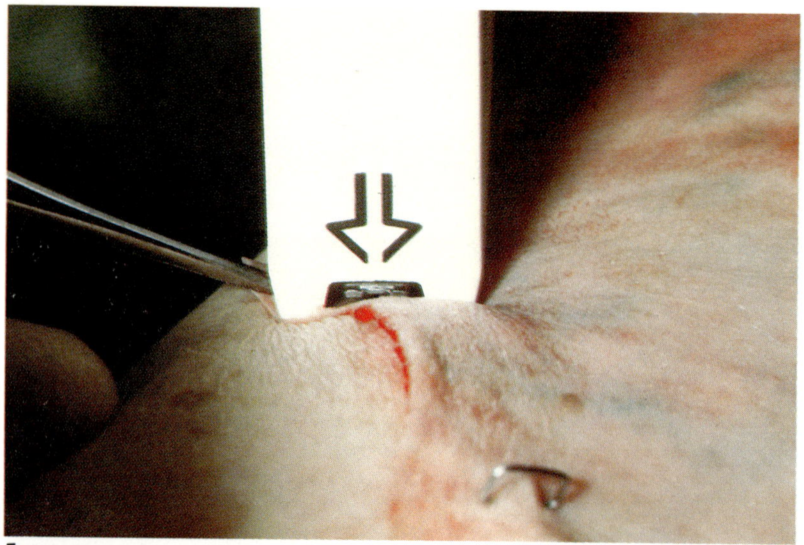

5

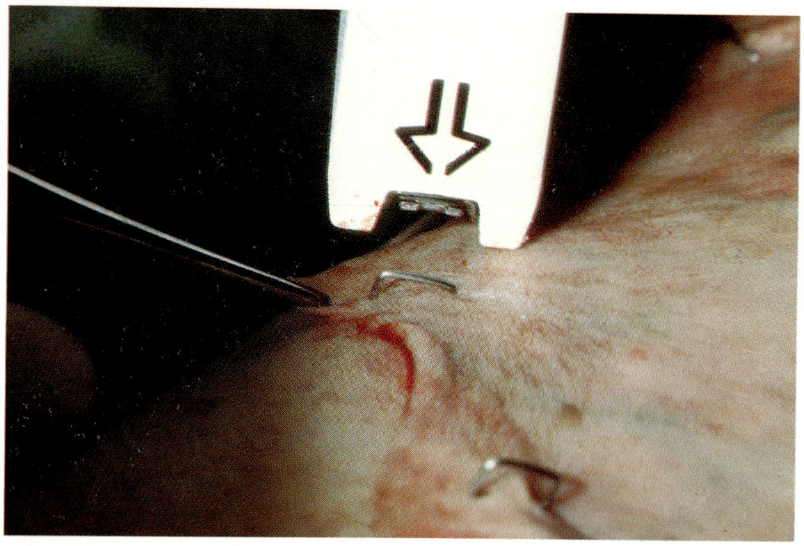

4 Surgical clips are applied to the graft. A large bolus dressing which might cause obstructive pressure to major vessels is impractical over a joint flexure. Fine interrupted sutures could be used if desired.

6

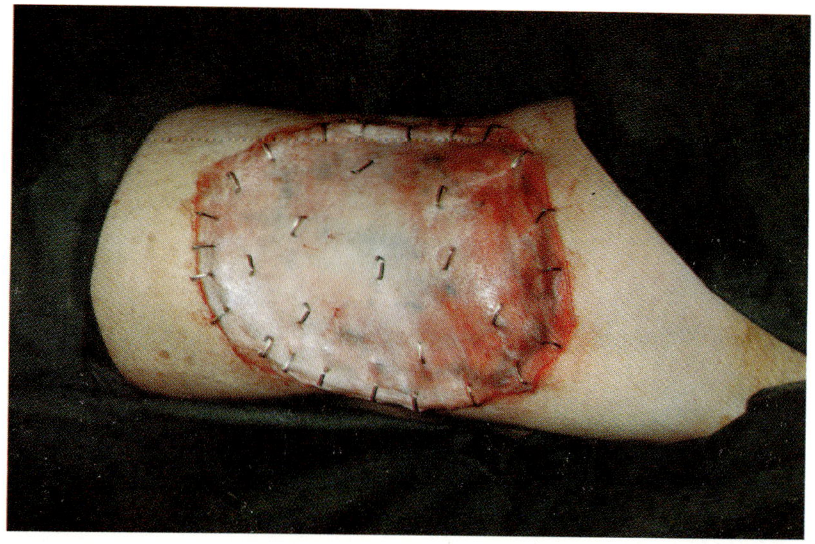

5 A double grip of the graft is taken in order to overlap the margin of the wound.

6 The fixation of the graft is completed. A carefully padded dressing is then applied, together with a Plaster of Paris splint and left in place for about a week. In certain patients, who are fit and able to cooperate, the graft can be treated exposed so that any haematomas can be expressed regularly towards the graft edge.

Full thickness skin graft to repair a defect from excision of a basal cell carcinoma of the eyelid

1

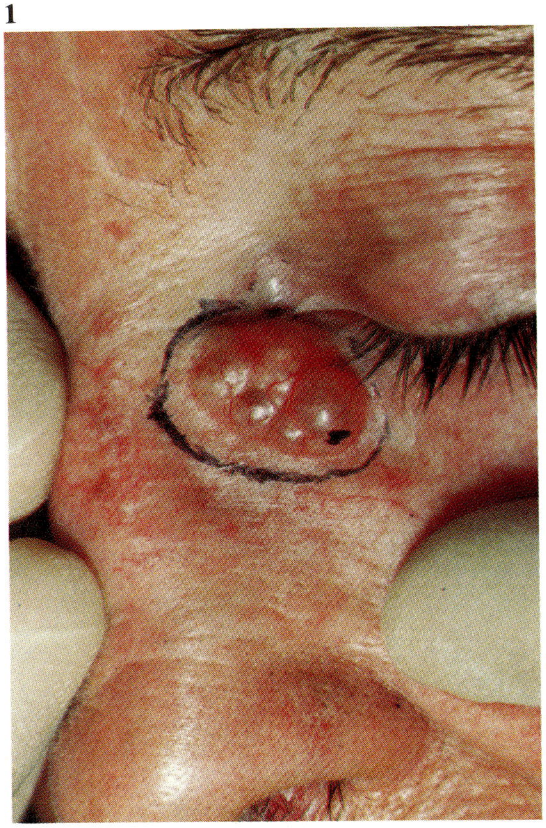

1 A basal cell carcinoma of the lower eyelid is marked prior to excision.

2

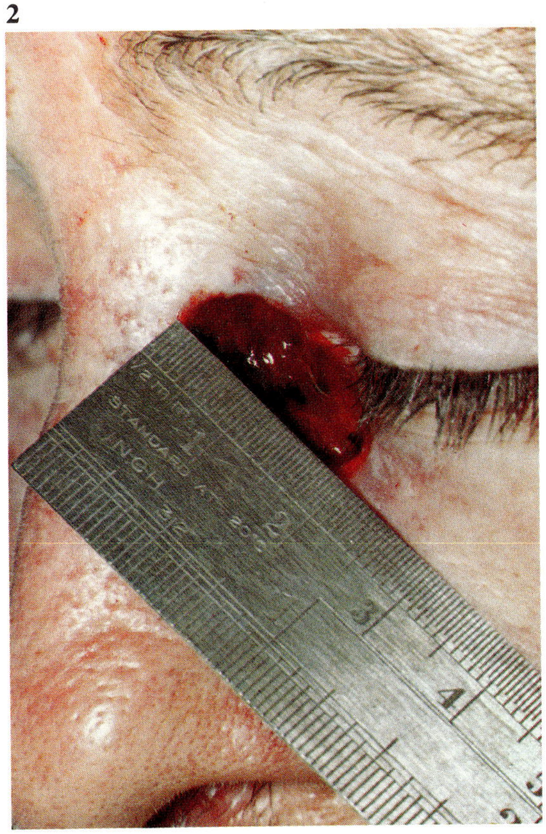

2 The resulting defect is measured.

3

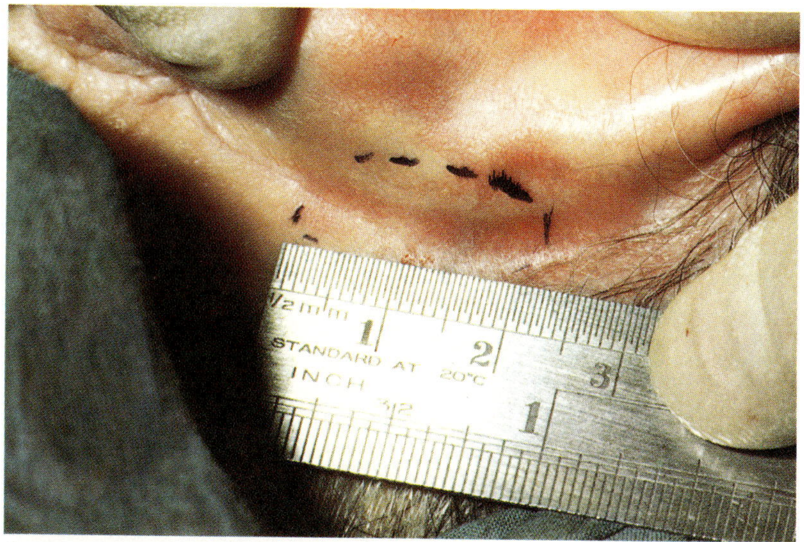

3 A similar sized area is marked out on the hairless postauricular skin.

4

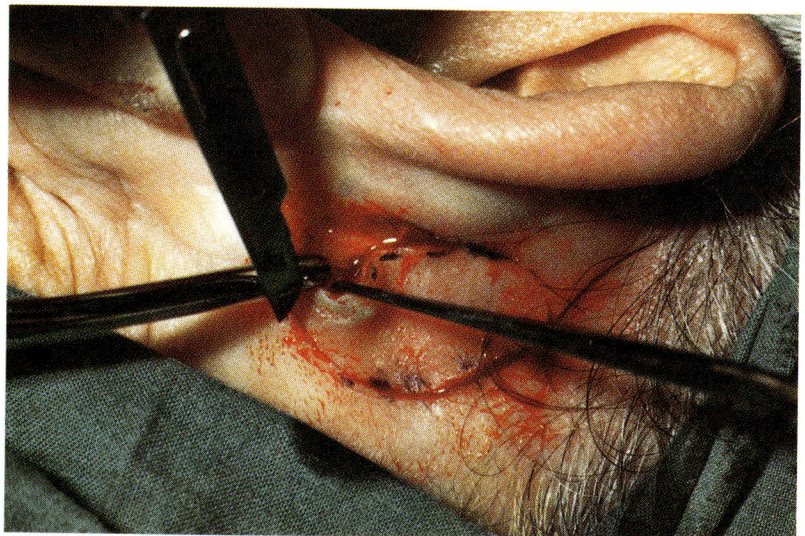

4 The postauricular full thickness skin graft is excised. The graft is held with a skin hook. The postauricular defect is closed by direct suture.

5 The fat is carefully trimmed from the deep surface of the graft, taking great care not to buttonhole it.

6 Defatted graft ready for application to the defect. The graft is kept moist with isotonic saline.

5

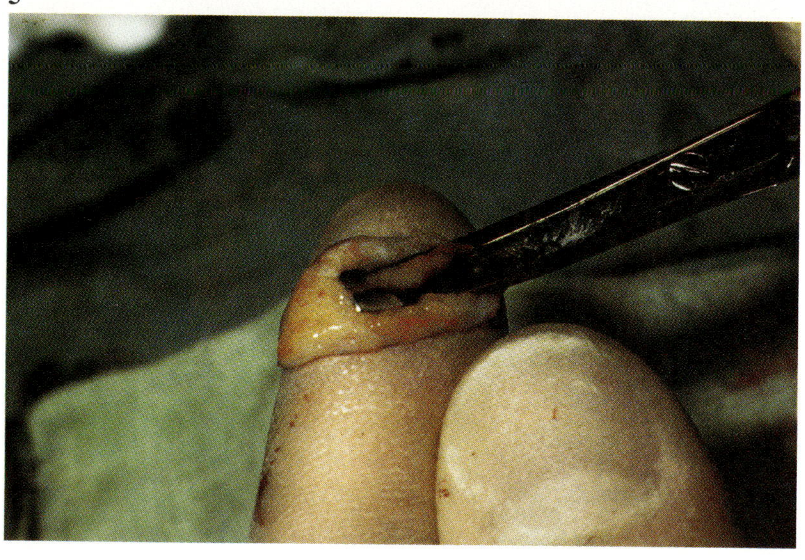

6

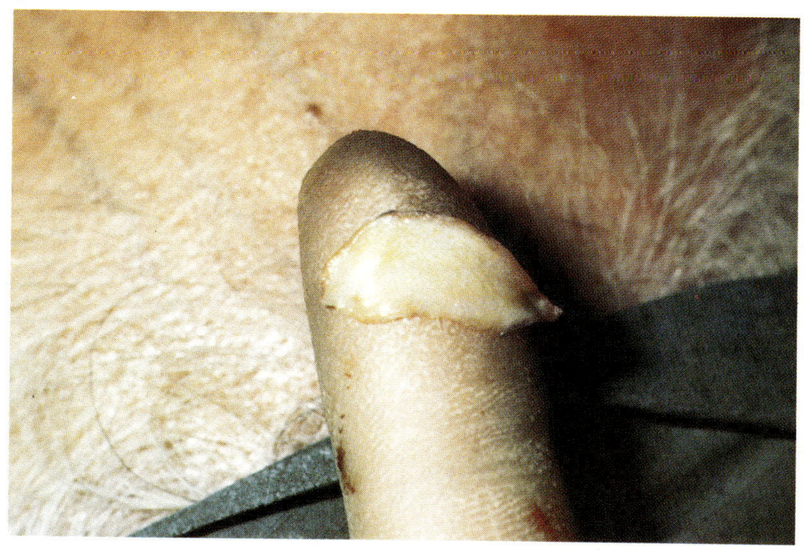

7

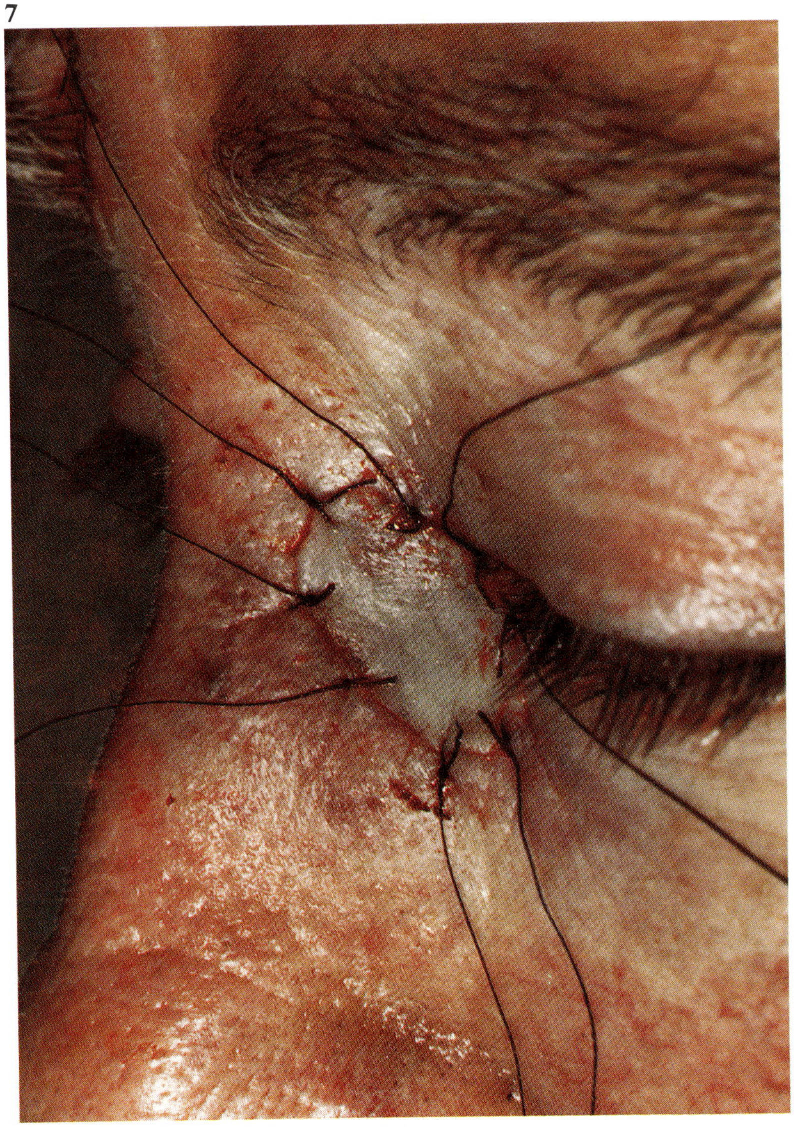

7 The graft is sutured carefully into the defect with accurate edge-to-edge apposition of the skin margin. Overlap at the edge should be avoided.

8

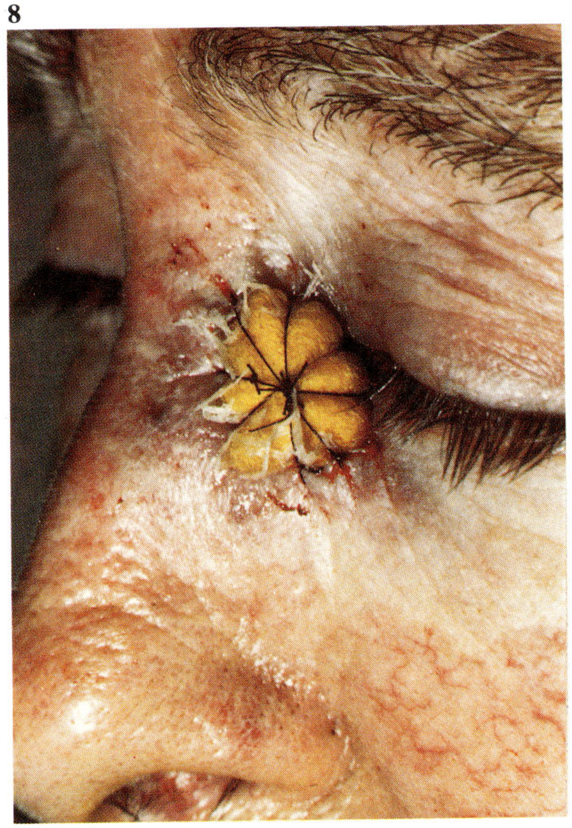

8 A tie over dressing is completed using silk sutures. This dressing is left in place for one week.

Local flap repair

1 **A cellular naevus of the nose** prior to excision under local anaesthetic.

2 **After excision of the lesion a local flap repair is planned.** The flap is centred over the nasolabial fold and the dog ear is also marked out for excision. An alternative method of repair would be a full thickness postauricular skin graft. Direct closure is not recommended as it would cause distortion of the nose.

3 **The skin flap is elevated** with a generous amount of subcutaneous tissue to preserve its blood supply. The flap is handled gently using a skin hook to avoid undue trauma.

4 **The flap is sutured into place** and the donor site then repaired using interrupted 5-0 Prolene sutures. Alternate sutures can be removed at four days but a few sutures must be left in place for at least a week.

1

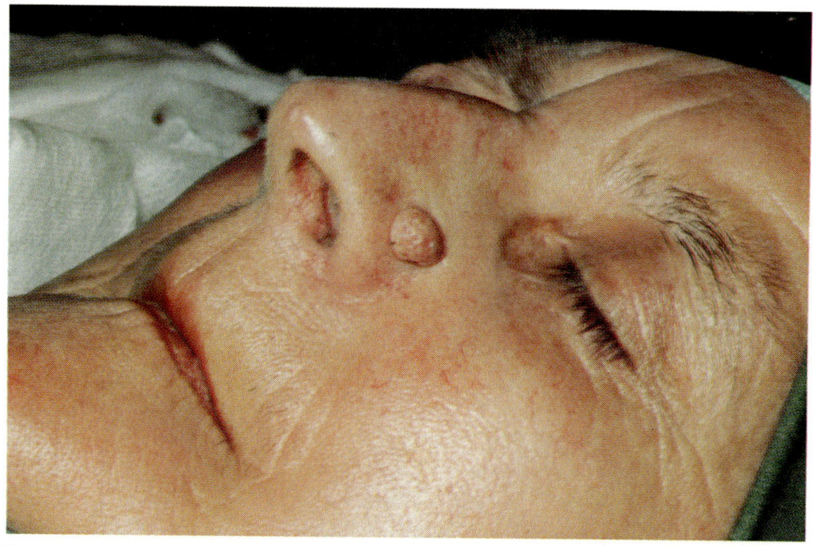

2

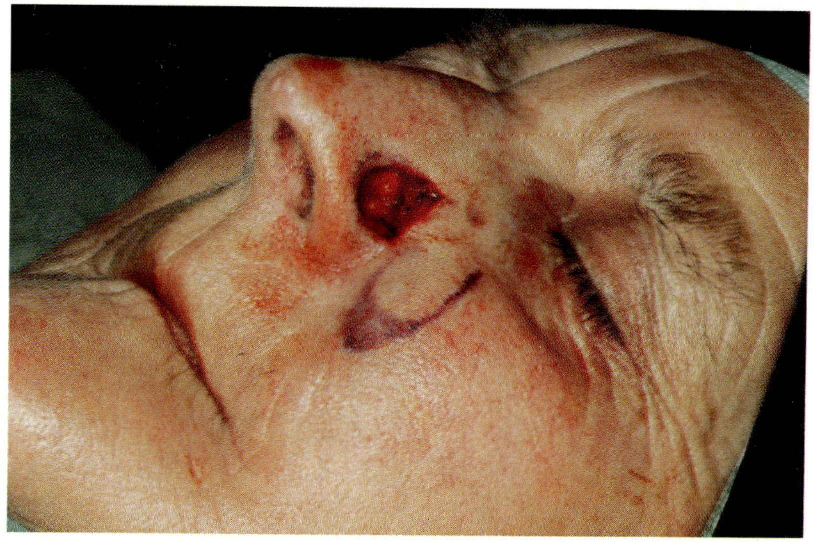

3

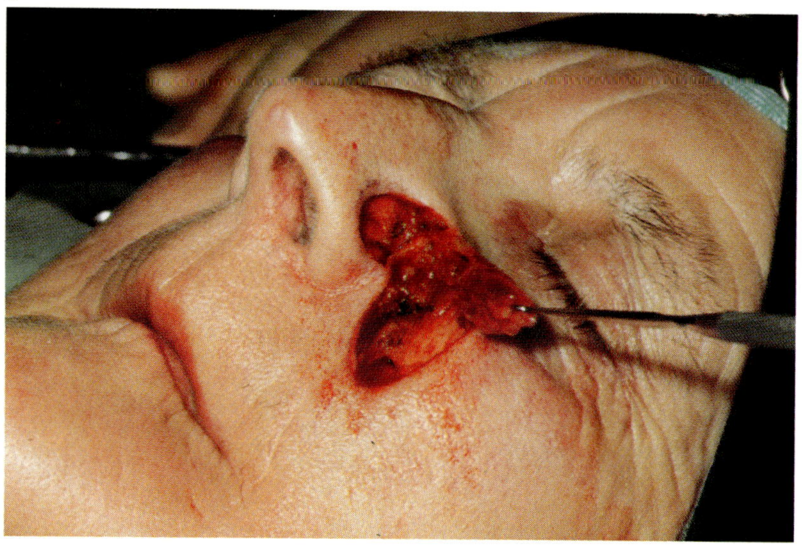

4

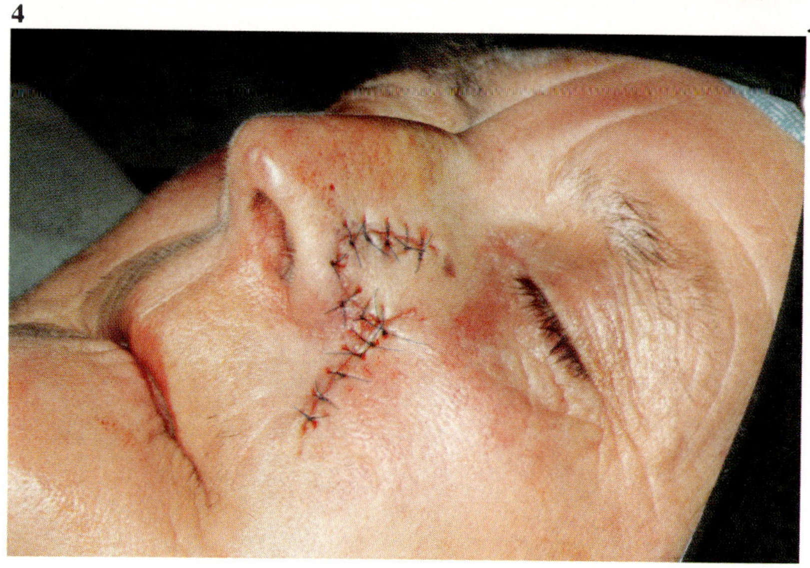

Cross finger flap

1

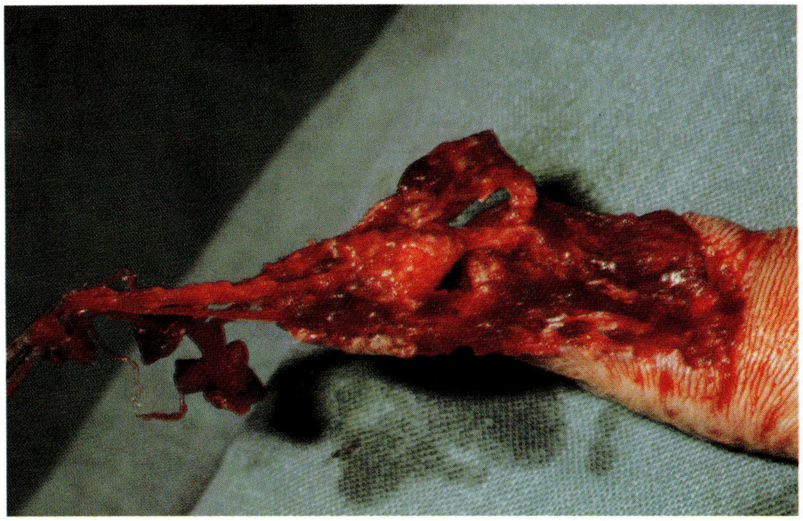

1 A severe crushing laceration of the left middle finger tip caused by a carding machine.

2

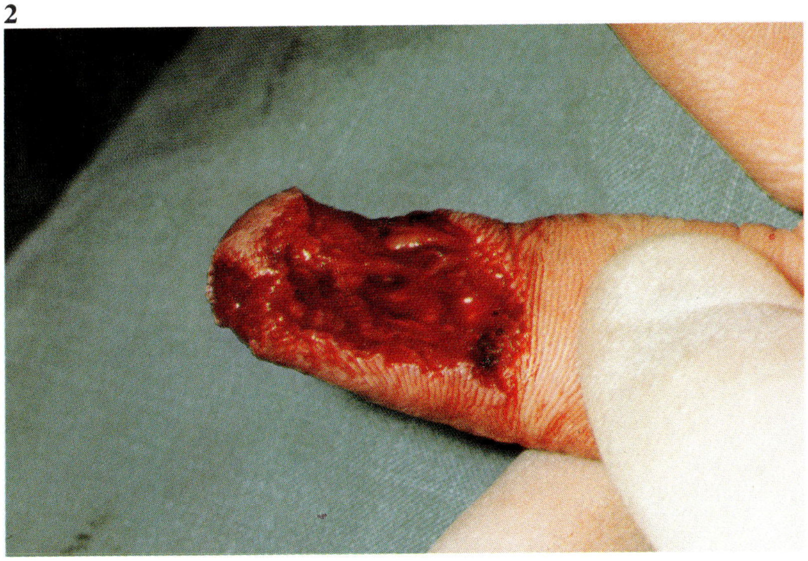

2 After thorough cleaning and debridement a neurovascular bundle and the flexor tendon is exposed. Flap repair of this defect is essential.

3

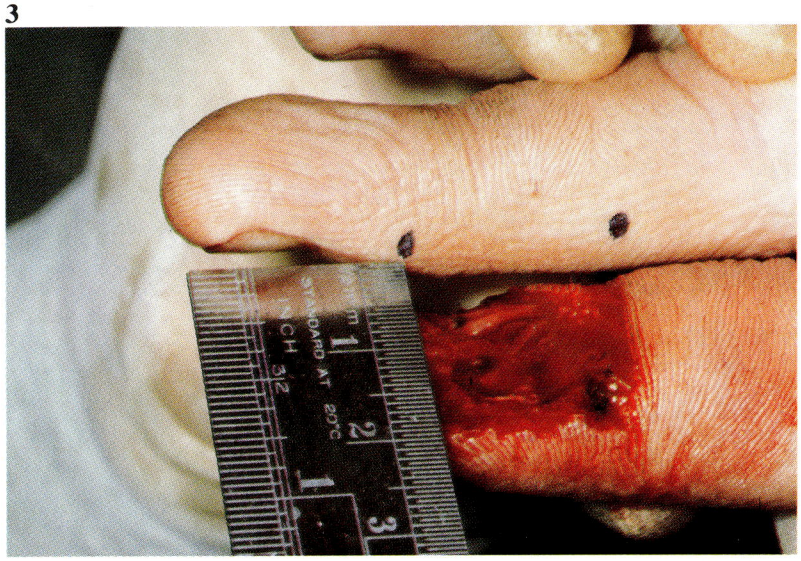

3 The donor finger is approximate, in a comfortable position alongside the defect. The ink spots mark the width of the flap which is to be used. The ruler is measuring the 2 cm length of flap required to cover the defect and bridge the section.

4

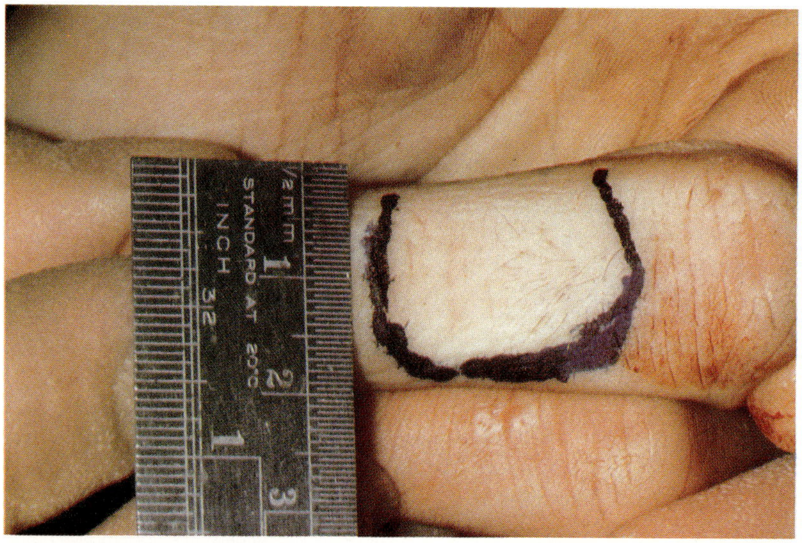

4 The flap is then marked out on the dorsum of the donor finger 2 cm in length (the curve of the finger gives the appearance that the flap is smaller than 2 cm). If possible the donor defect should be centred over a phalanx and not over a joint crease area.

5

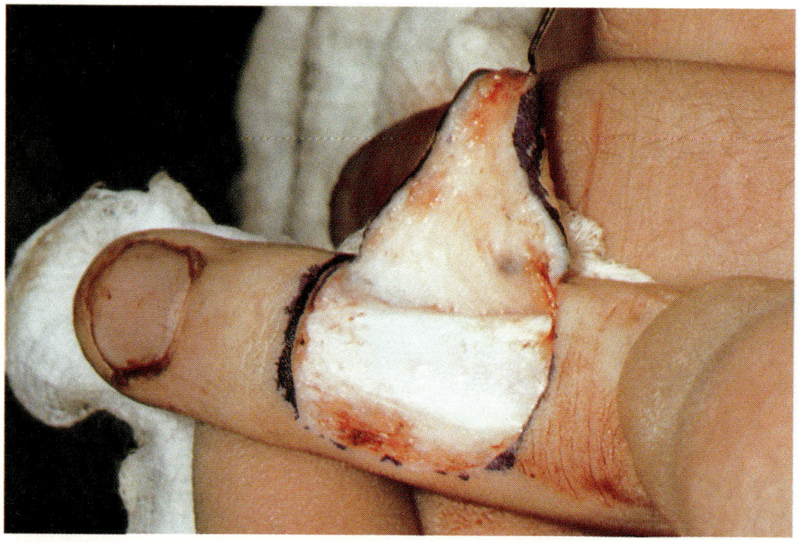

5 A tourniquet is then applied and the flap is raised. It is essential to leave paratenon over the extensor tendon to give a viable bed in the donor area for the application of a split thickness graft.

6 The flap held in skin hooks is folded over like the page of a book and a check is made that it will cover the defect.

7 The tourniquet is then released to check the viability of the flap and after haemostasis a split skin graft is applied to the flap donor site. The skin graft is left long at this stage to allow the bridge segment of the flap to be lined with a graft.

6

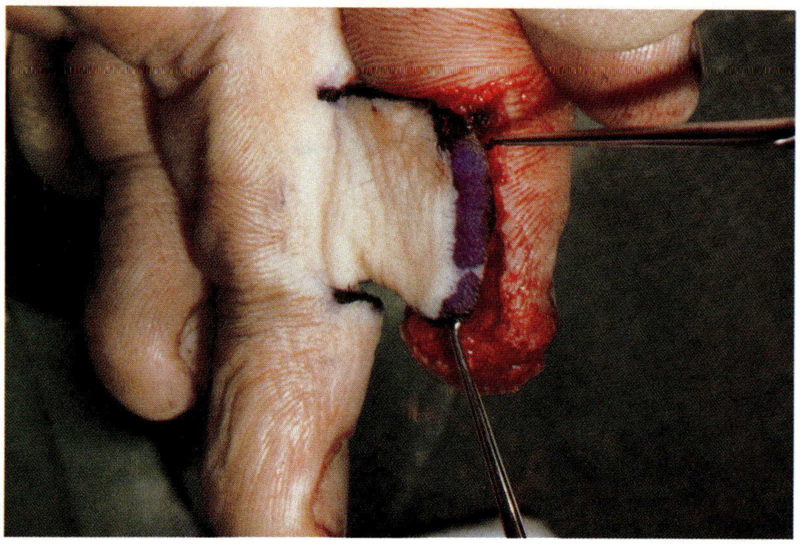

7

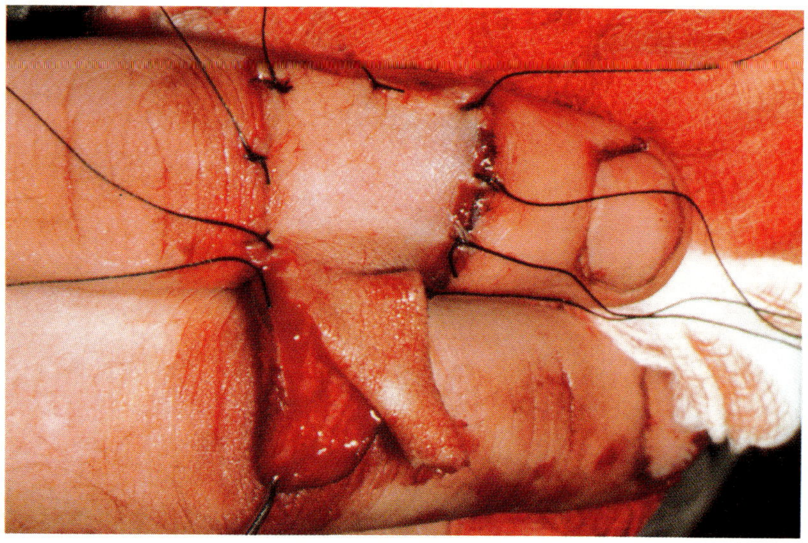

8

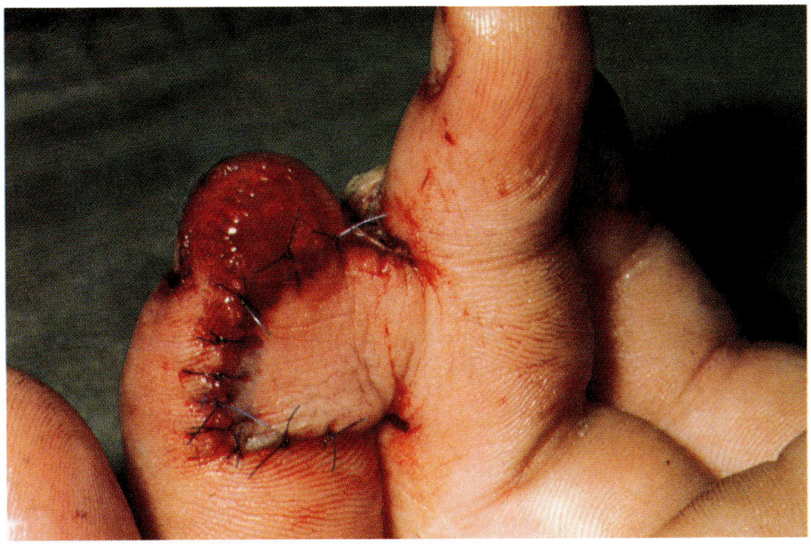

8 The flap is sutured in place.

9

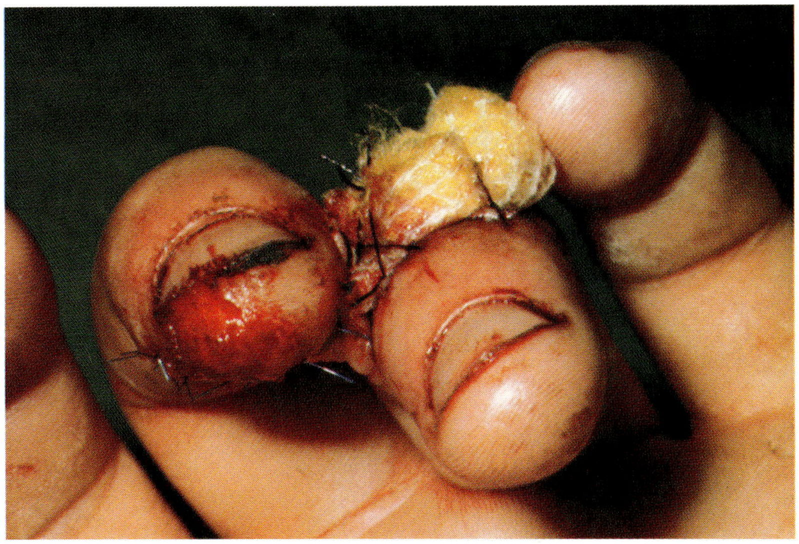

9 After applying a tieover dressing to the donor site, the redundant margin of split thickness skin graft is trimmed. The tie over dressing is removed one week later. The bridge of the flap is divided at two weeks if healing is proceeding satisfactorily by incising between the two fingers. It is not necessary to suture the divided edge of the flap in place. A light dressing is applied for a few days.

Wedge excision of a small lesion of the lip

1

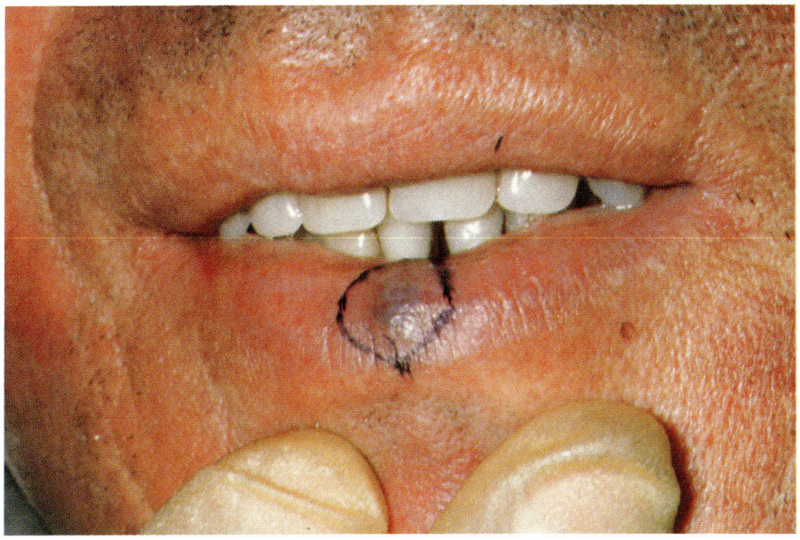

1 A haemangioma of the lip is marked for excision with the ellipse arranged at right angles to the lip margin. Local anaesthetic is then inserted.

2

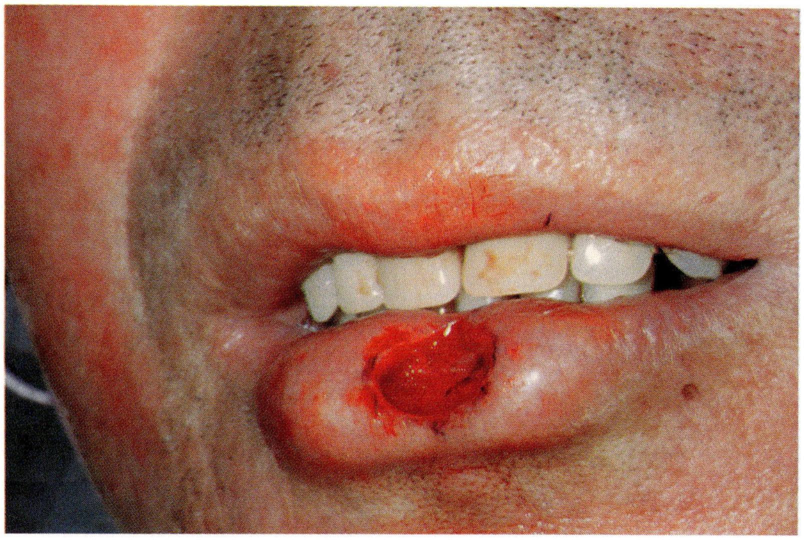

2 After excision the lip muscle can be seen running crosswise in the defect.

3

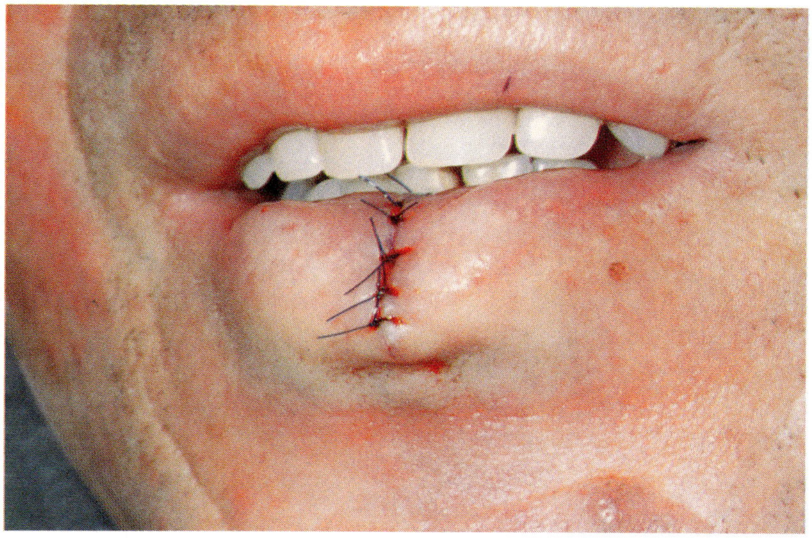

3 The repair is completed using simple interrupted sutures.

Vermillionectomy

1

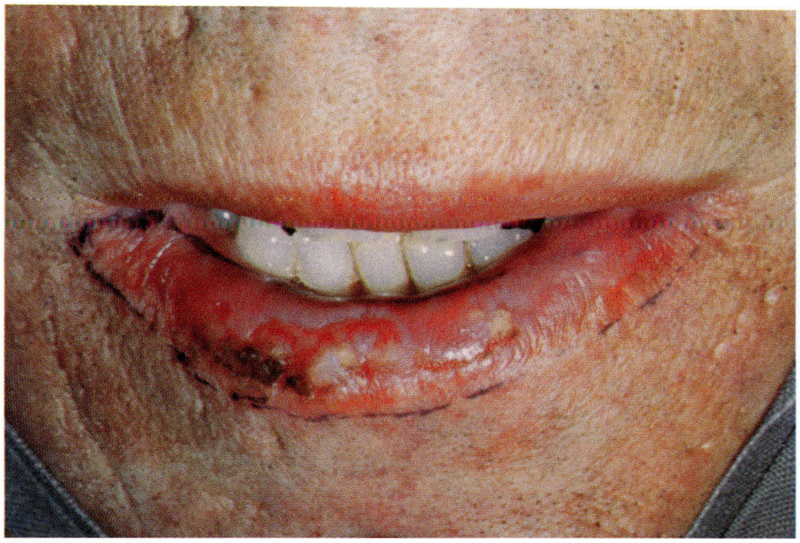

1 The excision biopsy for a diffuse premalignant change of the major part of the lower lip is marked out. It is important to carry the excision forward to include the red margin of the lower lip. Local anaesthetic 0.5% Lignocaine plain is then injected.

2

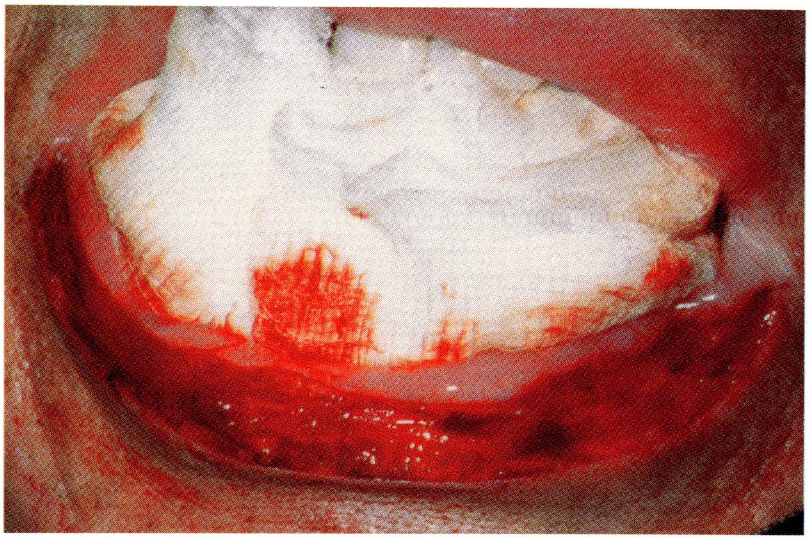

2 A moist swab is inserted in the mouth to collect any bleeding and the excision performed down to the muscle of the lip. Undermining is not usually required as the oral mucosa protrudes easily to close the defect. The specimen is sent for histological examination.

3 **The wound is sutured** with interrupted sutures, which are removed at one week.

3

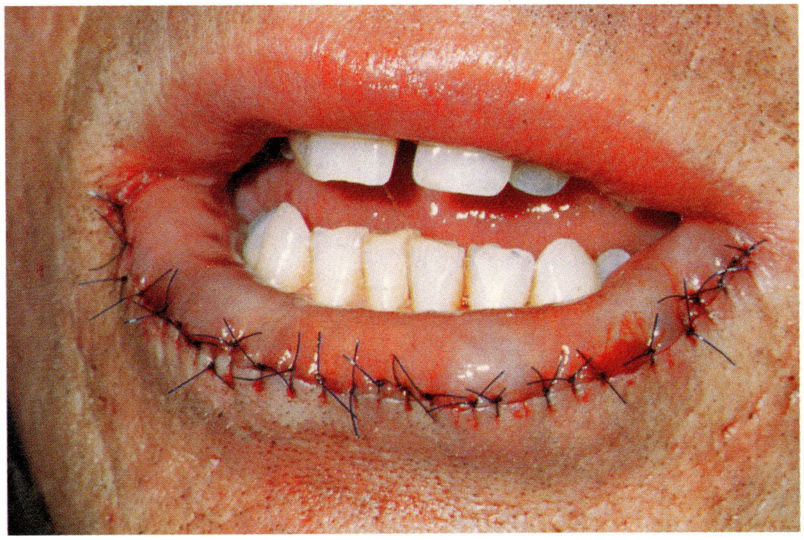

W wedge excision of a malignant lesion of the lower lip

1

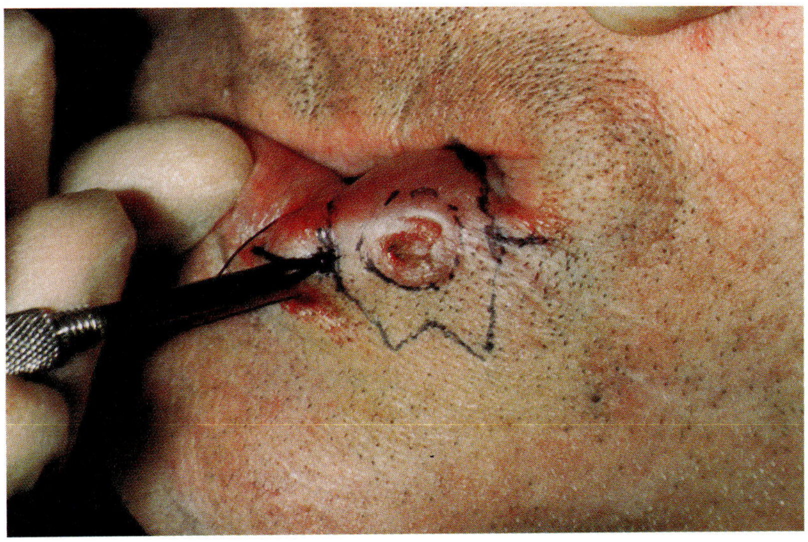

1 A small squamous cell carcinoma of the lower lip is marked prior to excision. The outer edge of the indurated area is marked and a further generous excision margin is allowed. The W shape of the wedge limits the extent of the scar to a small inverted Y. After local anaesthetic is inserted, the red margin of the lip is marked and tattooed with Bonney's blue ink to allow accurate alignment of the repair.

2

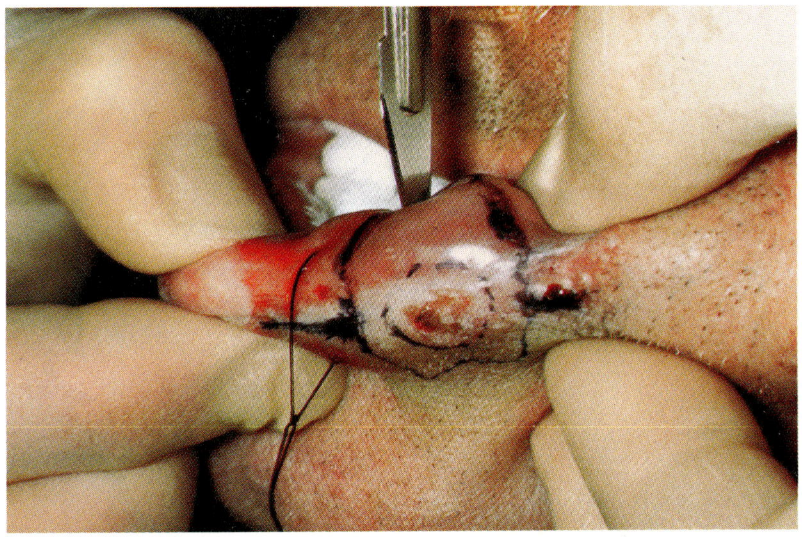

2 An assistant squeezes the lip to evert it and compress the labial artery for haemostasis. The lesion is excised as a full thickness wedge of lip margin. The specimen is sent for histological examination.

3

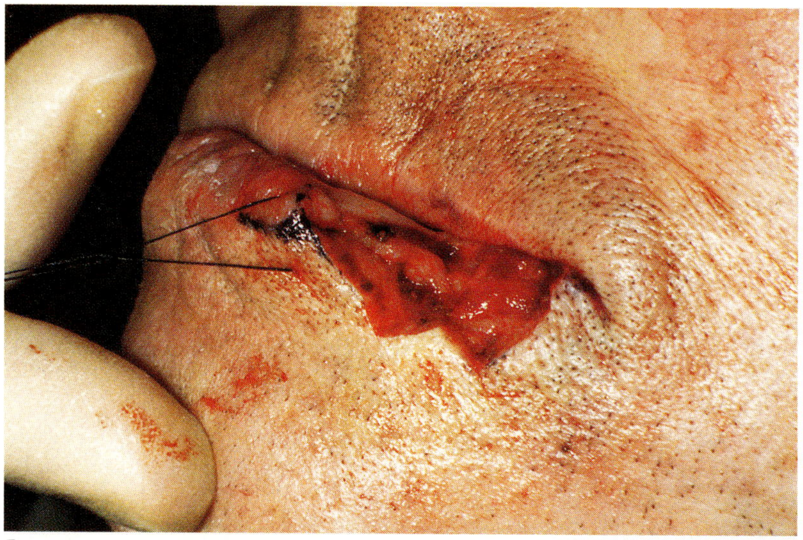

4

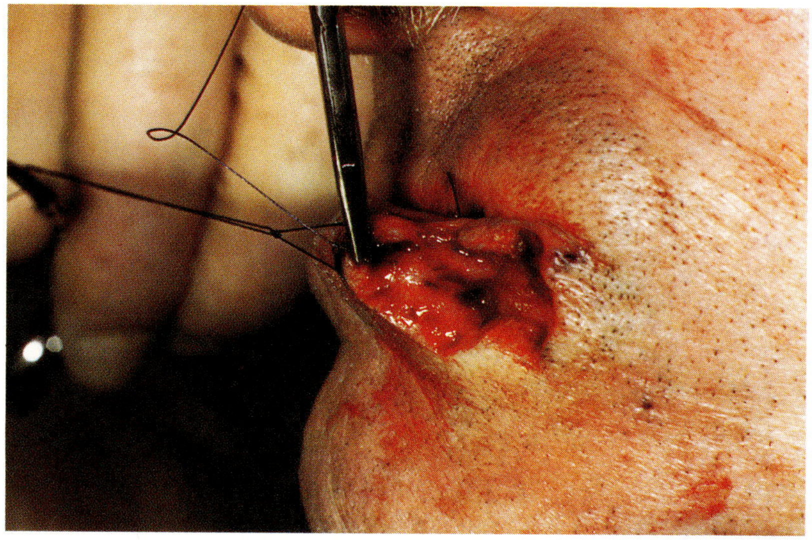

5

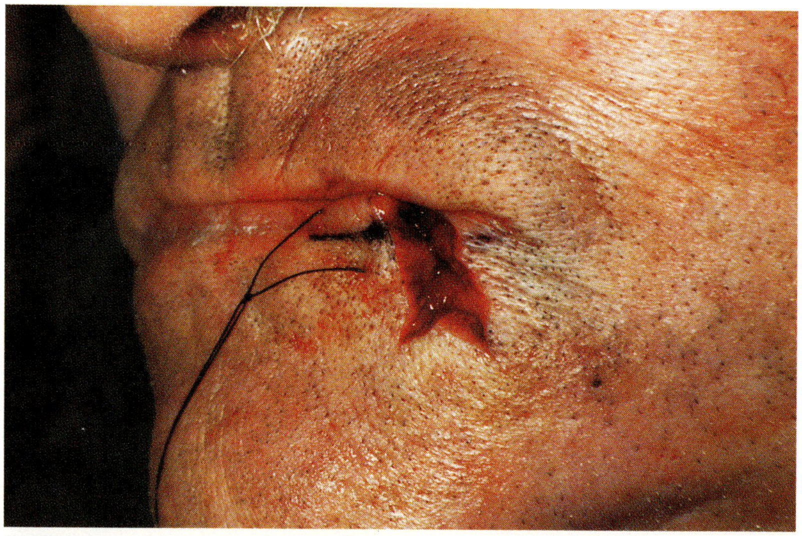

6

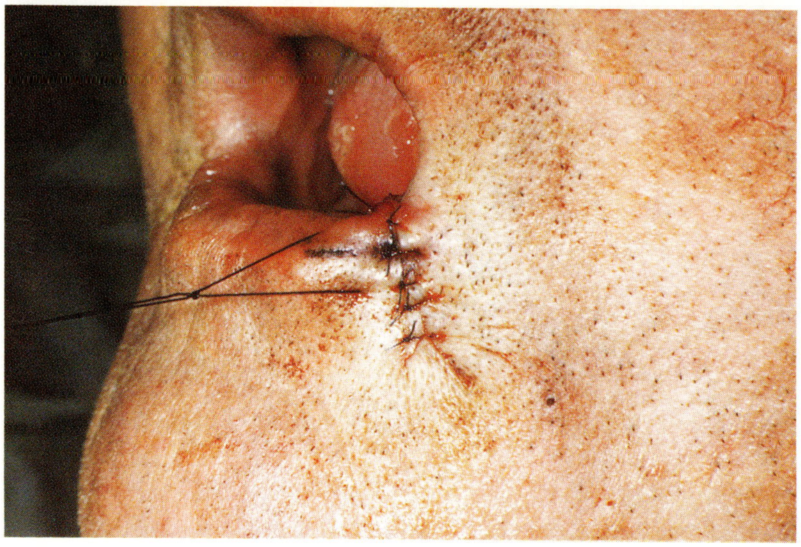

3 The defect springs open widely because the orbicularis muscle is divided. A transfixation stay suture gives easy control of the wound margin.

4 Buried absorbable sutures are used to repair the orbicularis oris muscle.

5 The mucosa inside the lip is sutured with a soft braided suture, such as Vicryl 4-0.

6 The repair is completed with interrupted skin sutures. One suture at the lip margin passes through the tattoo mark to ensure accurate alignment of the lip.

Triamcinolone injection of a hypertrophic scar

1 Local anaesthetic is injected through the hypertrophic scar into the subcutaneous tissue. This minimises the risk of further hypertrophic scarring developing from needle wounds. Triamcinolone is then injected into the scar in multiple small quantities. Considerable pressure is required to balance the scar. It is important that Triamcinolone is not injected into the subcutaneous tissue, as this causes severe atrophy of the subcutaneous fat and can produce a depressed scar.

Injection can be repeated at monthly intervals if necessary.

1

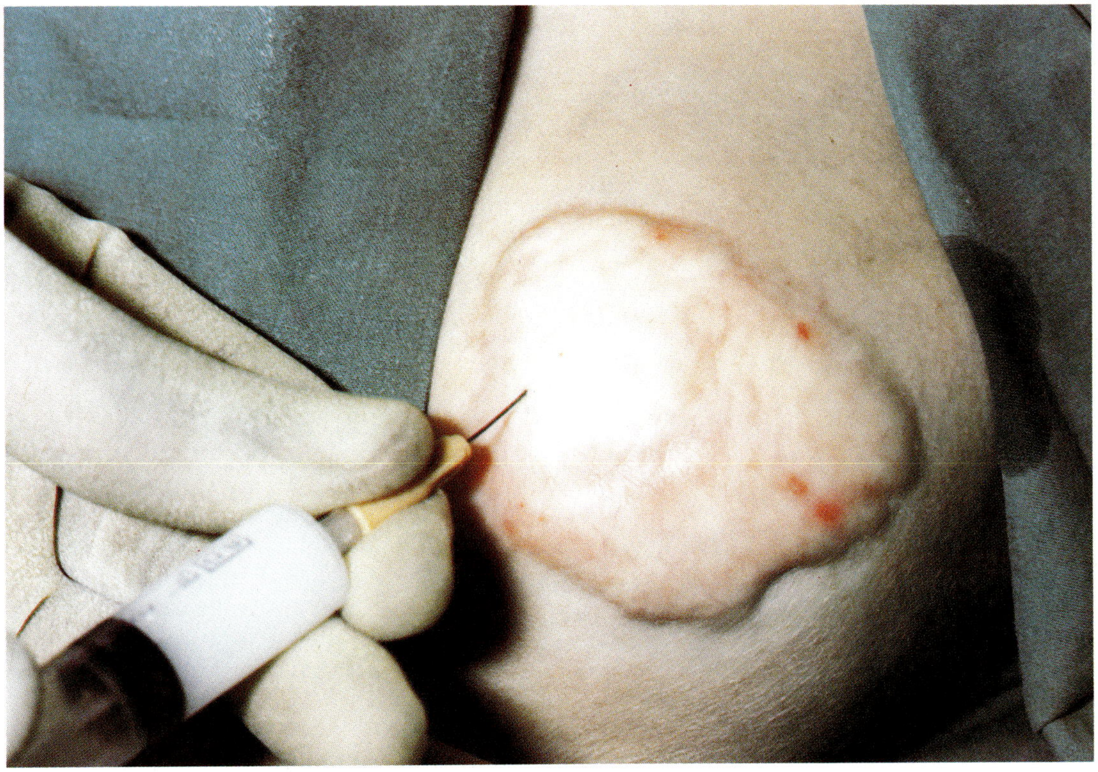

Scar revision – W plasty

1

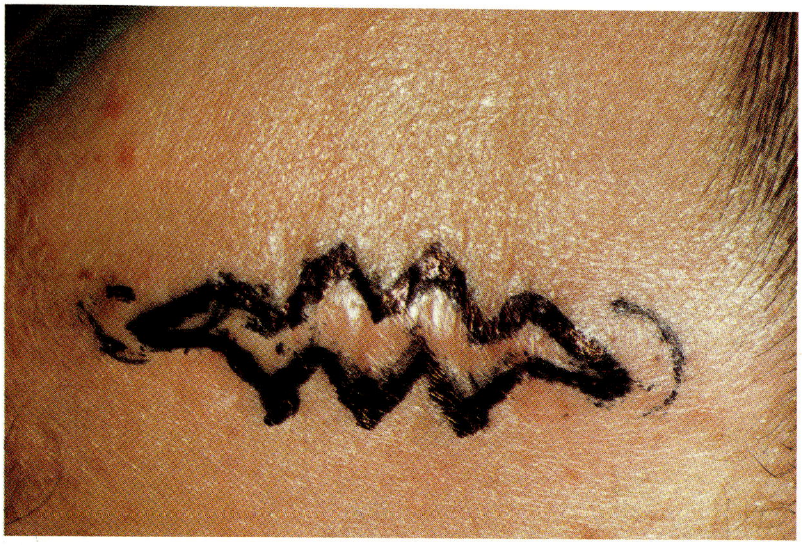

1 A prominent spread scar of the forehead is marked out for W Plasty. The interdigitating flaps are kept at less than 1 cm along each limb.

2

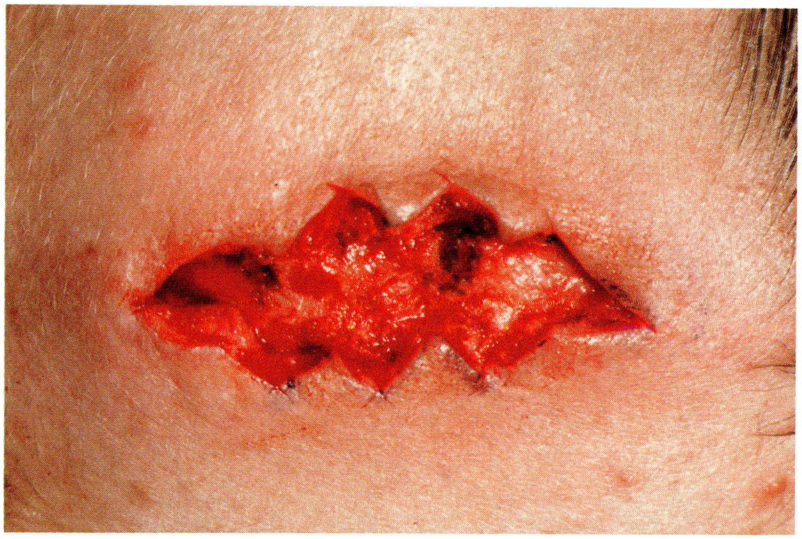

2 The scar is excised and the edges undermined to allow closure.

3

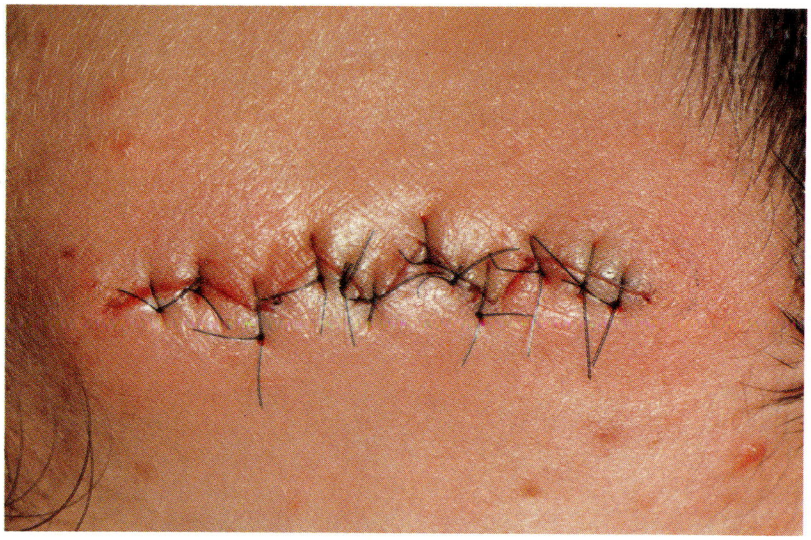

3 The wound is repaired using fine interrupted sutures. Some sutures are removed as early as two days and the wound is reinforced using skin tape. All the sutures should be removed by seven days.

Scar revision – Z plasty

1

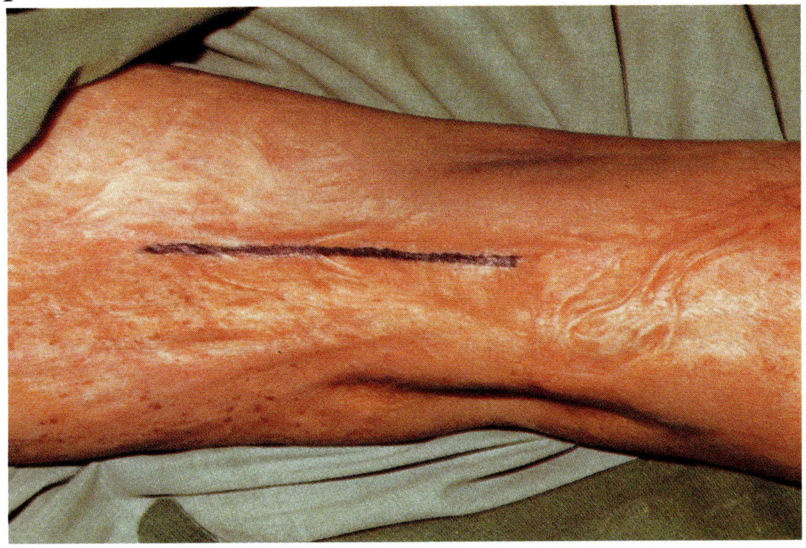

1 A tight scar of the ante cubital fossa is marked.

2

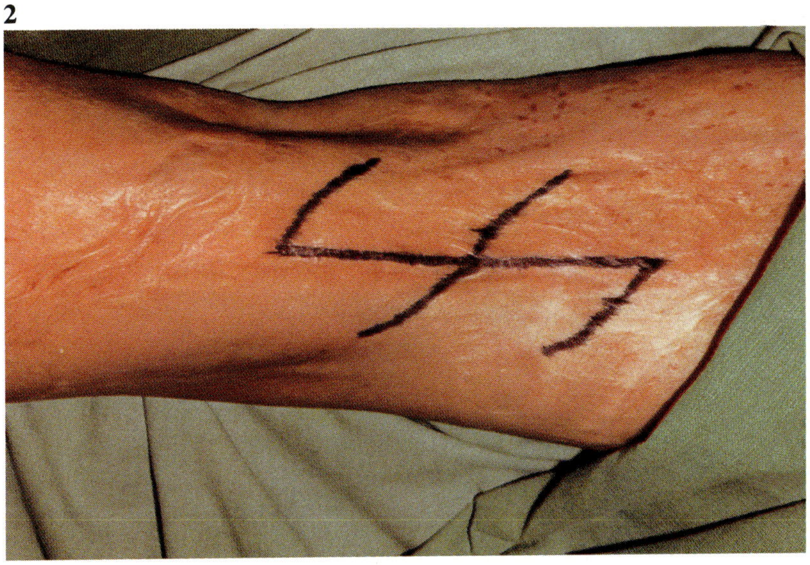

2 Two 60° Z plasty incisions are marked. If the scar is a long one several small Z plasties give greater release, without causing circumferential tightening, than one large Z plasty.

3

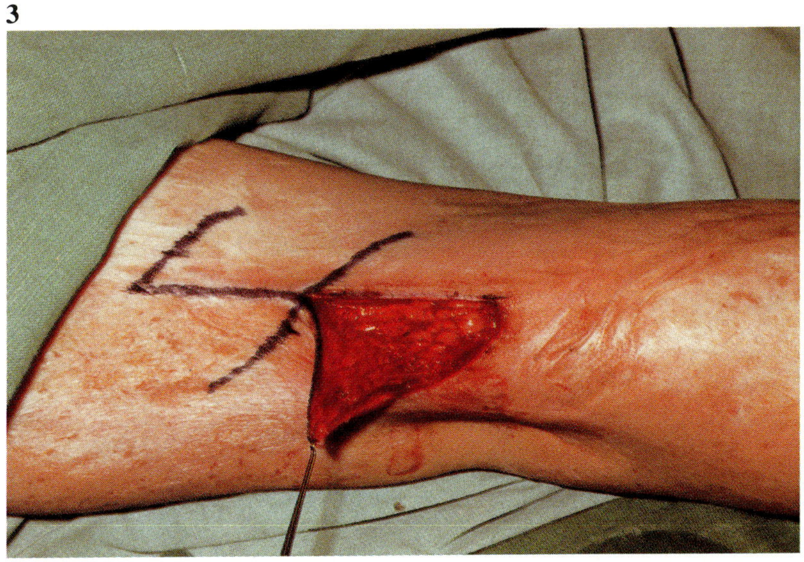

3 One of the flaps is incised and elevated, keeping a generous amount of subcutaneous tissue in the flap.

4

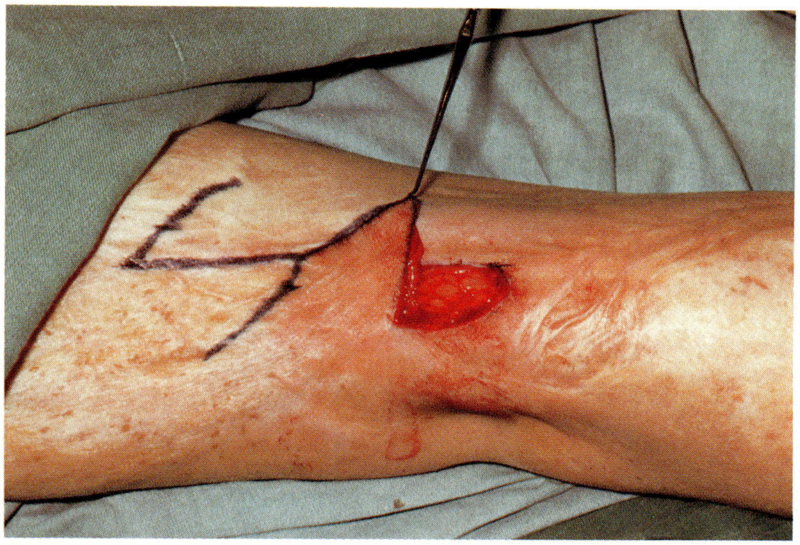

4 This flap is then transposed to check the new position prior to elevation of the second flap.

5

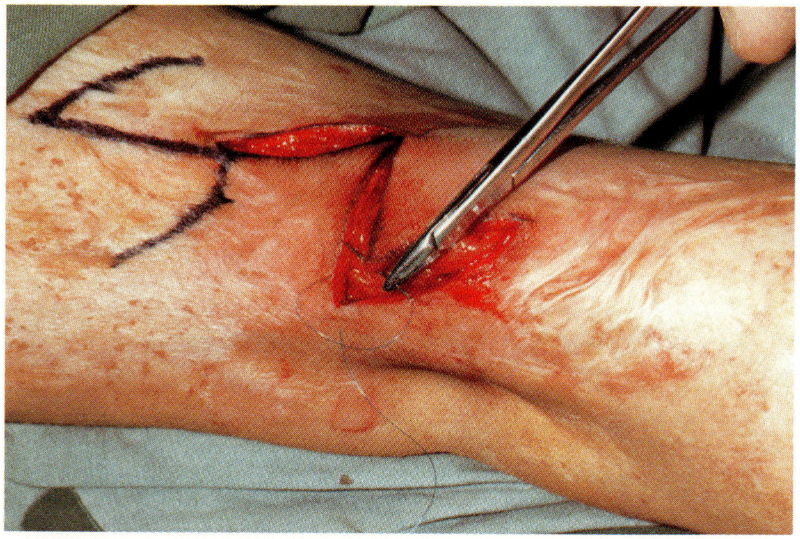

5 The apices of the flaps are sutured first using a horizontal mattress suture with a subdermal bite in the flap apex.

6 The suturing is completed with interrupted skin sutures. The elongation of approximately 50% can be seen by comparing the two Z plasties.

7 The second Z plasty is completed. Scarred skin is slow to heal and some sutures may need to be left in for approximately 10 days.

6

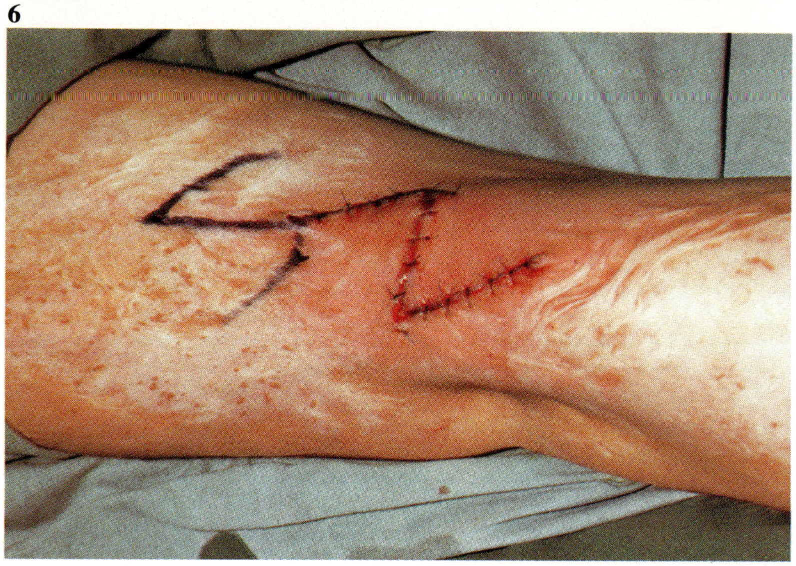

7

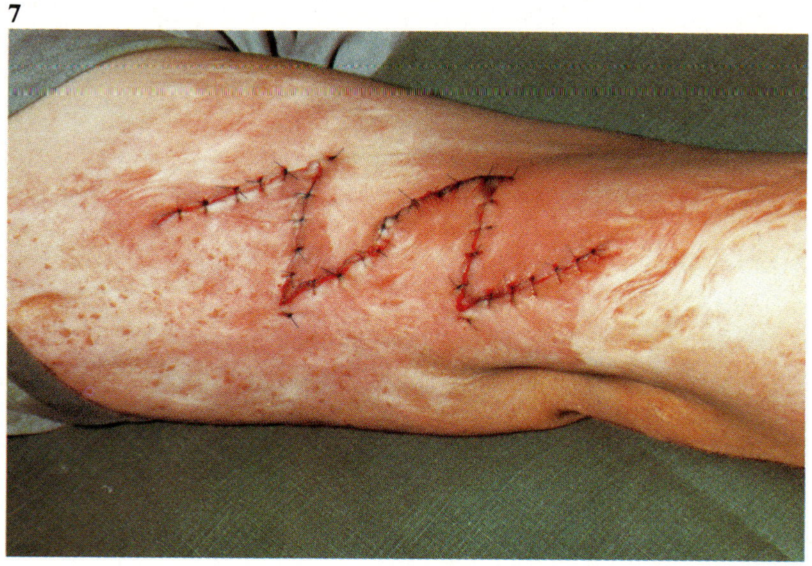

Scar revision – excision

1

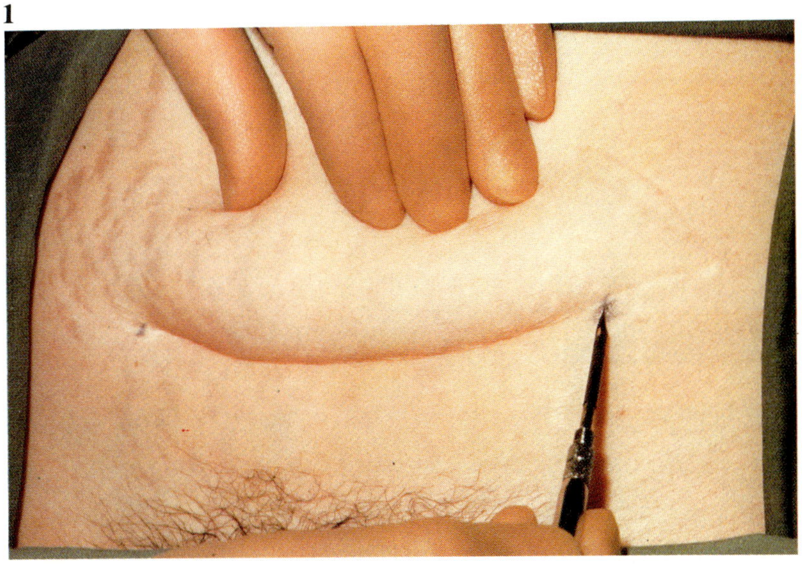

1 The extent of the tethering is marked. The non-tethered part is well healed and is left undisturbed.

2

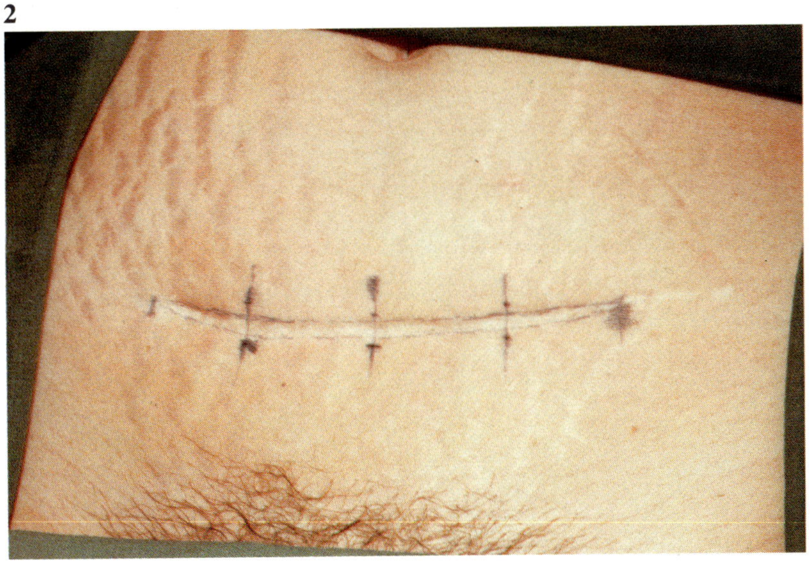

2 The area to be excised is marked and cross lines are placed to allow accurate alignment of the wound.

3

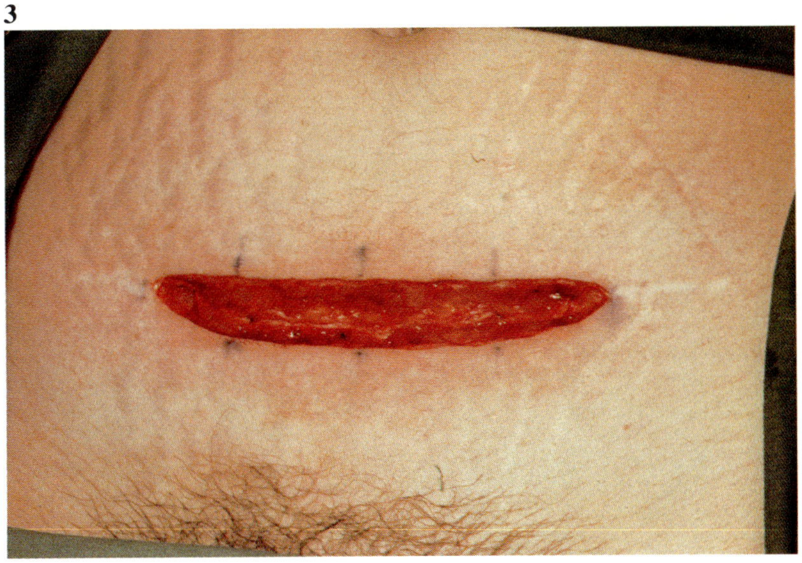

3 The skin scar is excised leaving the deep subcutaneous scarring.

4

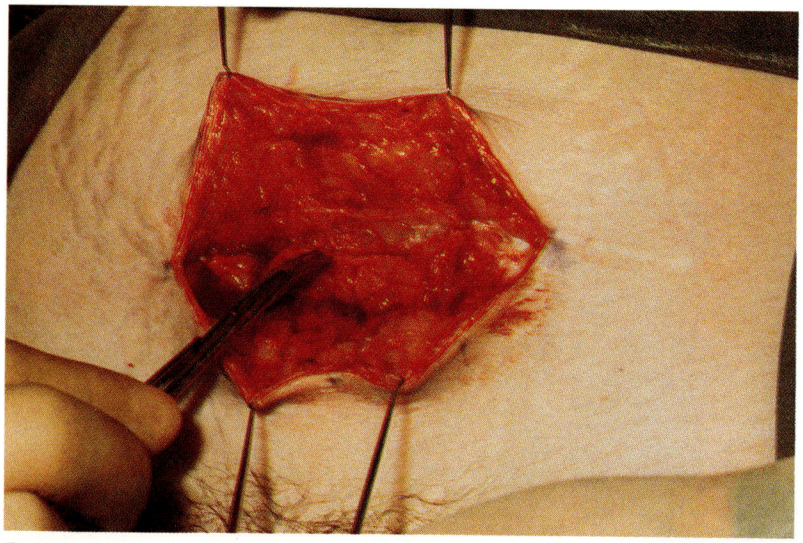

4 Traction applied on either side of the wound with skin hooks allows the deep tethering bands to be incised to give full release of the wound edges. If there is very dense subcutaneous scarring it may be necessary to excise some of it. If the area undermined leaves a large cavity a suction drain should be inserted for 24 hours.

5

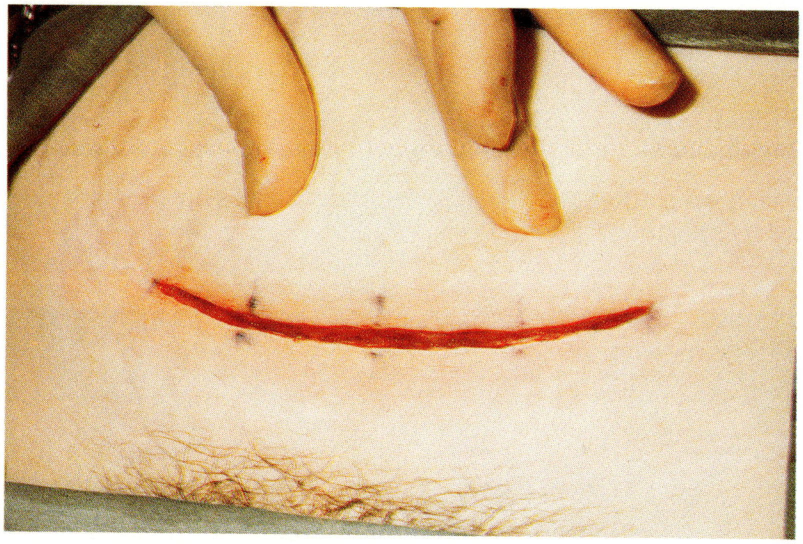

5 Tangential pressure across the wound after subcutaneous and subcuticular sutures of synthetic absorbable material have been inserted shows that all the tethering has been eliminated.

6

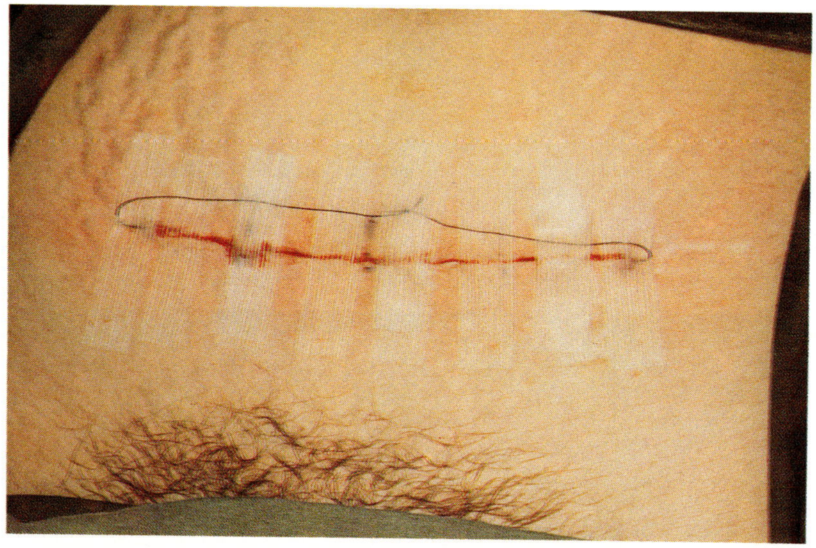

6 A subcuticular Prolene suture and steristrips complete the wound closure. This suture should be left in for at least three weeks.

Perineal warts

Perineal condylomata acuminata are viral in origin and are often associated with vaginal infection such as trichomonas vaginalis and monilia. Small perineal warts can be treated by application of Podophylline 25% or frozen CO_2 or by excision under local anaesthesia with adrenaline.

Large areas of perineal warts should be removed either by surgery or diathermy. The surgical removal is carried out using a scalpel and excising the warts. Care should be taken to make sure that the underlying skin is not extensively damaged.

The raw area after removal of the warts is covered with a dressing such as Sofratulle. If excision is necessary, suture with catgut may be required. The specimens removed should be sent for bacteriological and histological examination.

The dressing should be removed 24 hours later and no further dressing of the area may be required. The area should be kept dry and clean. Infection of the wound is the likely complication. Small areas of warts can be treated using cryosurgery probes. No anaesthetic is required.

1

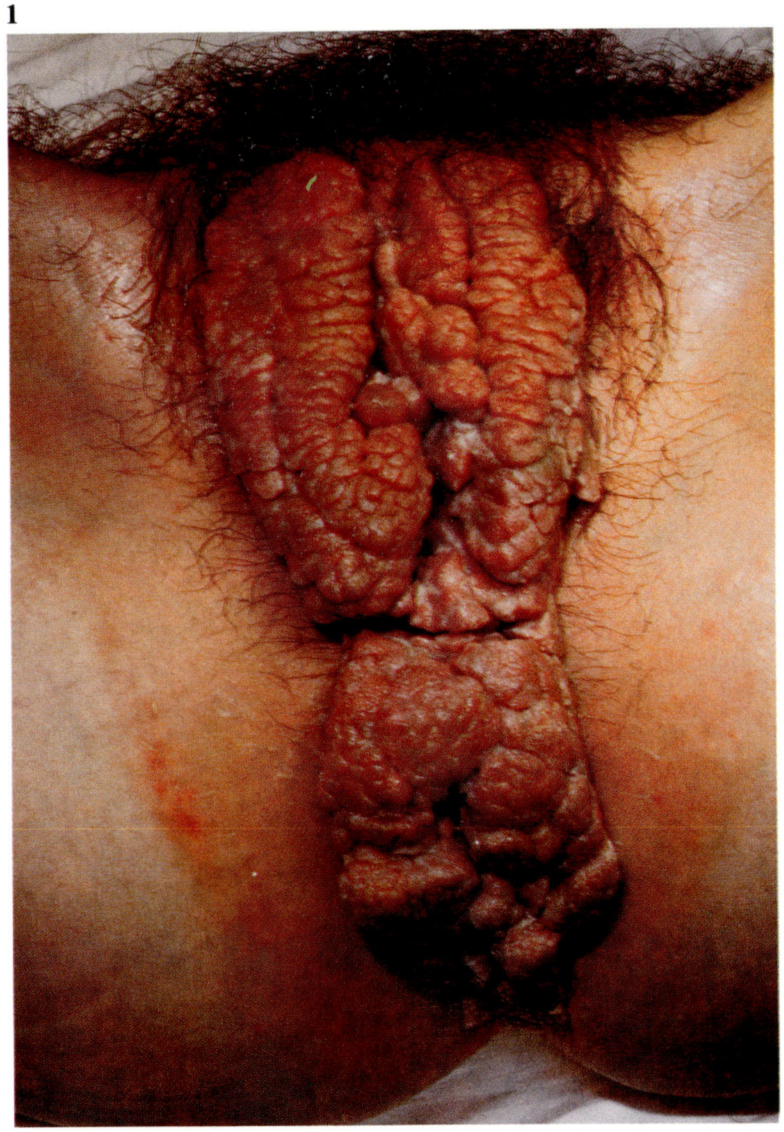

1 Mass of condylomata around the perineum and the anus.

2

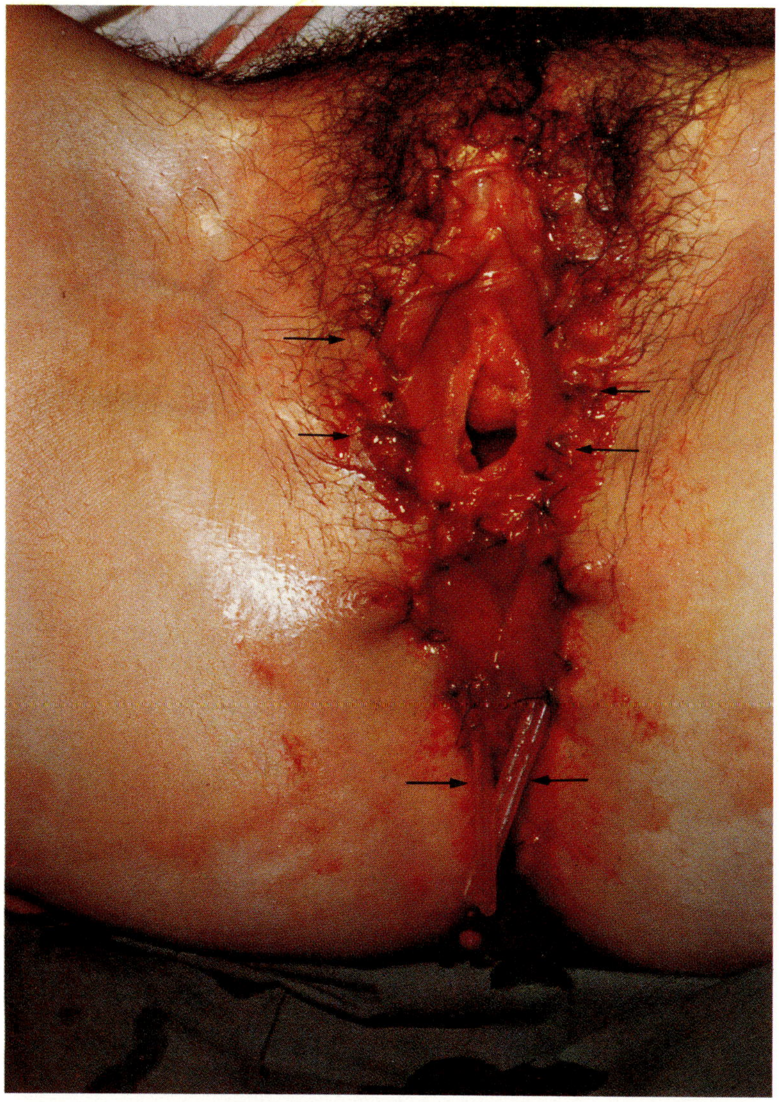

2 **Surgical removal of the warts.** The skin edges sutured with catgut (arrowed). Two small tube drains in situ (arrowed).

3

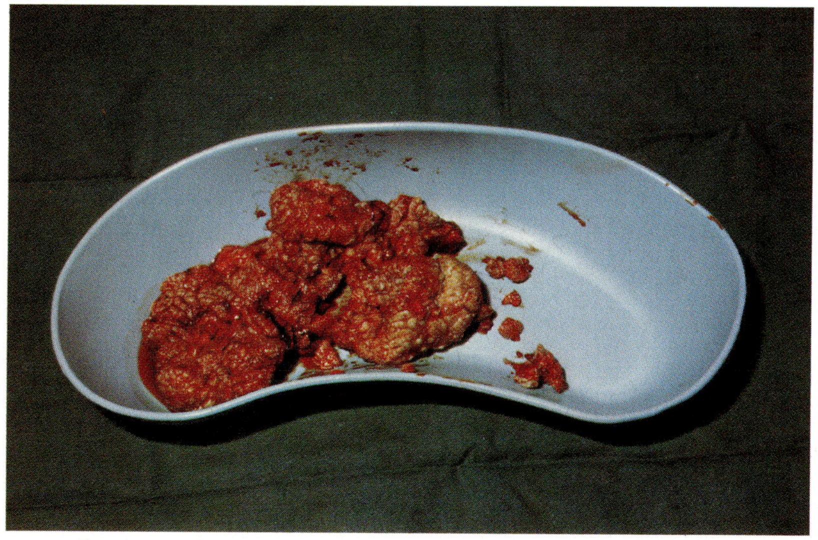

3 Removed warts – for histological and bacteriological examination.

Labial warts

Small areas of labial or vulval warts can be treated using cryocautery. The diagnosis is made from history and examination of the area concerned.

1

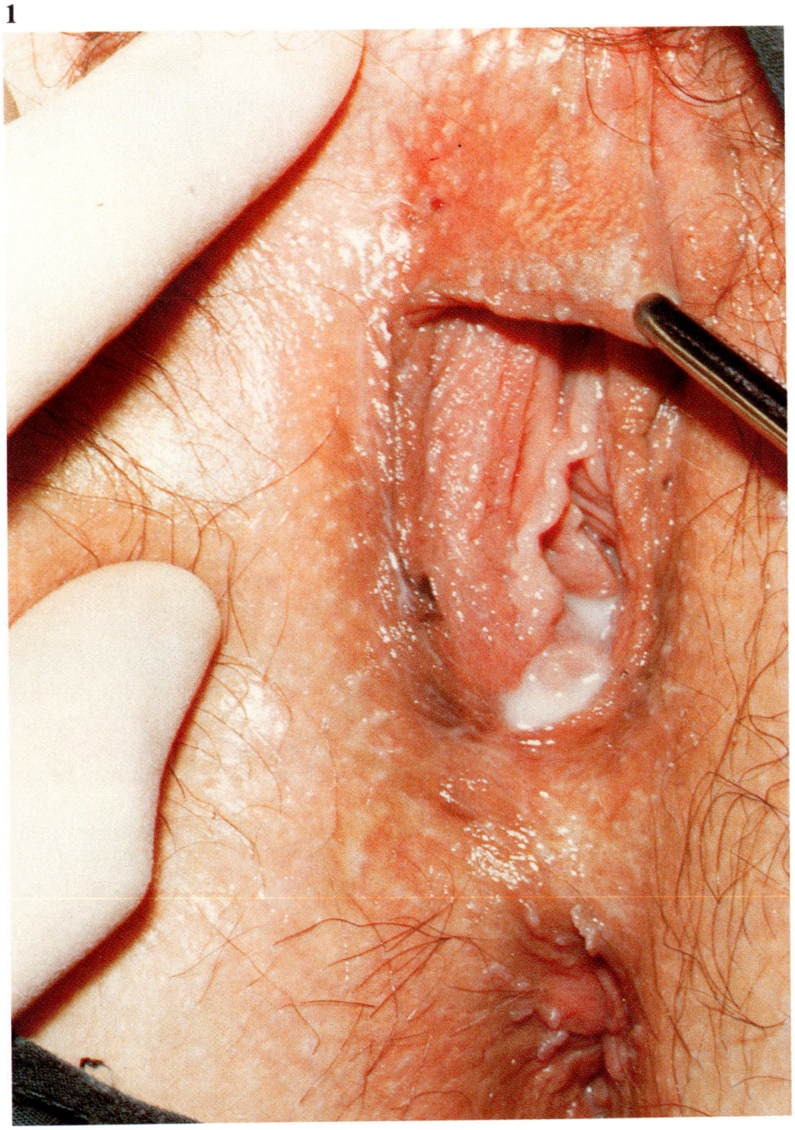

1 Small area of warts on left labia. Vaginal infection with candida is also seen.

2

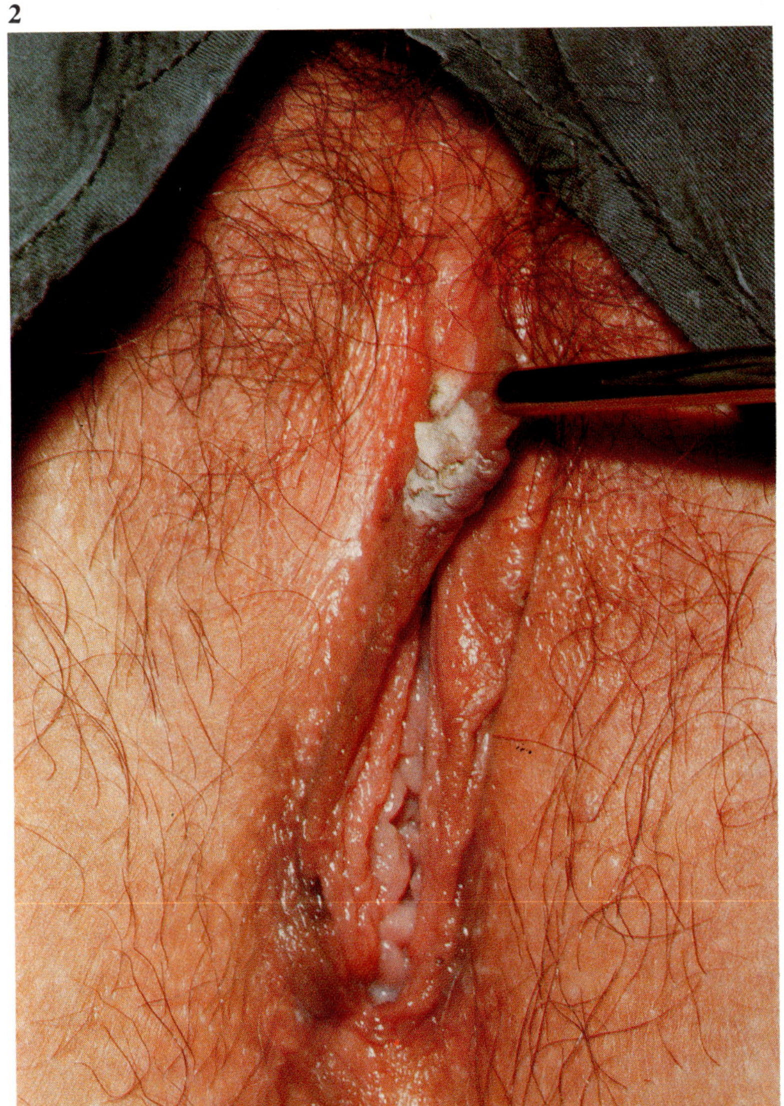

2 Area after treatment with cryocautery.

Excision of labial cysts

Cysts of the labia commonly occur in the region of the Bartholin's gland and can become infected. The common organisms are coliform. Bartholin's abcess involves both gland and duct. Surgical treatment of a cyst can be either by marsupialisation or excision of the cyst. Treatment of certain abscess is by drainage.

Apart from keeping the area dry and clean there may not be any need to apply any further dressing.

1

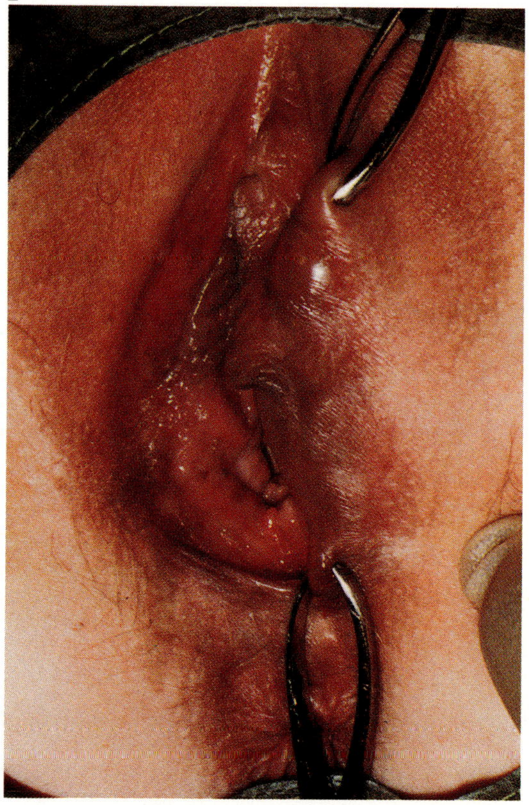

2

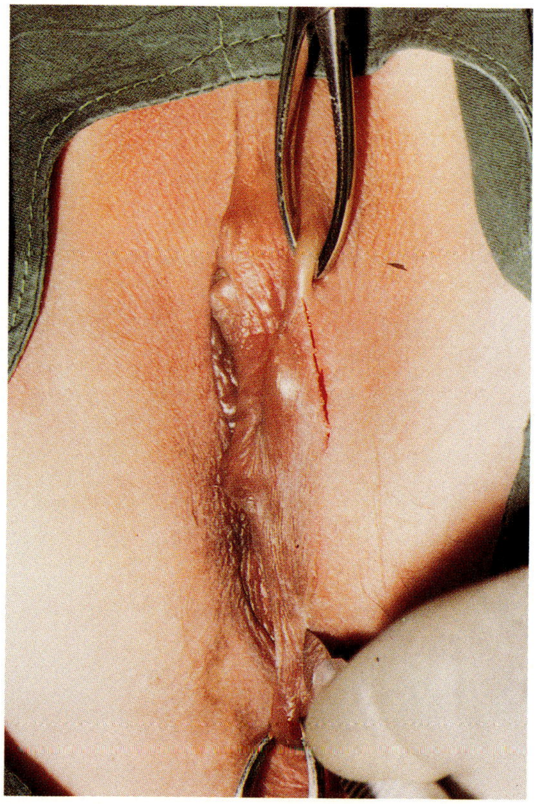

3

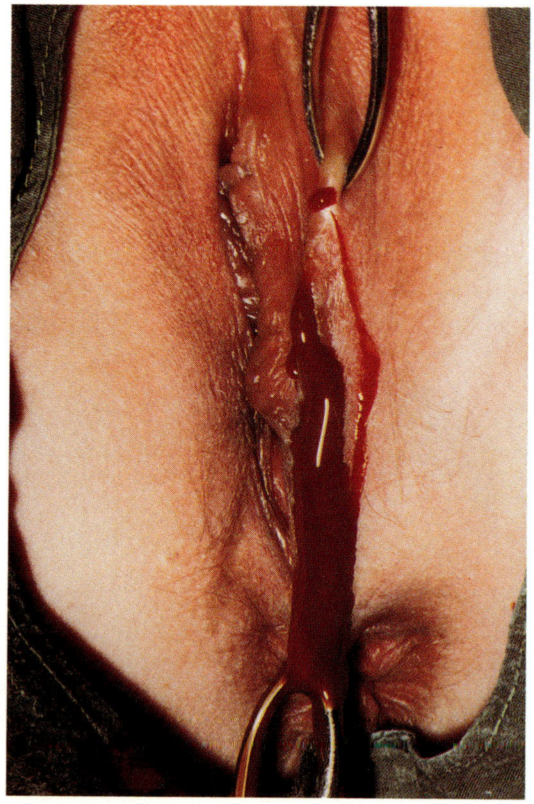

1 Left sided labial cyst. Marsupialisation of cysts.

2 and 3 Labia is excised, using scalpel, around the edge of the cyst. Occasionally there is considerable bleeding from the edges.

4

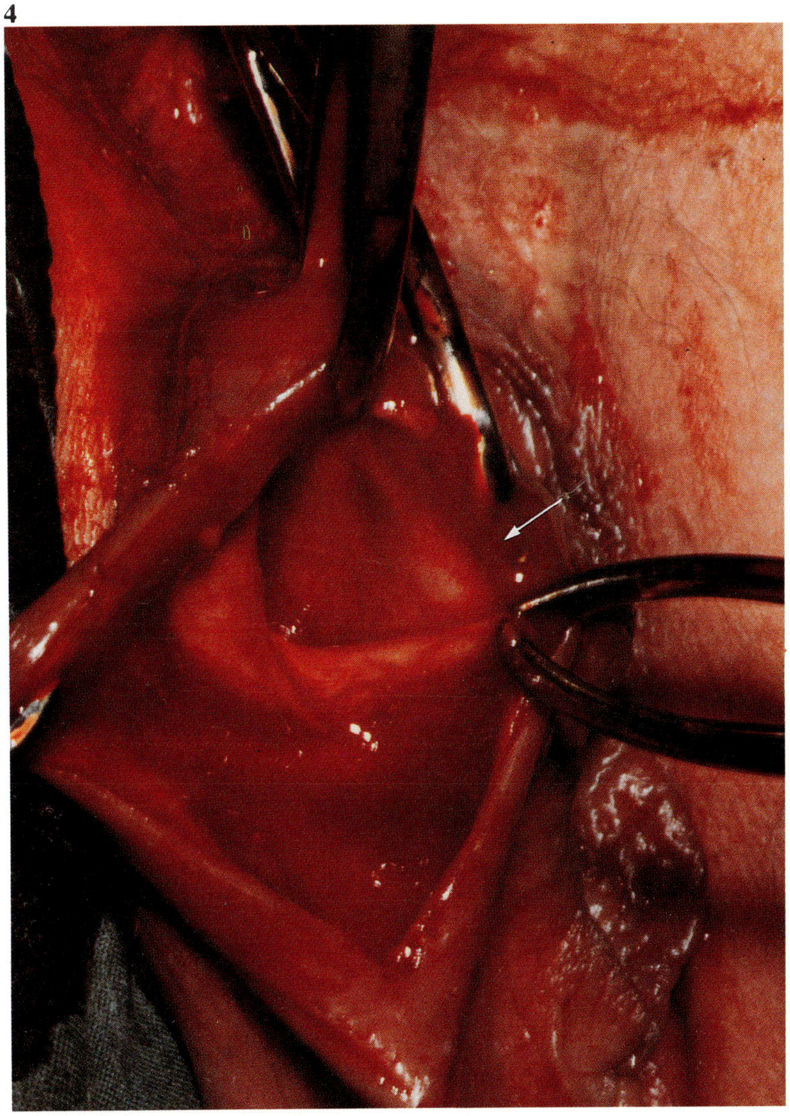

4 The cyst cavity is opened (arrowed). Swab should be taken for bacteriological examination.

5

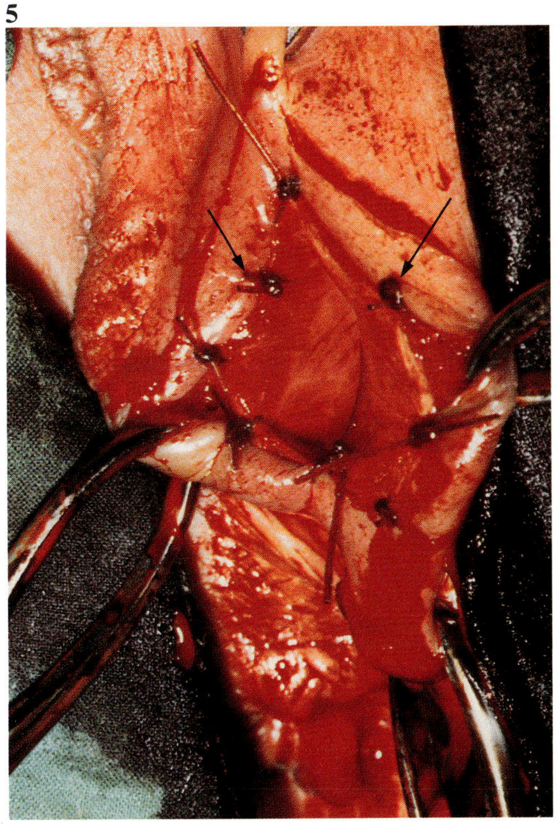

5 The cyst wall and the skin edges are sutured together (arrowed) using no.491 2 chromic catgut sutures. Interrupted catgut sutures are inserted. This way a stoma is created.

There is no need for any dressing. The area should be kept dry and clean.

Bartholin's cyst

Bartholin's cysts can be the result of scarring from episiotomy.

1 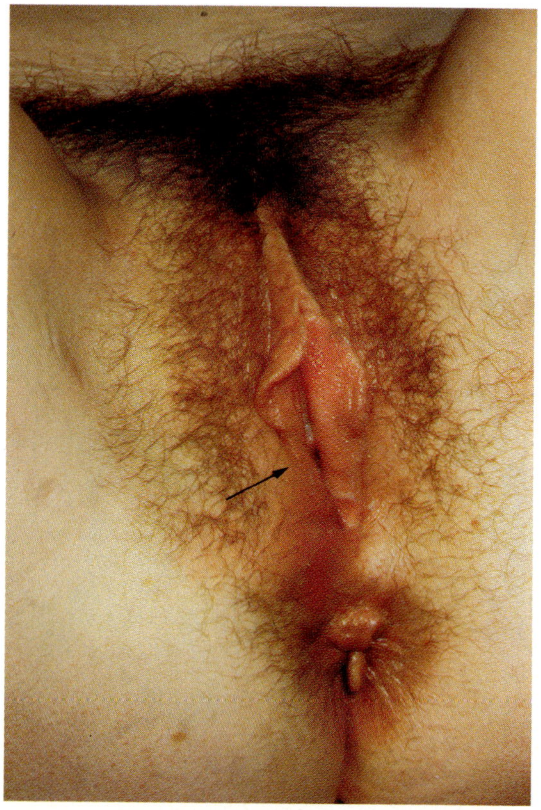

1 The diagnosis is made on examination when a swelling, which may be tender, is found in the Bartholin's area (arrowed).

2 An incision is made over the cyst using a scalpel and the cyst wall is excised.

3 If the cyst is infected, pus is released and a swab should be taken for bacteriological culture.

4 After evacuation of the cyst, the cyst cavity is packed using a gauze wick soaked in Milton solution or cream of Proflavine.

2 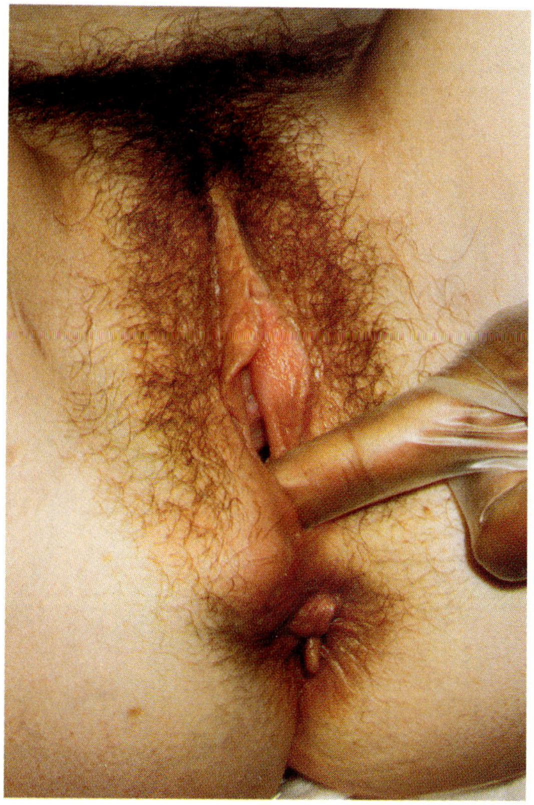

3 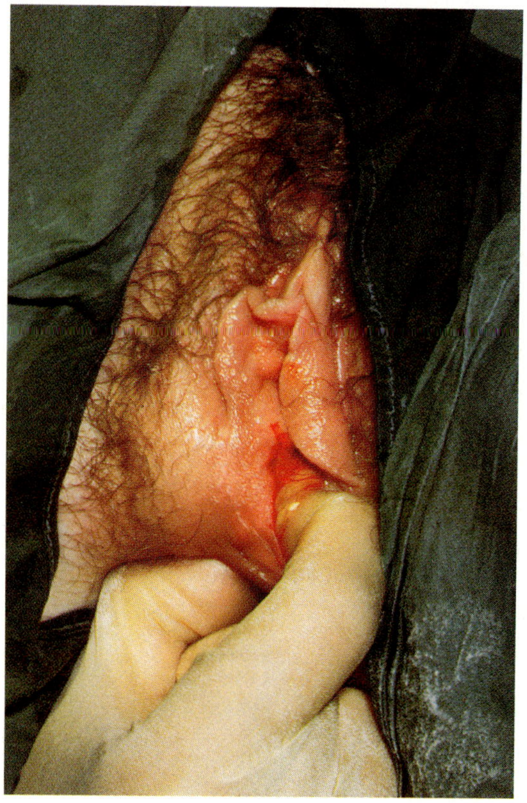

4 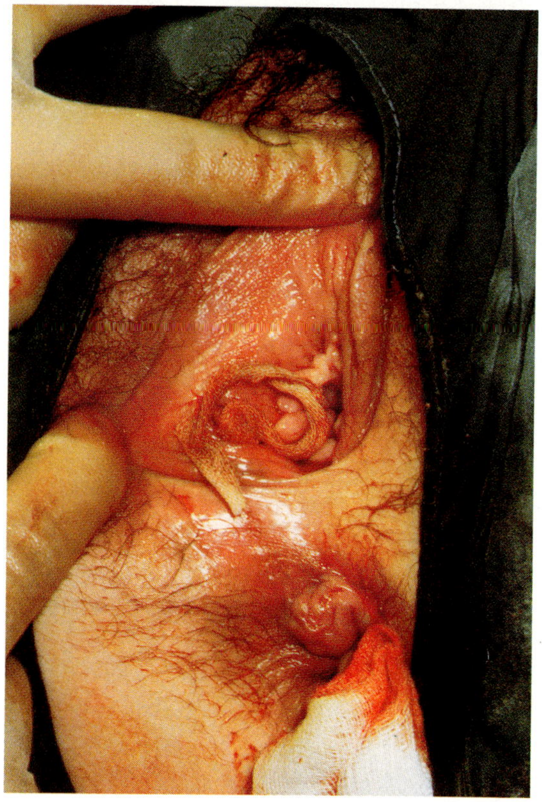

Acute Bartholin's abscess

1

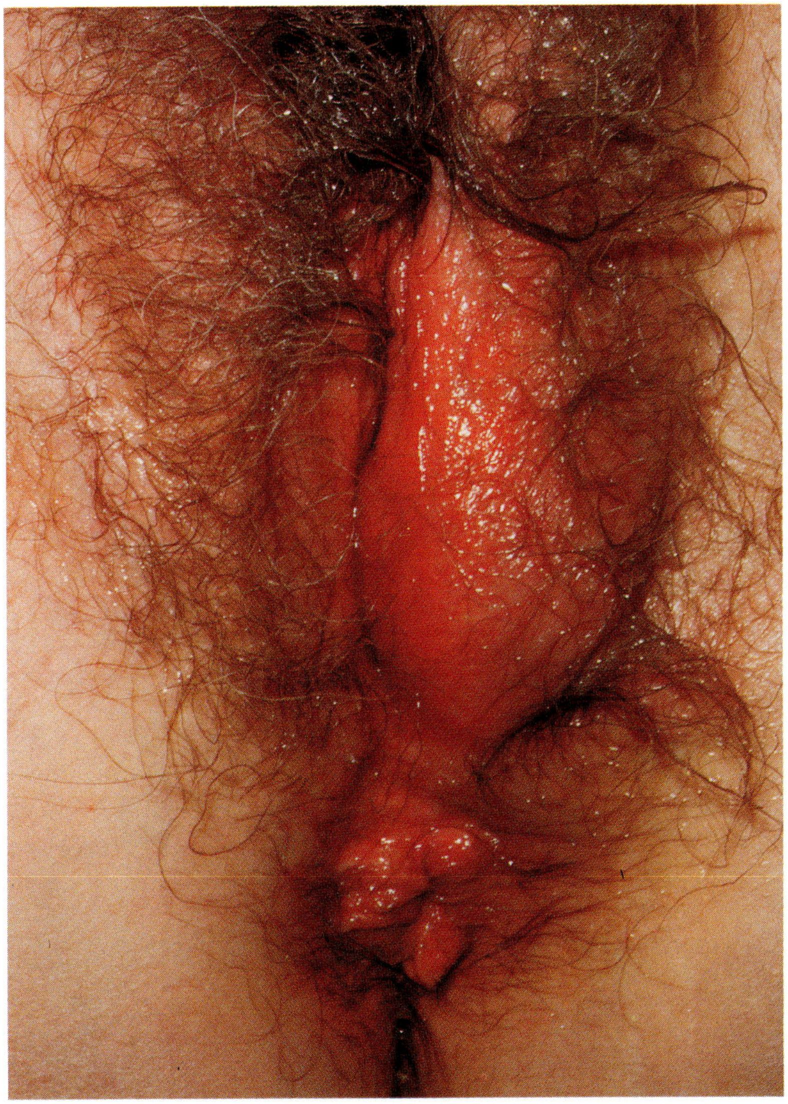

1 The Bartholin's cyst may become infected and may become an abscess. The condition is acute; the patient presents with a swelling and internal pain.

2

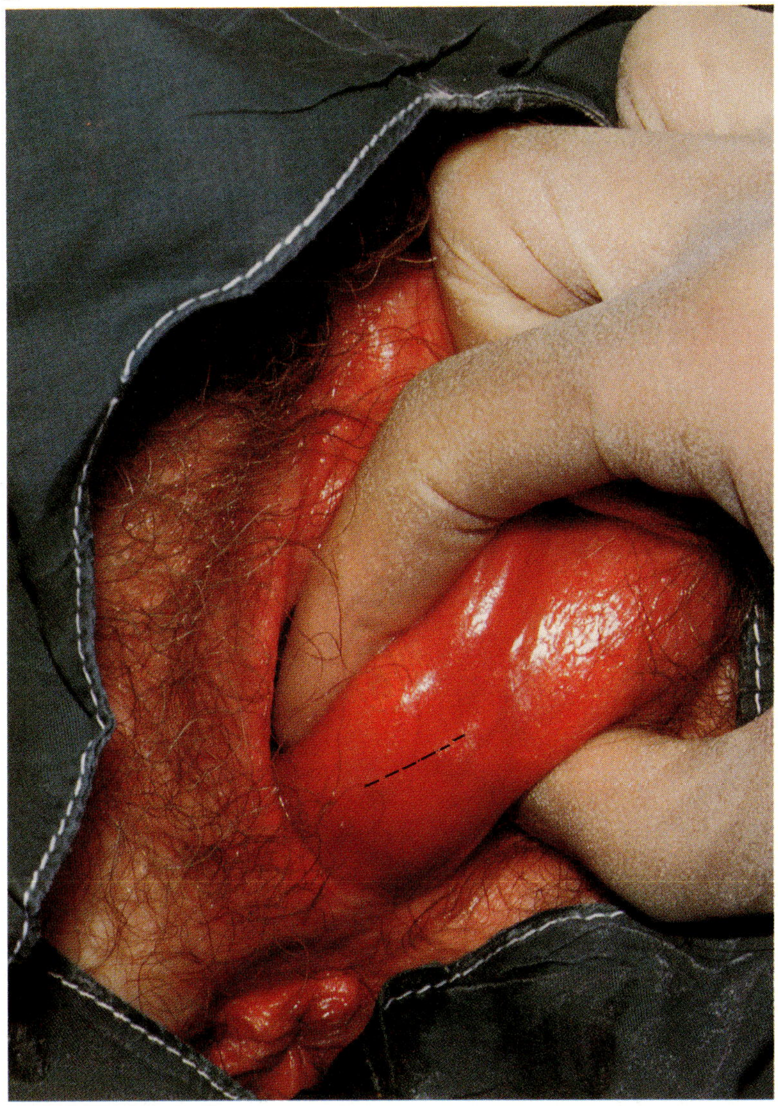

2 The diagnosis is made by examination of the labial area where an inflamed swelling is observed.

3

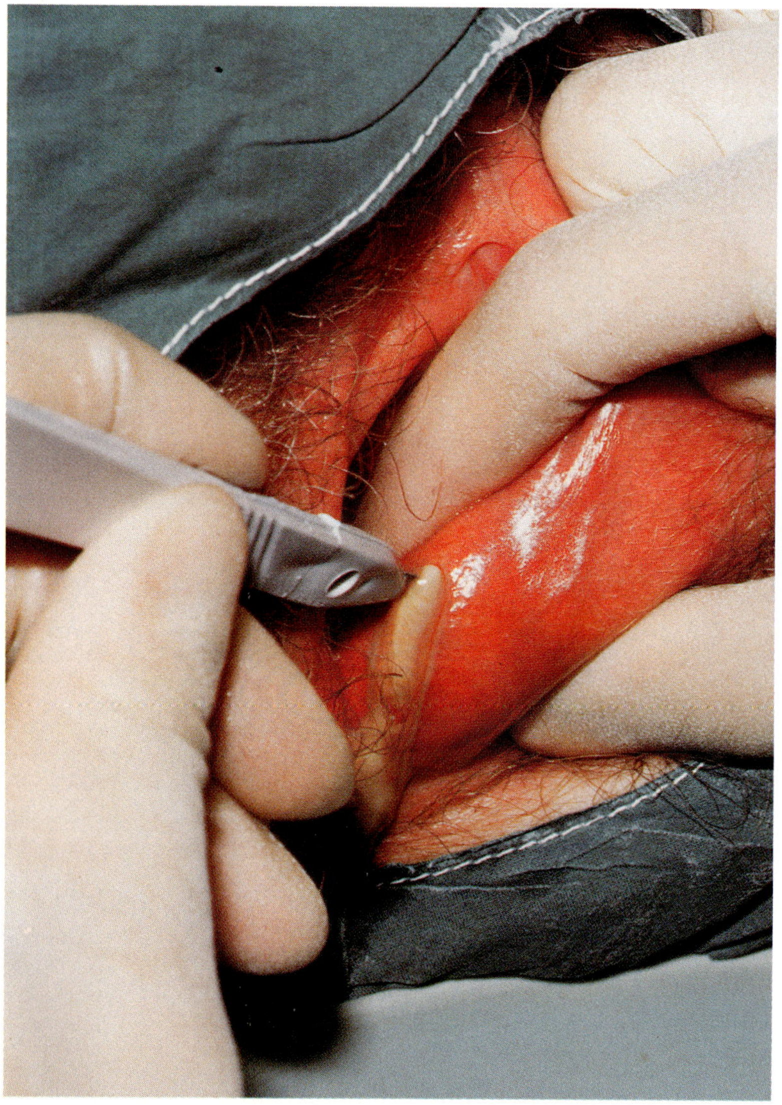

4

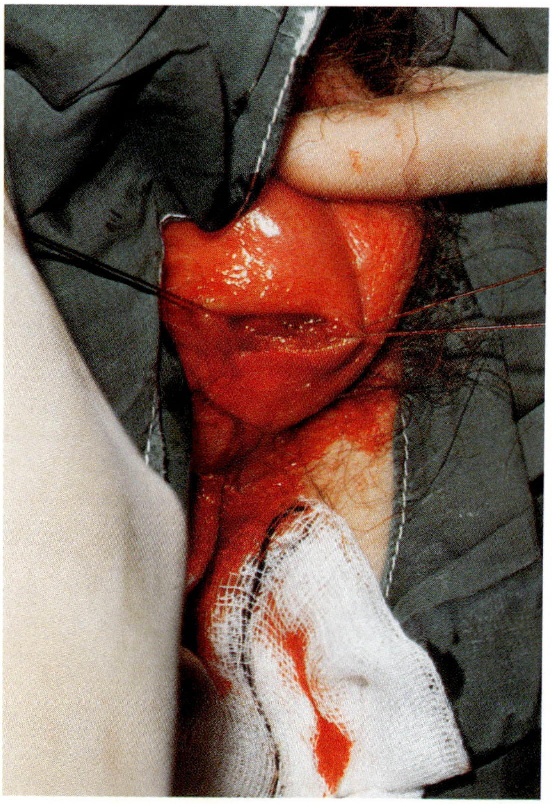

5

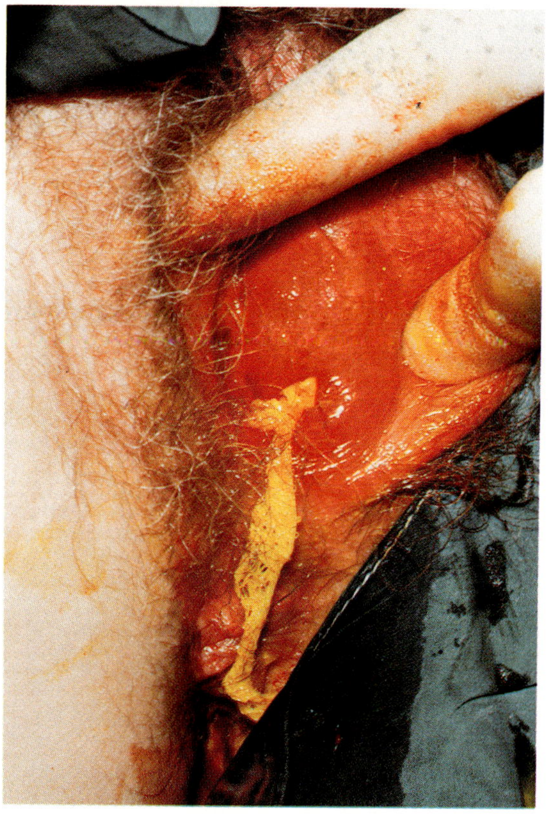

3 Under general anaesthetic the labial skin over the abscess is incised with a scalpel letting out the pus. A swab is taken and put into Stewart's medium for transportation to the bacteriology department for culture.

4 After drainage of the pus the abscess cavity is exposed.

5 The cavity is packed with gauze soaked in cream of Proflavine for 24 hours. The pack is removed and the area is then kept dry and clean and if necessary cleaned using Milton solution.

Excision of vaginal cyst

A vaginal cyst is relatively uncommon but may produce vaginal discharge or dyspareunia. The diagnosis is usually made on examination with a speculum.

1

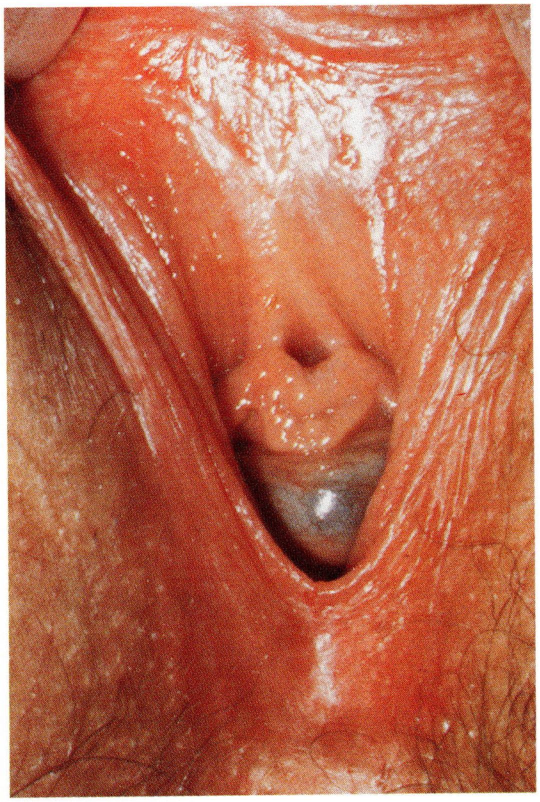

2

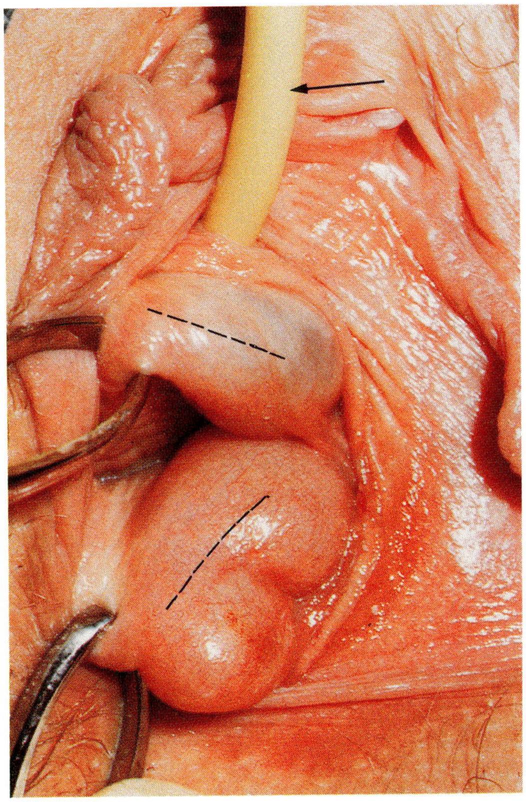

1 and 2 Sub-urethral and anterior and posterior vaginal cysts. Sub-urethral cysts could occasionally originate from the urethra and therefore care should be taken when excising. A Foley's catheter (arrowed) is inserted into the bladder and an incision is made in the vaginal skin over the cyst: shown by dotted line.

3

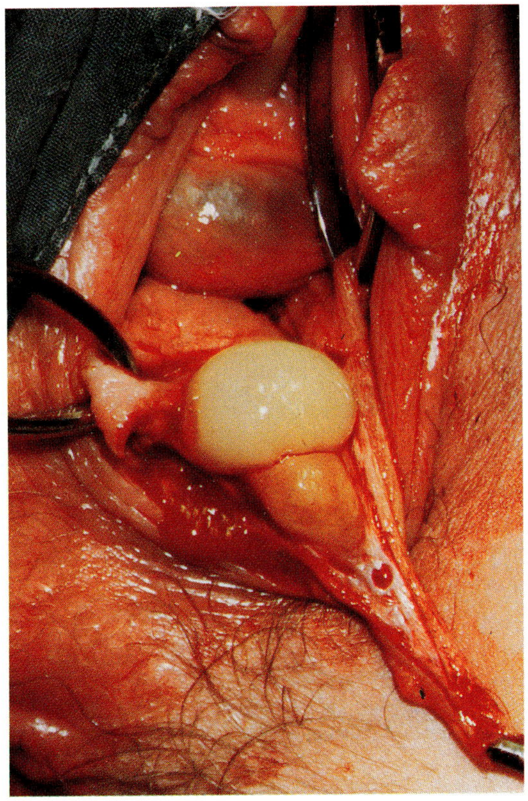

3 On opening the cyst using a scalpel either cyst fluid or sebaceous material is released. If the cysts are found to be infected, a bacteriological swab should be taken and sent for culture.

4

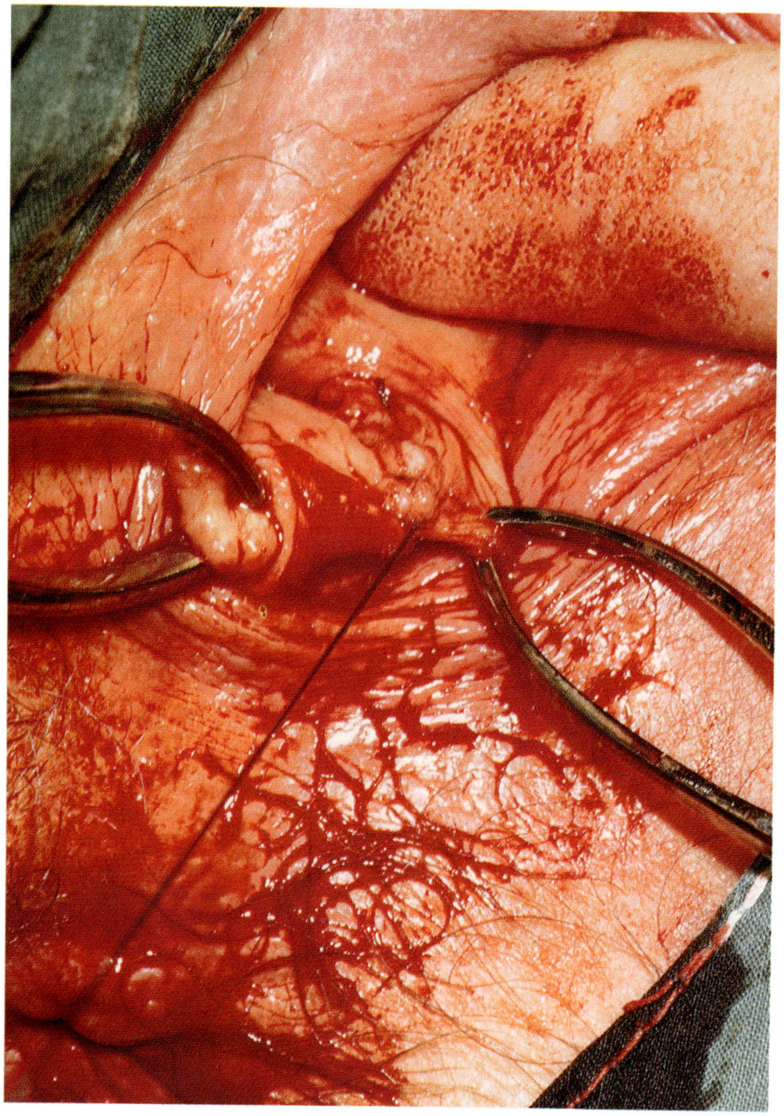

5

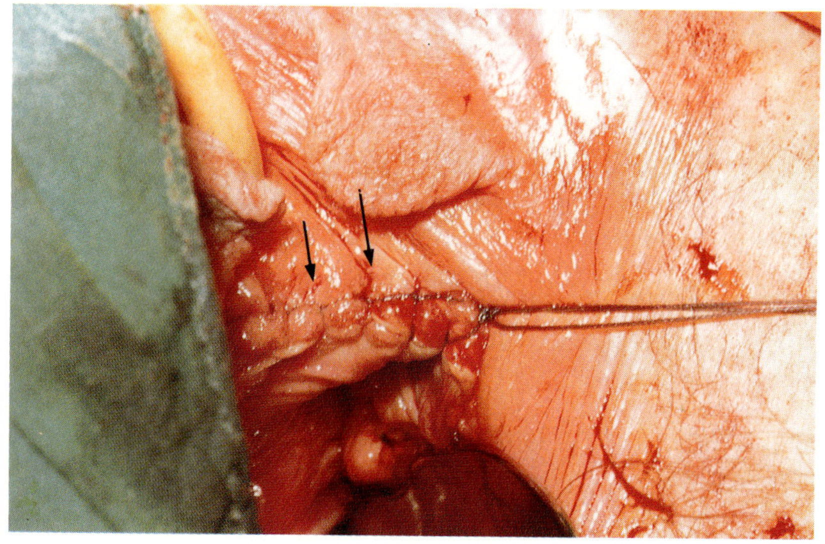

4 and 5 After evacuation of the cysts, the vaginal skin is closed using no. 491 2 chromic catgut with a taper point needle and interrupted catgut suture (arrowed). Apart from occasional bleeding which can be easily controlled there are no other complications.

Cervical cysts

Large cysts of the cervix requiring surgical treatment are uncommon. Nabothian follicles which are commonly found are easily treated by using diathermy or cryocautery. Cervical cysts may cause vaginal discharge or lead to dyspareunia. **Diagnosis is usually made on examination using a speculum. A cervical smear should be taken for cytology at this stage.**

1

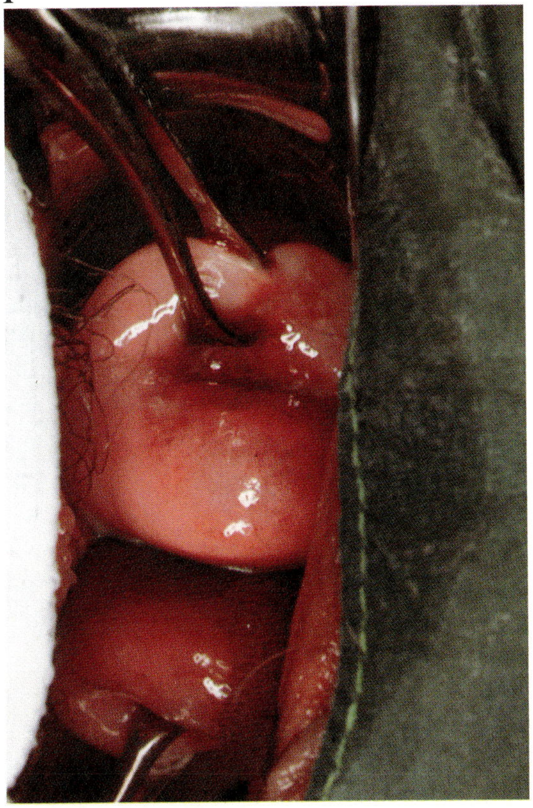

1 The posterior lip of the cervix is grasped with a Volsellum forceps. A Sim's speculum is inserted into the posterior fornix and posterior vaginal wall, allowing easy access to the cervix.

2 Using the scalpel an incision is made on the cervix over the area of the cervical cyst (dotted line).

3 and 4 The cyst is then removed by careful dissection using the dissecting forceps and scissors. If the cyst is incised, there is often a release of mucinous material. The cervical incision is then sutured using no. 491 2 chromic catgut. Usually no more than two catgut sutures are required.

2

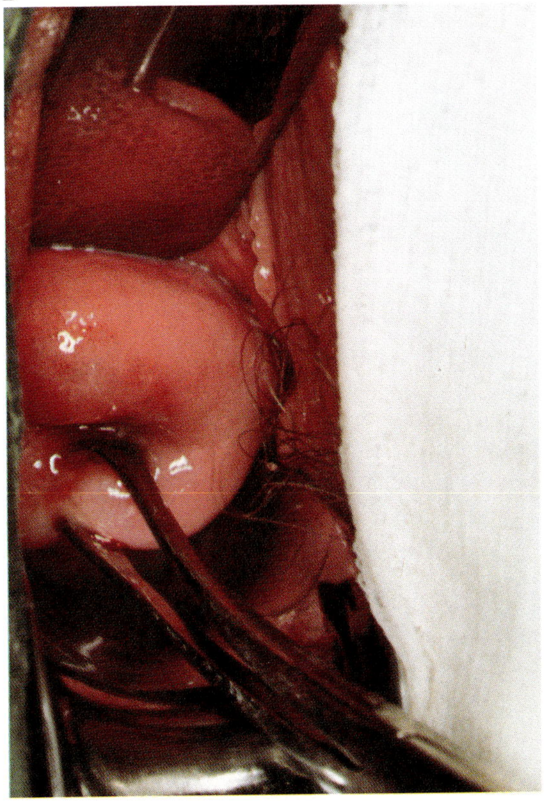

3

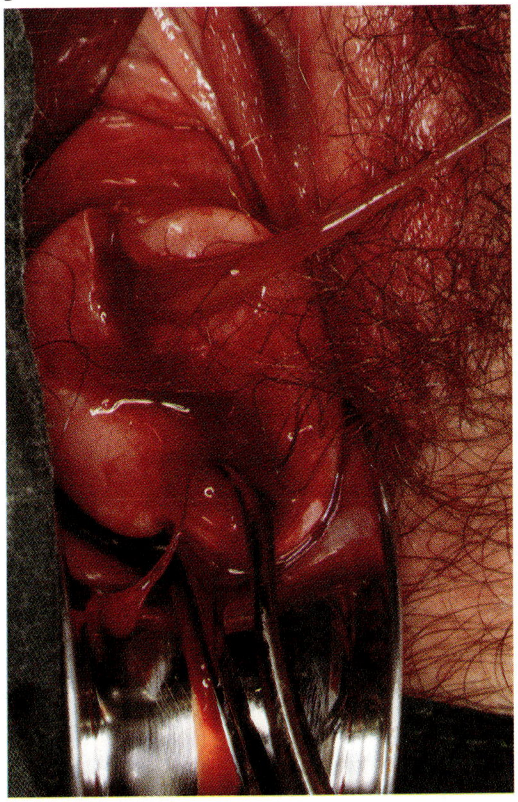

4

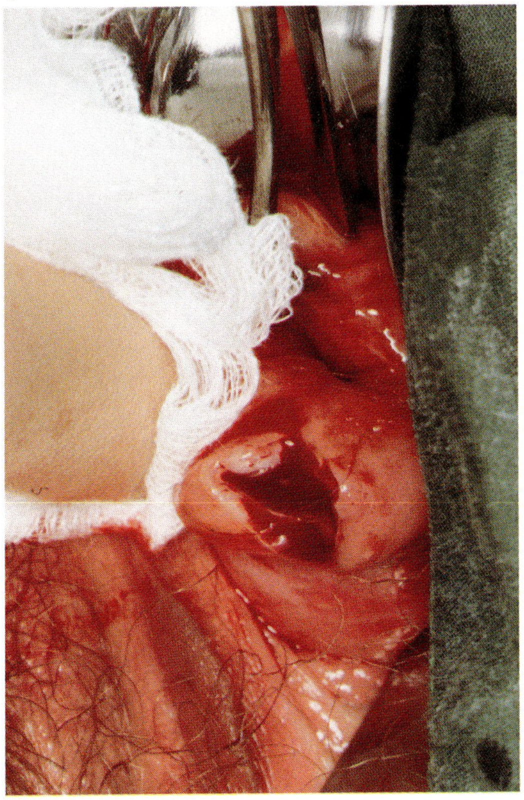

Pedunculated labial and vulval benign tumours

Pedunculated labial fibroma

1

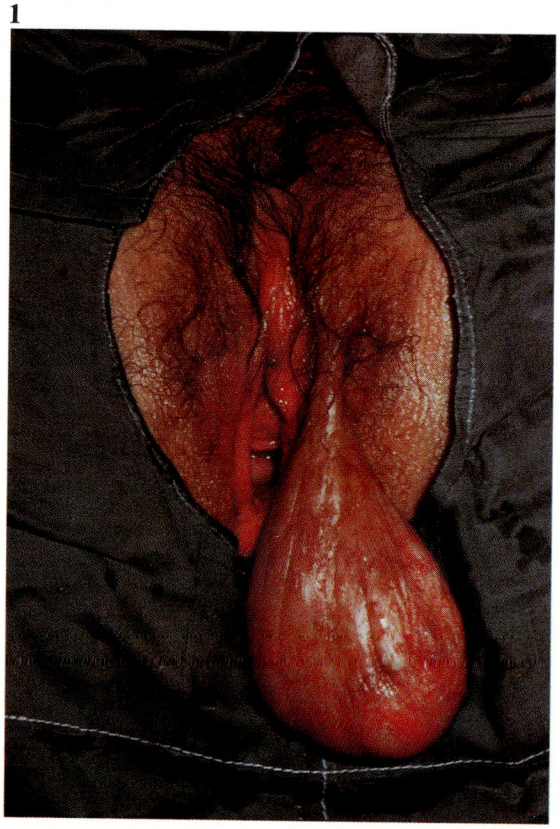

2

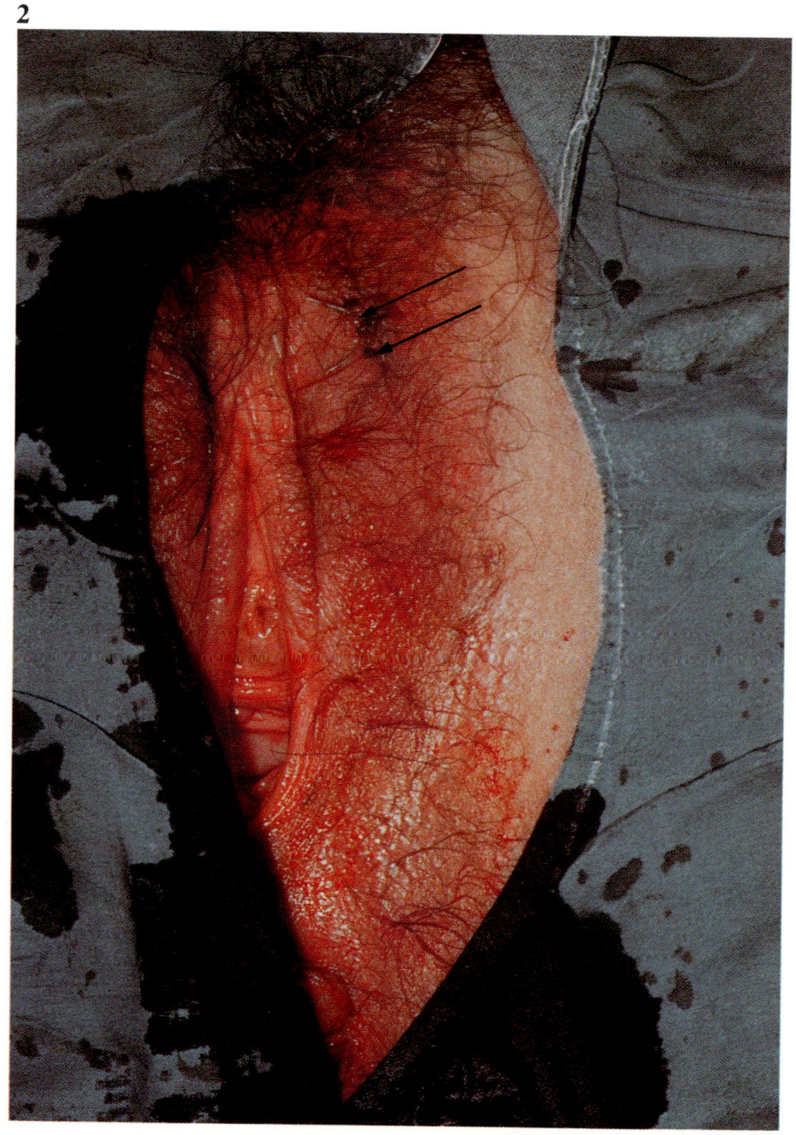

1 The benign pedunculated tumours of either labia or vulva are usually small and are either sebaceous cysts or fibromas.

2 They are easily removed by excision. With a scalpel an incision is made at the base, close to the vulval or labial skin. The incision is then closed using catgut sutures with chromic catgut (arrowed). The specimen should always be sent for pathological examination.

Cervical polyp and cervical erosion

The symptoms related to these conditions are cervical discharge and or irregular vaginal bleeding.

1 The diagnosis is made on speculum examination of the cervix. Cervical smear for cytology should be taken initially.

2 The small cervical polyps could be removed by grasping the base of each polyp with a Mayo's forceps and twisting it off.

3 Usually there is no troublesome bleeding, but if this occurs it can be treated using diathermy.

4 Cervical erosion should be treated using unipolar diathermy, strength 5 (arrowed) or cryocautery.

1

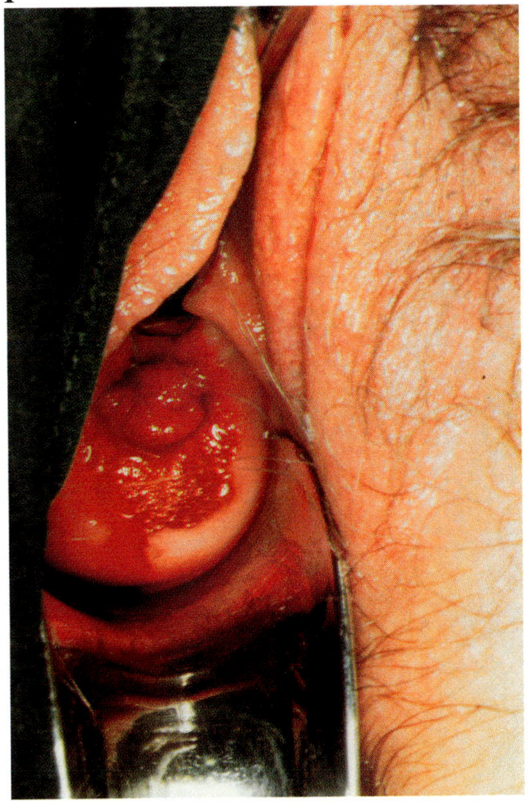

2

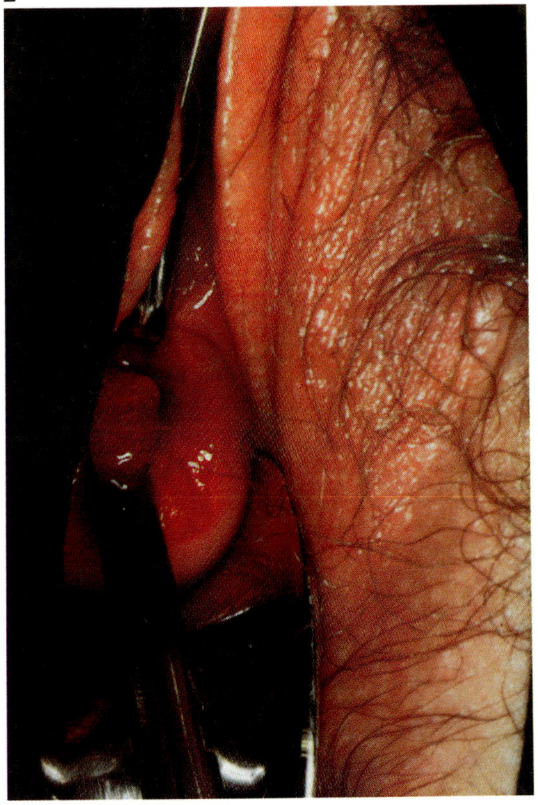

3

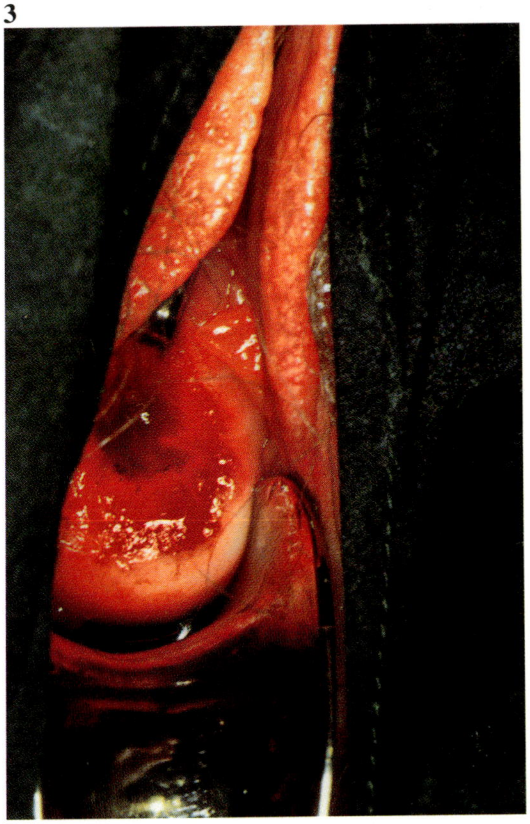

4

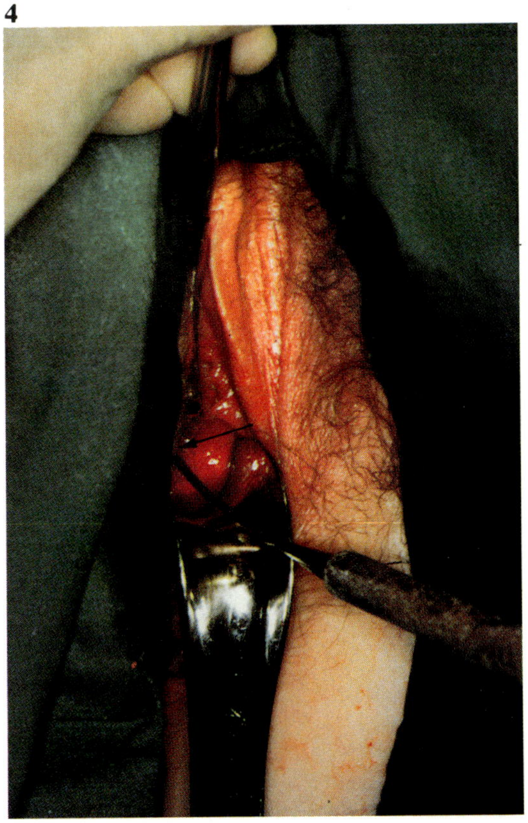

Removal of large cervical polyps

Large cervical polyps are removed by surgical excision.

1

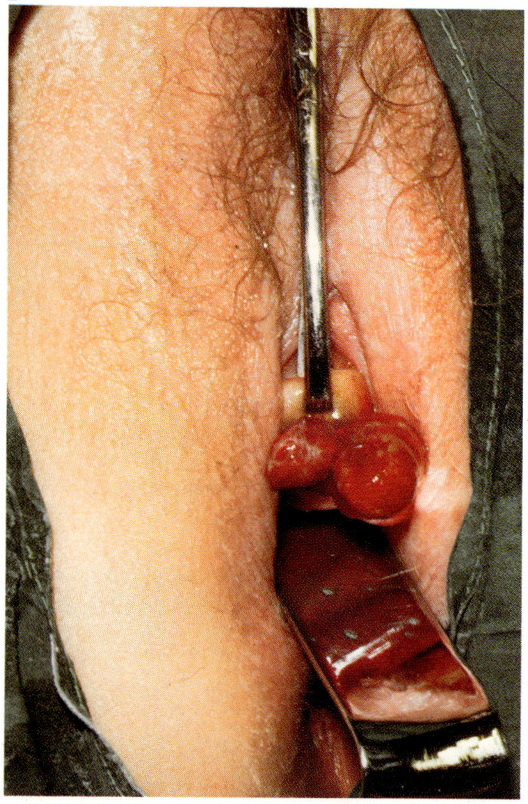

2

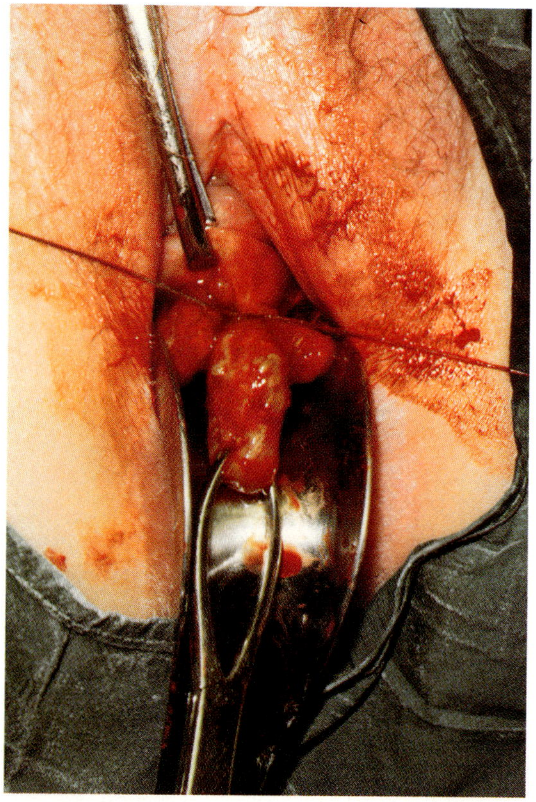

3

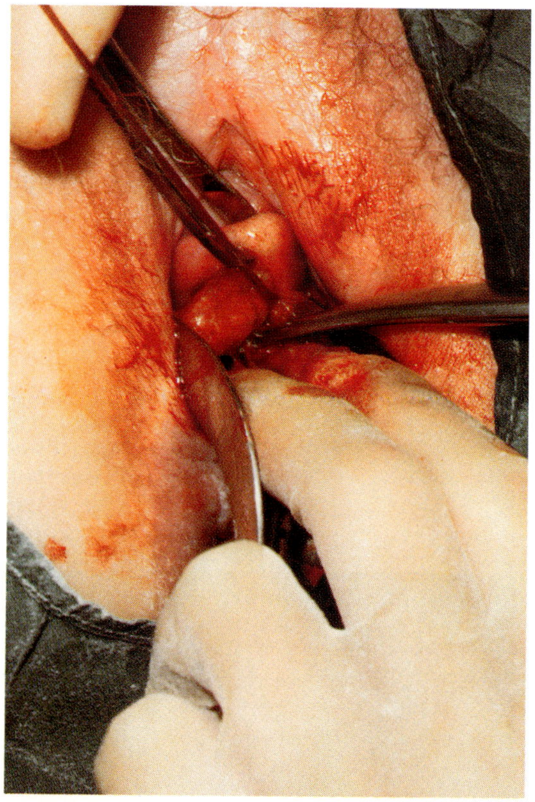

1 The anterior lip of the cervix is grasped with a Volsellum forceps, exposing the cervical polyps.

2 The polyps are grasped with a Littlewood's forceps. The base of the polyp is ligated with no. 2 chromic catgut.

3 and 4 The polyps are then excised with a pair of scissors.

4

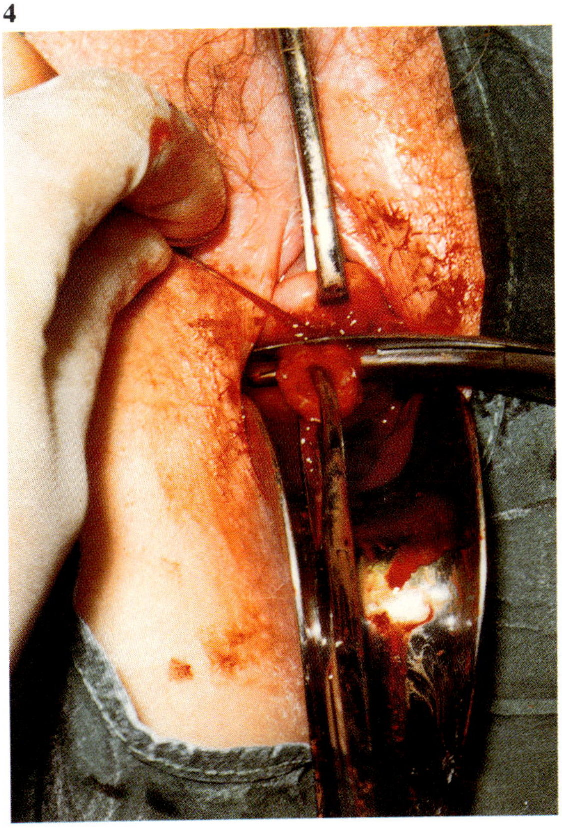

5

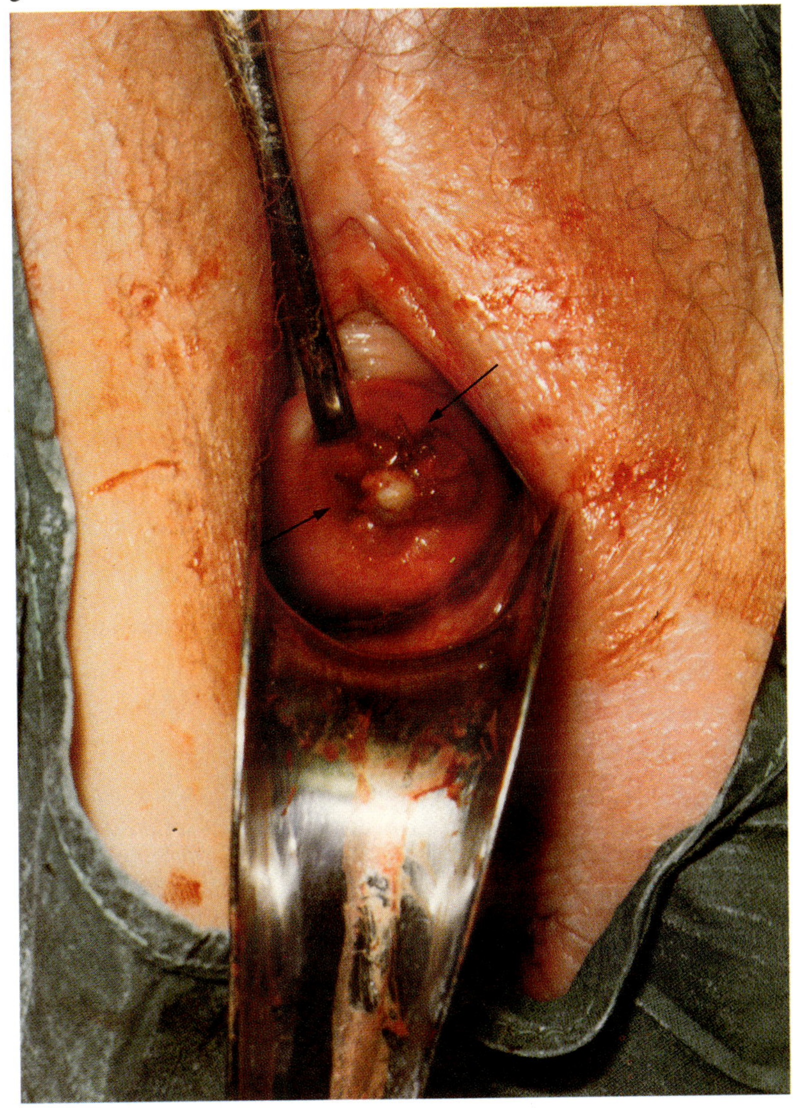

5 The base of the polyps can be seen, following ligation. No troublesome bleeding occurs following this, but if there is some it can be treated using diathermy or cryocautery. The polyps should be sent for histological examination.

Dilatation and curettage

Dilatation of the cervix and Curettage of the uterus is carried out for diagnostic and histological examination of the endometrium. Two of the common indications are for menstrual irregularity and post menopausal bleeding.

1

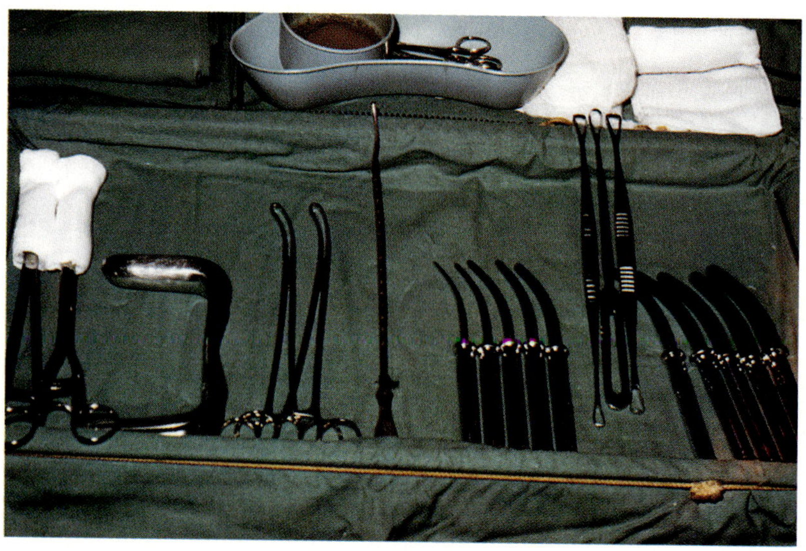

2

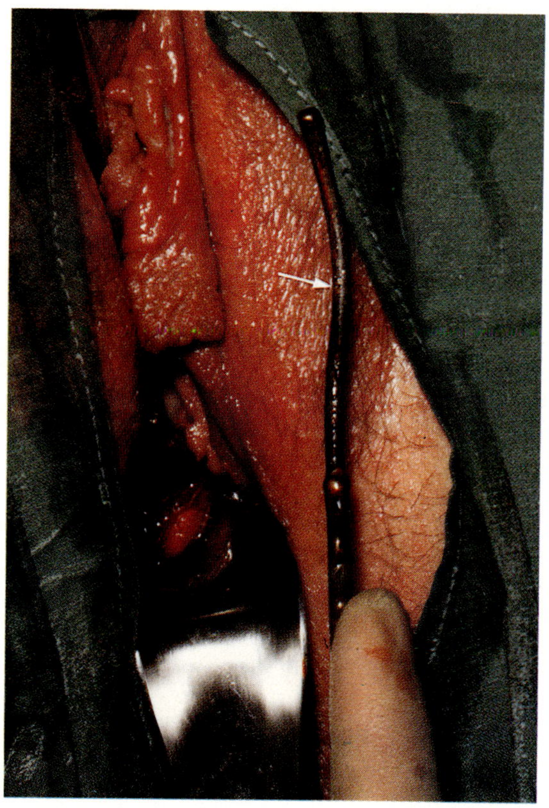

1 A tray showing the instruments required.

2 A Sims speculum is inserted into the posterior fornix of the vagina, exposing the cervix. The anterior lip of the cervix is grasped with a Volsellum forceps. A uterine sound (arrowed) is used to assess the uterine size.

3

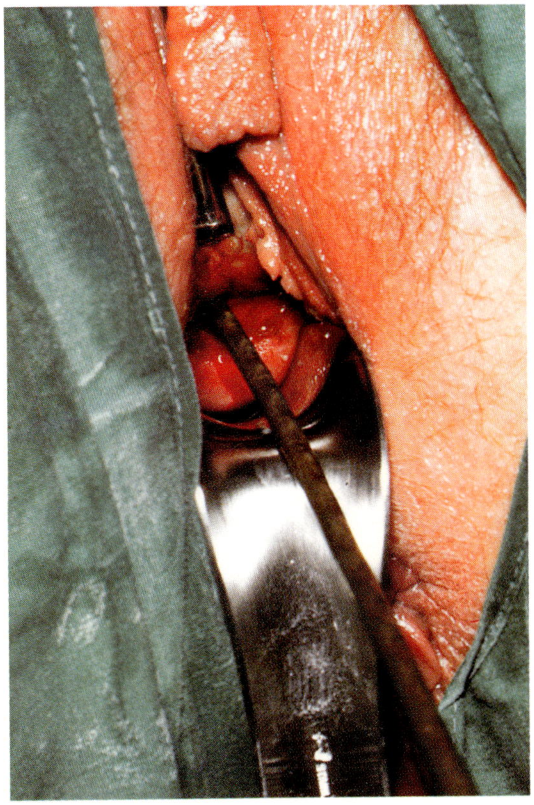

3 Having checked the position of the uterus by bimanual examination, the size of the uterine cavity is measured using uterine sound.

4

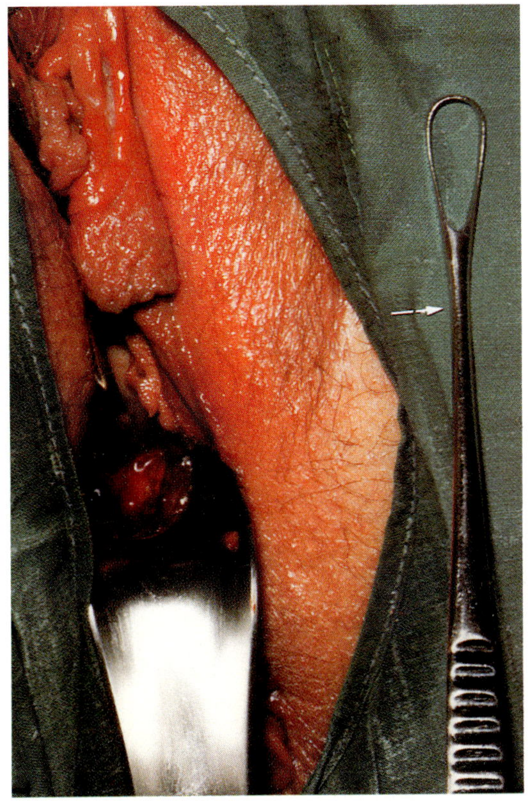

4 After dilatation of the cervix with Barker's cervical dilators – usually up to 8 to 10 mm, curettage of the uterine cavity is carried out using uterine curette (arrowed).

5

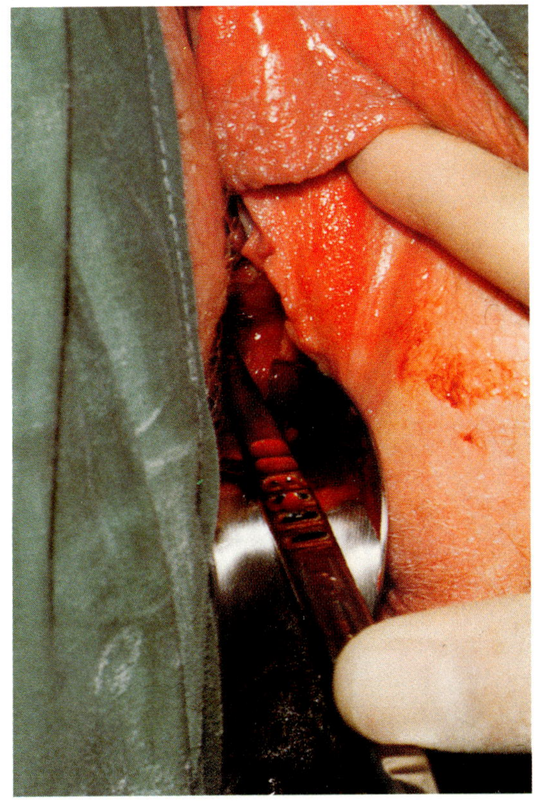

5 A sharp curette is introduced into the uterine cavity. The whole area of the uterine cavity should be covered, so as not to miss an endometrial polyp or a small area of endometrial carcinoma.

The uterine curettings obtained should always be sent for histological examination.

Pilonidal sinus

These occur commonly in areas of hair growth. Usually a chronic condition causing discharge and pain.

1

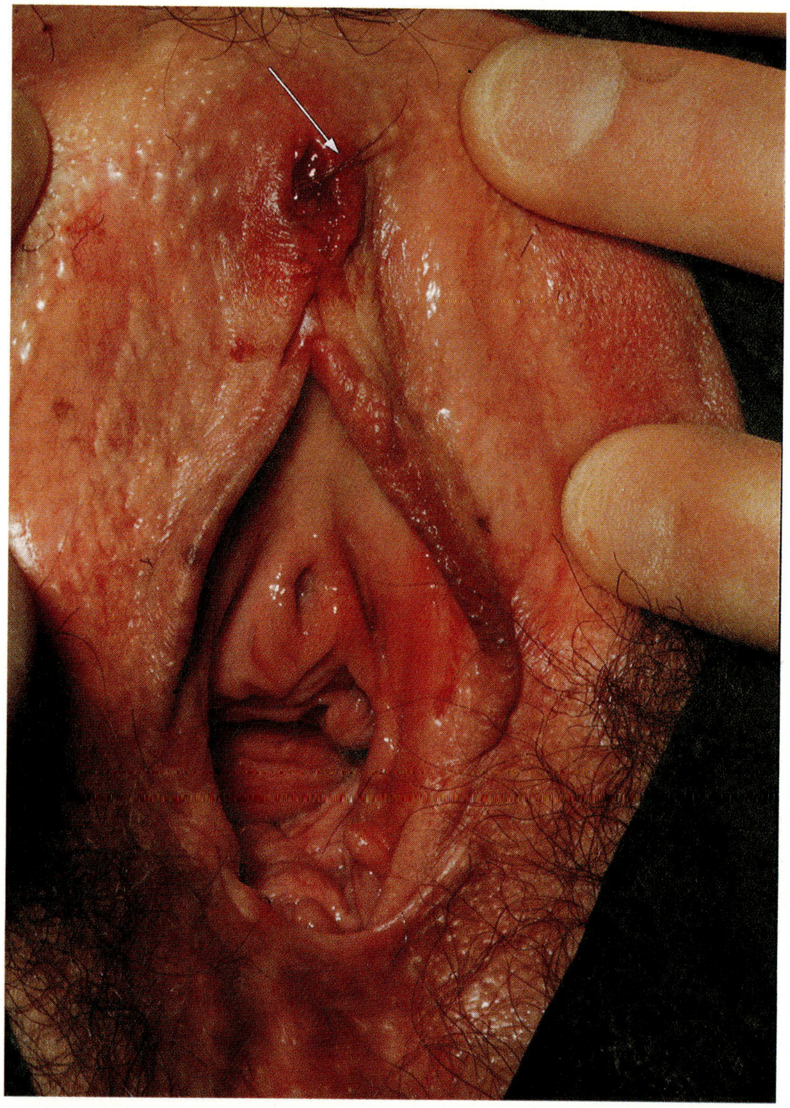

1 Pilonidal sinus in the region of the clitoris, with hair growing out (arrowed). Treatment is by excision of sinus and removal of hair. If there is evidence of infection, a bacteriological swab should be taken. Wound closed with interrupted catgut sutures.

Lichen sclerosis

1

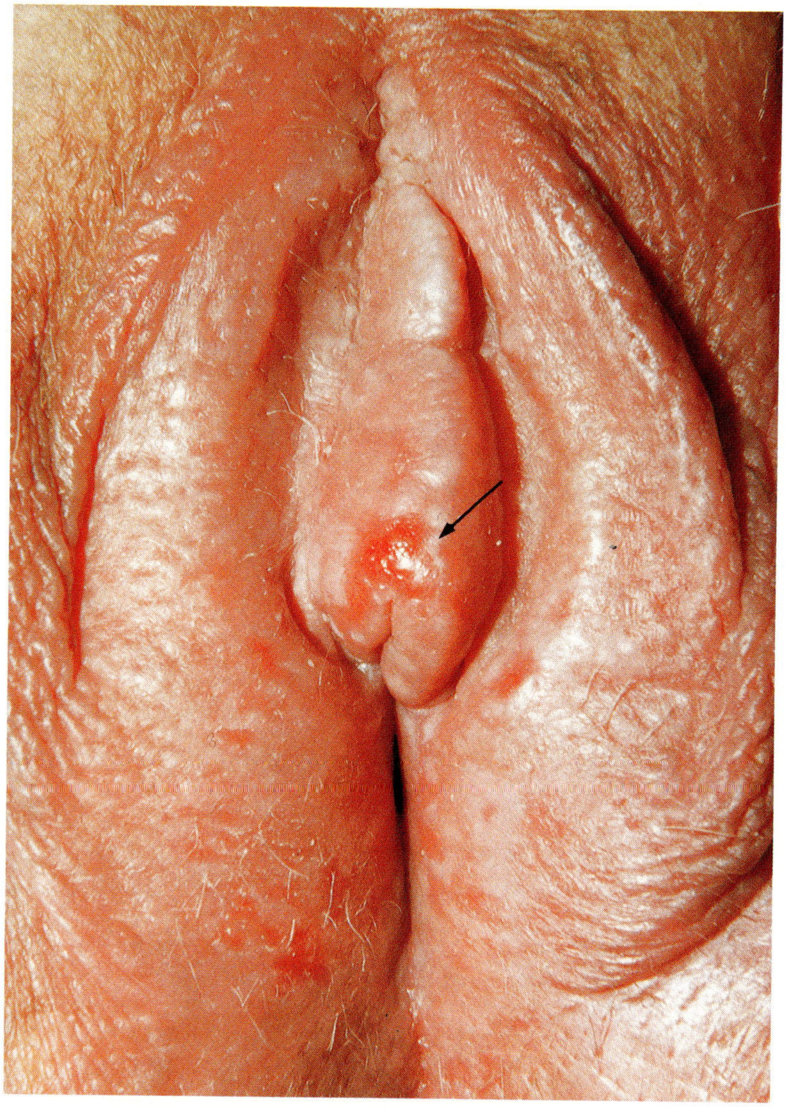

1 The common presenting complaint is that of pruritus. On examination, there is atrophic vulvitis and oedema. Presence of ulceration may signify malignant change (arrowed). A biopsy should be taken using biopsy forceps and sent for histology.

Leukoplakia

1 Presenting complaint is of pruritus and occasionally discharge. When it is extensive, the treatment is by local excision (marked with dotted line). Suture using interrupted catgut suture.

1

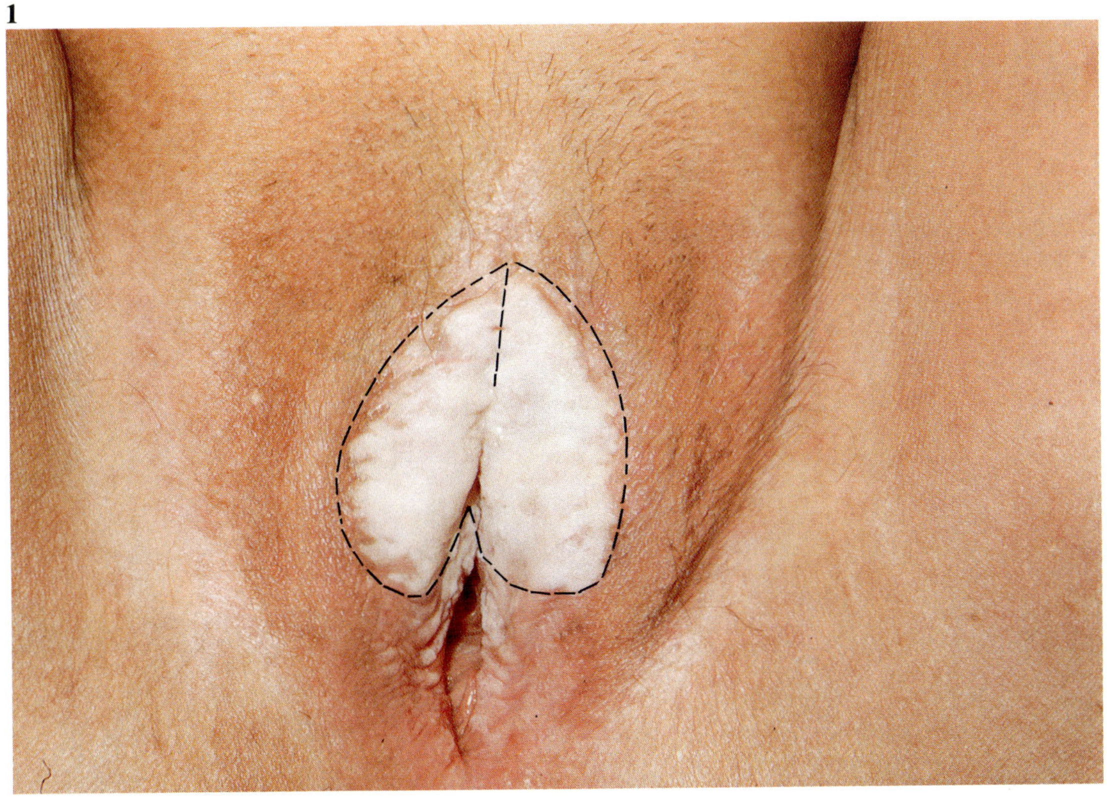

Leukoplakia of cervix

The presenting complaint is of vaginal discharge or irregular vaginal bleeding, or both. On examination, marked cervicitis with erosion is noted. A cervical smear should be taken.

1 Colposcopic examination shows extensive leukoplakia. Several punch biopsies should be taken to exclude cervical intraepitheal neoplasia (CIN) disease. Following this, the area should be treated with Semm Coagulator at 100° for 20 seconds.

1

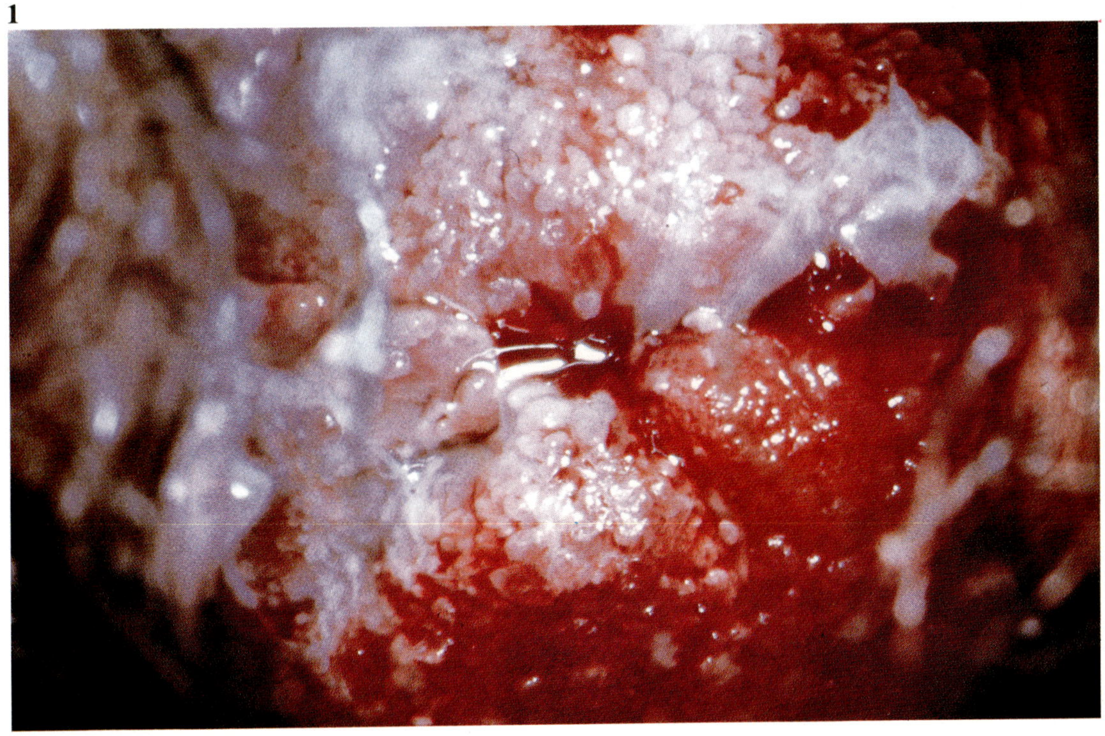

Cervicitis

The patient presents with vaginal discharge which may be bloodstained. A cervical smear should be taken.

1

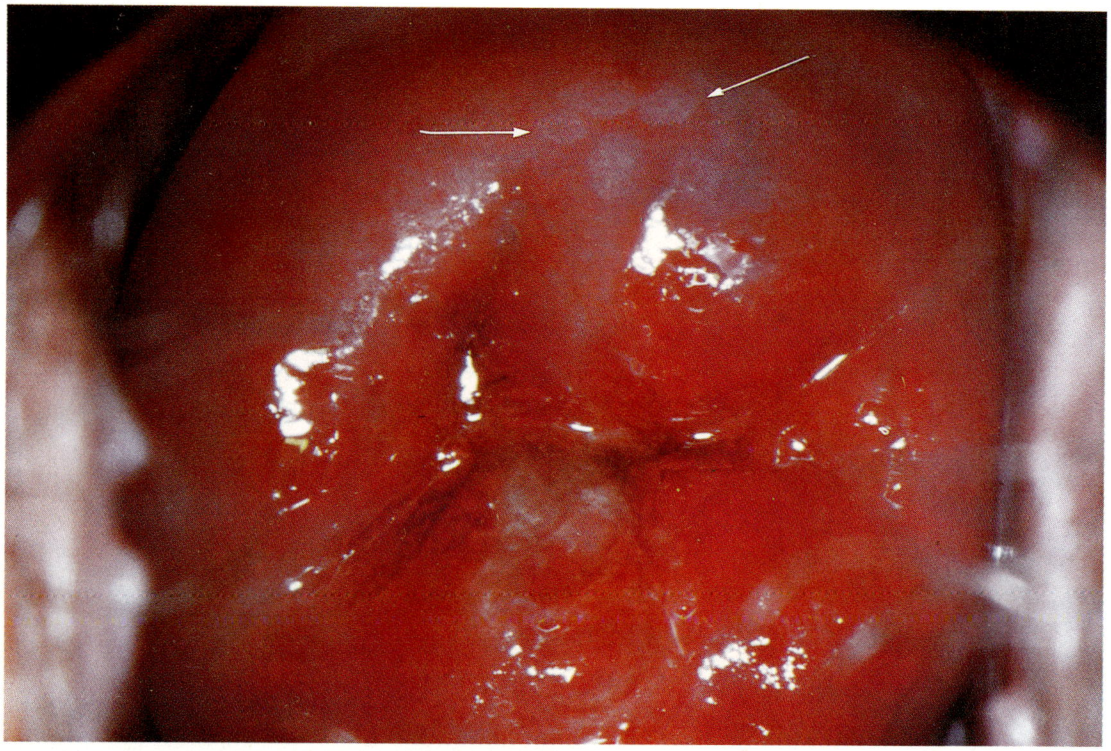

1 Colposcopic examination shows cervicitis with 'viral' plaques (HPV – human pappiloma virus). Arrow shows area to be biopsied.

2

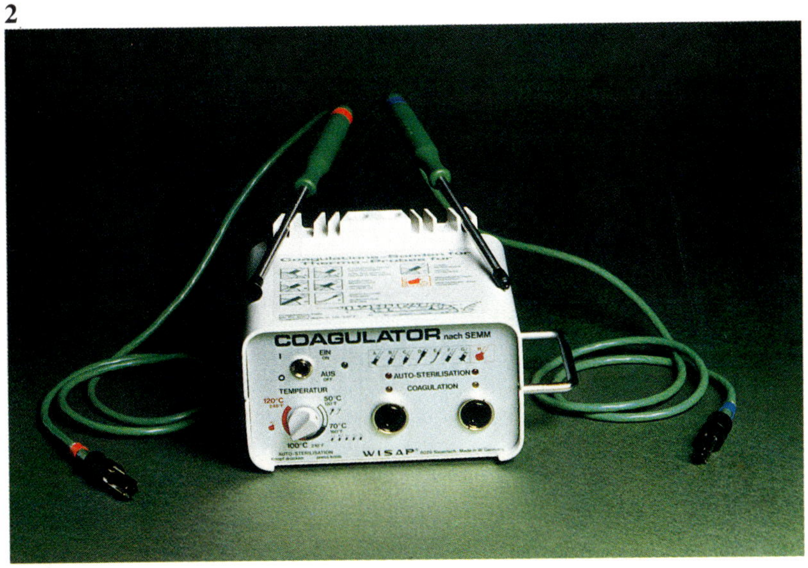

2 and 3 The area is then treated using Semm's coagulator and the appropriate probe. The whole area of the external os should be treated, with the temperature set at 100°C.

3

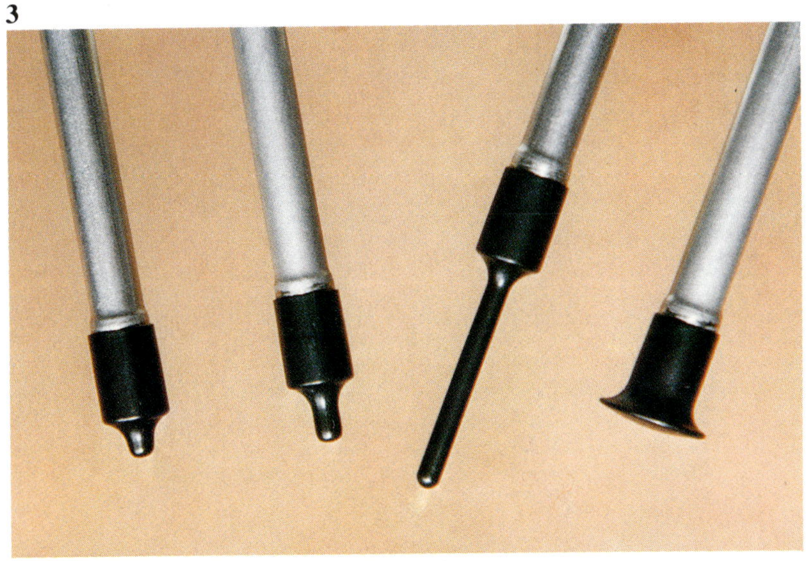

4 Application should be for 20 seconds. The patient should be warned that the vaginal discharge may be worse for a few days. Vaginal antibiotic cream such as Sultrin could be prescribed. Patient should be reviewed 6 weeks later.

5 The cervix should be healed. The photograph also shows threads of intrauterine contraception device.

4

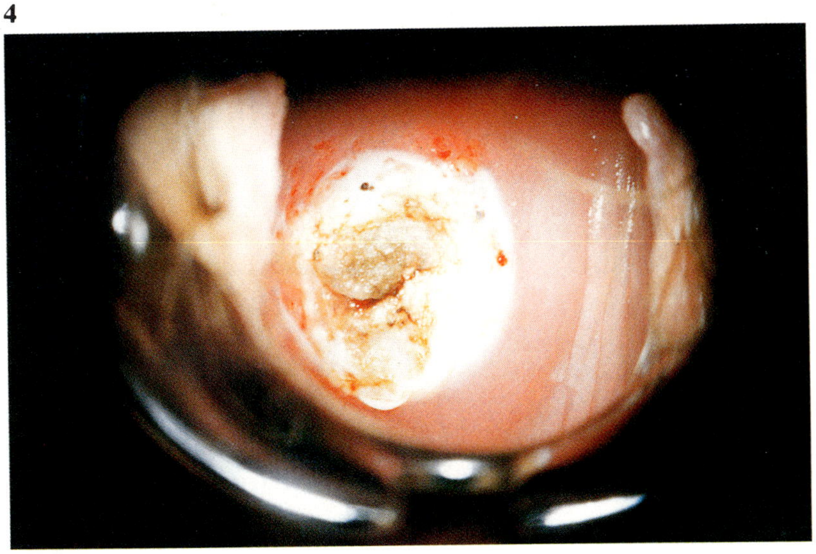

5

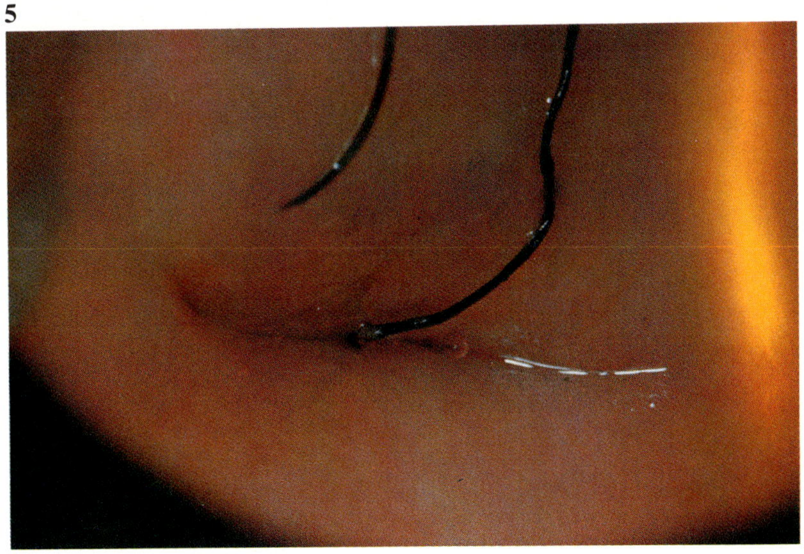

Laparoscopy

Laparoscopy is a relatively simple technique which is useful for both diagnosis and treatment of certain gynaecological conditions. The most common indication is for female sterilisation. In patients referred with infertility and pelvic pain, laparoscopy is helpful in diagnosing pelvic disease and tubal patency.

Prior to the procedure, the bladder is catheterised. Pneumoperitoneum is induced by insufflation with carbon dioxide. To allow uterine manipulation a Spackmann cannula is attached to the uterus. Methylene blue dye can also be injected through the cannula to check for tubal patency.

1

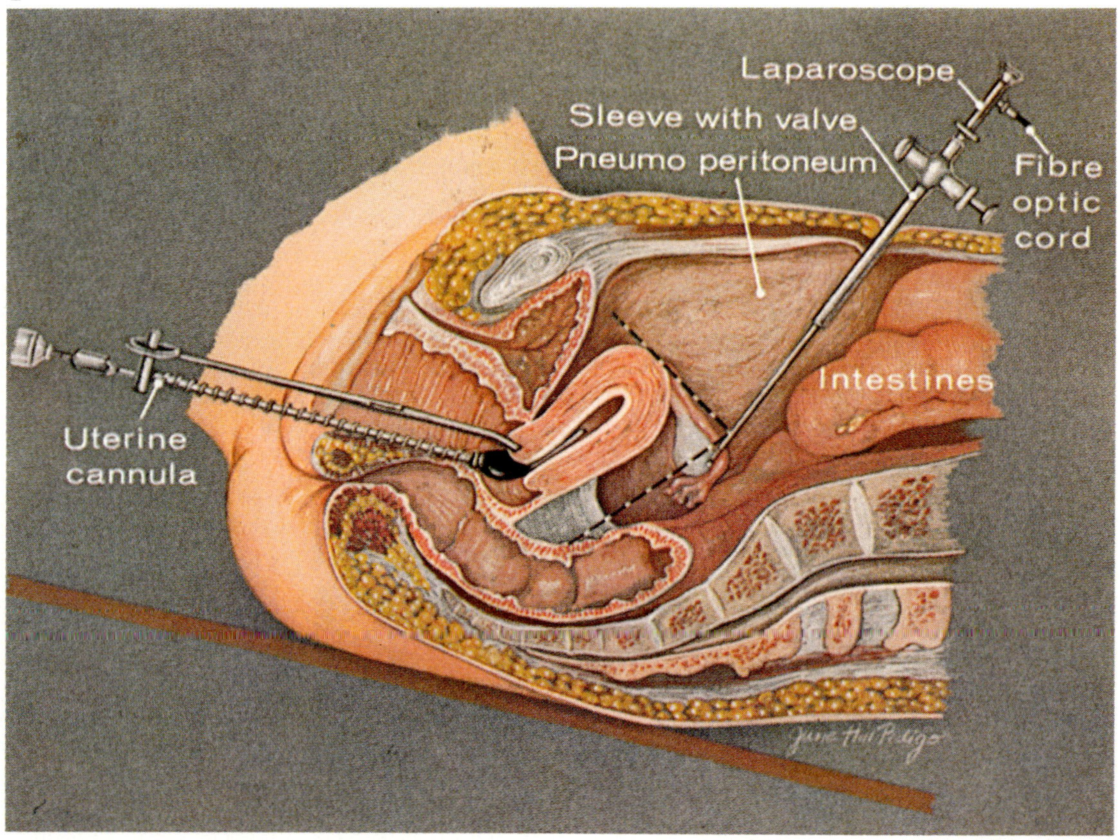

1 Prior to the introduction of the laparoscope, a trocar is introduced at the level of the umbilicus – directed at 45° angle in the direction of the uterus. Extreme care should be taken if complications such as vascular and bowel damage is to be avoided. Obese patients or patients with multiple scars may not be suitable for this procedure. Vascular damage of pelvic blood vessels has been reported. Extreme care must be taken. The following pictures show pelvic organs as seen through the laparoscope.

2

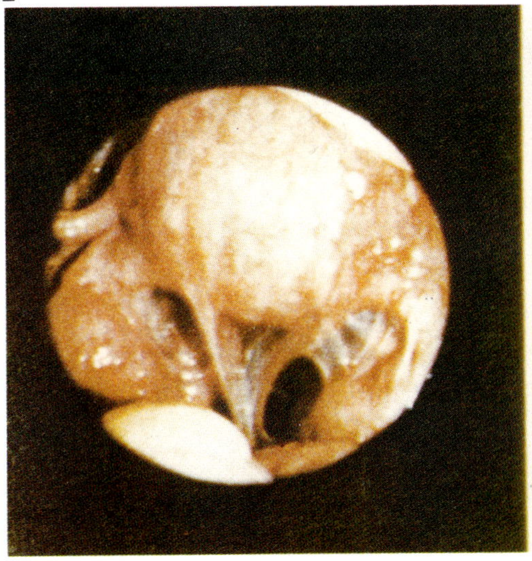

3

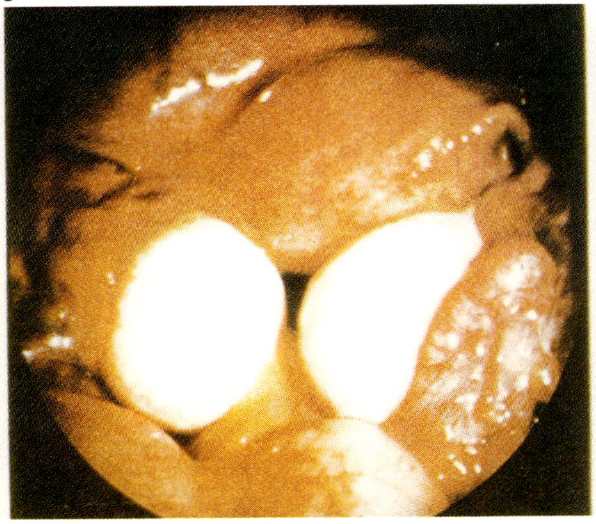

4

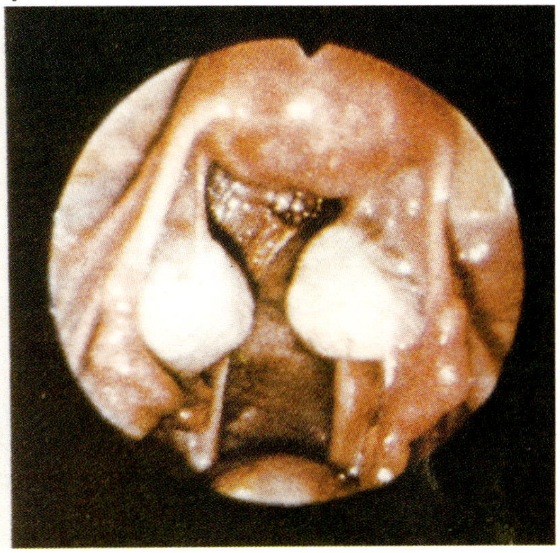

2 shows normal pelvic organs. The uterus, fallopian tube and ovaries are clearly seen.

3 shows enlarged ovaries that are white in appearance with thickened tunica seen in polycystic ovarian disease.

4 shows adhesion of uterus to pelvic organs. Fine adhesion can be divided using scissors. These are usually the result of pelvic inflammatory disease.

Index

All figures refer to page numbers

A
Abscess
– Bartholin's 179-180
– Breast 87
Anaesthesia
– Local 5, 7, 58-60
Anatomy 5
Appendicectomy 62-65
Artery
– Temporal 17
Arthroplasty
– Keller's 112-113
Aspiration
– Breast cyst 81
– Epididymal cyst 41
Axillary clearance 100-102

B
Bartholin's
– Cyst 178
– Abscess 179-180
Biopsy
– Lesion of face 141
– Lesion of leg 138
– Lichen sclerosis 190
– Needle biopsy breast 83-84
– Open biopsy breast 85
– Pyogenic granuloma 148
– Temporal artery 17-19
Breast 81-101
– Lesions 97-99
– Open biopsy 85-86
Bone
– Hyoid 23
Bunionectomy 109-111

C
Cannula
– Lacrimal 130
– Carcinoma
– Sin 144-145
– Eyelid 157-159
Cautery
– Ectropion 128
– Erosion 185
Cervical cyst 183
– Polyp 185-187
Cervicitis 192-193
Cervix
– Leukoplakia 191
Chalazion 121
Cheek
– Laceration 146-147
Circumcision 30-33
Colostomy closure 71-72
Contracture – Dupuytren's 103-105
Corneal foreign bodies 120
Cross finger flap 161-163
Cyst
– Bartholin's 178
– Breast 81
– Cervical 183
– Epididymal 41-42
– Labial 176-177
– Meibomian 121
– Sebaceous back 9-10
– Sebaceous neck 11-12
– Scalp 11-12
– Thyroglassal 22-24

D
Dartos-muscle 39-40, 46
De Quervain's stenosing teno-vaginitis 106
Dilatation and curretage 188-189
'Dog ears' – excisions 144
Drugs (local anaesthetic) 7
Duct
– Breast 88-90, 92-96
– Thyroglossal 23
– Parotid 25
Dupuytren's contracture 103-105

E
Ectropion 128-129
Epididymis cyst 41-42
Epigastric hernia 52
Entropian 123, 125
Excision impalpable breast lesion 97-99

Eye – foreign body 120
Eyelid – Cancer excision and graft 157-159

F
Fascia
– Scarpa's 38
– Palmar 103-105
Fertility 41
Fibroadenoma breast 85-86
Finger – trigger 118
– Crush injury 161-162
Fistula in ano 66
Foreign body – eye 120
Frenulum 34
Frenuloplasty 34-35

G
Ganglion 13-14
Gland of neck – excision 20-21
Granuloma – pyogenic 148

H
Haemorrhoidectomy 67-70
Hernia
– Epigastric 52-54
– Inguinal
– direct 57-61
– indirect 47-51
Hydrocele 43-45
Hyoid – bone 23
Hypertrophic scar 167

I
Ingrowing toe nail 115-117

K
Keller's arthroplasty 112-113

L
Labium – cyst 176-177
Laceration of cheek 146-147
Lacrimal cannula 130
Lacrimal duct, syringing 130
– Three-snip procedure 133
– Probing
Laparoscopy 194
Leg – biopsy excision 141
Leukoplakia 191
Lichen sclerosis 190
Lip
– Vermillionectomy 164-165
– Wedge excision 163
– Wedge excision cancer 165-166
Lipoma of back 15-16
Liposarcoma 15
Local anaesthetic drugs 7
Lord's operation 43
Lower axillary clearance 100-102

M
Meibomian cyst 121
Melanoma 144, 153-157
Mole – excision 139, 141
Microdochectomy 92-96

N
Naevus – nose 160
Neck – excision of gland 20
Needle biopsy of breast 83-84
Nerves – intercostobrachial 102
– Genitofemoral 60
Nerves – intercostobrachial 102
– Ilioinguinal 58-60
– Ilionypogastric 58
– Latissimus dorsi 102
– Serratus anterior 101
Nose – naevus 160

O
Operation – Lord's 43
Open biopsy of breast 85-86

P
Palmar facciectomy 103-105
Parotid
– Duct 25-26
– Stricture 25
Perineal warts 173-175
Phimosis 30
Pilonidal sinus 73-76
Pilonidal sinus vulva 190
Plastic surgery 134-172
Prepuce 30
Phenolisation 115
Phimosis 30

R
Radius – excisions of head 107-108

S
Scalp cyst 11-12
Scar excision of 171-172
– Revision 135
– Triamcinolone injection 167
– W-plasty 168
– Z-plasty 169-170
Scrotum 42
Sebaceous cyst 9-10
Syringing lacrimal duct 130
Skin carcinoma 144-145
– Dog ears 144
– Flaps 160-163
– Grafting 150-159
– Scar placing 136-137
Skin-crease lines 134
Stricture parotid duct 25
Sutures – removal 137
– Synthetic 134

T
Tarsal cyst 121
Tarsectomy 127
Tattoo excision of 149
Tear duct procedures 130-133
Temporal artery biopsy 17
Temporal arteritis 17
Tenovaginitis stenosing 106
Testis – undescended 38-40
Thyroglossal cyst 22-24
Thyroglossal duct 23
Toenail – ingrowing 115-117
Tourniquet 103
Tracheostomy 27-29
Trendelenburg operation 77
Trigger fingers 118-119

V
Vagina cyst 181-182
Vas deferens 36
Vasectomy 36-37
Vasoconstrictor 7
Varicose veins surgery 77-80
Vermillionectomy 164
Vulva
– Leukoplakia 191
– Lichen sclerosis 190
– Pilonidal sinus 190
– Tumour – benign 184

W
Warts
– Labial 175
– Perineal 173-175
Wedge resection extropion 129
W-plasty scar 168
Wedge excision cancer lip 165-166
Wheeler's procedure 125-127
Wies procedure 123
Wound repair – check 146-147

Z
Z-plasty 135, 169-170
Zadik's operation 115-117